ALLOGRAFTS IN ORTHOPAEDIC PRACTICE

ALLOGRAFTS IN ORTHOPAEDIC PRACTICE

EDITORS

ANDREI A. CZITROM, MD, FRCS(C), PhD

Clinical Associate Professor
Department of Orthopaedic Surgery
University of Texas Southwestern Medical Center
Humana Advanced Surgical Institutes
Dallas, Texas

ALLAN E. GROSS, MD, FRCS(C)

A. J. Latner Professor and Chairman
Division of Orthopaedic Surgery
University of Toronto
Mount Sinai Hospital
Toronto, Ontario, Canada

WILLIAMS & WILKINS
BALTIMORE · HONG KONG · LONDON · MUNICH
PHILADELPHIA · SYDNEY · TOKYO

Editor: Timothy H. Grayson
Managing Editor: Marjorie Kidd Keating
Copy Editor: Shelley Potler
Designer: Dan Pfisterer
Illustration Planner: Lorraine Wrzosek
Production Coordinator: Susan S. Vaupel
Cover Designer: Dan Pfisterer
Medical Illustrator: Mary-Anne Williams

Copyright © 1992
Williams & Wilkins
428 East Preston Street
Baltimore, Maryland 21202, USA

Printed in the United States of America

Library of Congress Cataloging-in-Publication Data

Allografts in orthopaedic practice / editors, Andrei A. Czitrom, Allan
  E. Gross.
        p.   cm.
    Includes bibliographical references and index.
    ISBN 0-683-02300-4
    1. Bone-grafting.   2. Joints—Transplantation.   3. Homografts.
  I. Czitrom, Andrei A.   II. Gross, Allan E.
    [DNLM: 1. Bone Transplantation.   2. Orthopedics.
  3. Transplantation, Homologous.   WE 190 A441]
  RD123.A44   1992
  617.4'710592--dc20
  DNLM/DLC
  for Library of Congress   91-30321
                                                          CIP

                        92   93   94   95   96
              1   2   3   4   5   6   7   8   9   10

FOREWORD

This book is a review of the fundamentals of musculo-skeletal allogeneic transplantation and its clinical application. It is authored by an experienced group of orthopaedic surgeons. The editors, Andrei A. Czitrom and Allan E. Gross, are both academic clinicians who have a broad perspective of the fundamentals of tissue transplantation.

The opening chapter is a brief review of the biology and repair of allogeneic bone transplants by Victor M. Goldberg and Sharon Stevenson from Case Western Reserve University. They are the senior investigators in a laboratory that has long focused on the study of various aspects of bone grafts in experimental animals. On the basis of this background, they present a brief, understandable discussion comparing the cellular mechanisms of repair in cancellous and cortical autogenous and allogeneic bone. This is followed by a chapter by Andrei A. Czitrom that is devoted to the role of immunology in the allotransplantation of connective tissues. This material is presented in depth and consists of a sophisticated discussion of the immunologic responses to allografts, the immunogenic components of bone and cartilage, and the approaches for modifying the deleterious effects by host immunosuppression, histocompatibility matching, and graft alteration. These two chapters provide the reader with the understanding to apply these principles to clinical situations.

In Chapter 3, C. Elizabeth Musclow presents the elements of establishing and operating a connective tissue bank. She discusses the various types of banks, donor selection, tissue recovery and its processing, storing, and distribution. This chapter will be of particular interest to tissue bankers and paraprofessionals concerned with tissue banking.

The remainder of the book is devoted to the clinical application of these principles. Whereas the first three chapters emphasized the broad spectrum of the field, the clinical chapters recount, in detail, the experiences of the Toronto group over the past two decades. While there, occasionally, is a somewhat unilateral view of controversial areas, the extensive experience of the Toronto group is a valuable guide through their methods of solving clinical problems. This is particularly appealing in that, for a variety of reasons, they have, for many years, emphasized the use of fresh, nonbanked allografts and have the largest experience in the modern era with these techniques.

The various chapters are authored by different senior clinicians in the form of reviews of the Toronto experience. Andrei A. Czitrom, in Chapter 4, provides the indications and uses of morsellized and small-segment allografts in general orthopaedics. He compares allografts with autografts and gives indications for the use of each in cavity-filling and buttressing. Clinical results and discussion follow. Chapter 5, by Allan E. Gross, is a report of his experience with more than 100 fresh osteoarticular allografts in managing traumatic joint defected. In this unique experience, he emphasizes that the limited indications (younger patients with unicondylar defects) and patient selection were vital in achieving the 75% satisfaction rate. The need for "decompressing" the repairing graft from undue stress by osteotomy and the importance of continuous passive motion in the rehabilitative management are clearly brought out.

The next two chapters concern the use of allografts in tumor surgery. In Chapter 6, Andrei A. Czitrom deals with lesions of the extremities. After a brief discussion of the principles of tumor surgery, he details the Toronto group's experience in the use of intercalary, osteoarticular, and composite allograft/prostheses at various sites. Several of the techniques described have been modified or refined in Toronto and are not widely practiced elsewhere. In Chapter 7, another tumor-related chapter, Robert S. Bell and Cameron B. Guest present their experience of allograft reconstruction after resection of pelvic neoplasms.

Chapters 8 and 9, by Allan E. Gross and Ian Stockley, deal with the use of allografts in revision surgery for failed hip and knee prostheses. In Chapter 8, regarding the hip, a useful classification of acetabular and femoral defects furnishes a guide to their indications. A detailed analysis of the experience with an extensive follow-up of a large series will be of particular interest to revision hipsters. Chapter 9, dealing with revision of total knee arthoplasties, involves a smaller series (22 patients) but contains some very useful tips.

Chapter 10, by Douglas W. Jackson and his colleagues, concerns the use of ligamentous allografts, particularly the cruciate ligament in the knee. Because the recipient population is younger (with normal life expectancy) and the potential donors come from a group in which risk factors for the HIV virus are higher, this chapter reiterates, in some detail, the need for donor screening. This is emphasized because secondary sterilization with either ethylene oxide or γ-irradiation has had deleterious effects on these soft tissue transplants. The authors discuss their preference for using patellar tendons or Achilles tendons to replace anterior cruciate ligaments because of the need for stronger transplants and the effect of "noncrimp" collagen on the function of the transplants. A major portion of this chapter is given to a detailed description of the authors' arthroscopic operative technique.

This book is a useful addition to the literature on allografted connective tissues, both as a primer on the basic sciences of allogeneic transplantation and as a detailed account of the somewhat unique clinical experiences of the Toronto group. We are all in their debt for the prodigious effect this book has required. Clearly, one of its most appealing aspects is the diversity of a multiauthored volume combined with a commonality in style, approach, and philosophy. It provides the breadth of experience and exposure without the oft-found contradictory and confusing differences in uncoordinated multiauthored works. To this end, we are particularly indebted to the editors, Andrei A. Czitrom and Allan E. Gross.

William F. Enneking, MD
Distinguished Service Professor Emeritus
Department of Orthopaedics
University of Florida College of Medicine
Gainesville, Florida

PREFACE

The field of orthopaedic surgery is currently inundated by textbooks and reviews summarizing advances in various surgical techniques and aiming at educating practicing clinicians in areas of subspecialties of orthopaedic surgery. *Allografts in Orthopaedic Practice* does not intend to address subspecialists but, rather, it hopes to fulfill the needs of all community and academic orthopaedic surgeons. It presents a methodology that is applicable to a diverse field of orthopaedic reconstruction procedures where the need arises to replace lost tissues by biological means using allogeneic transplants. Is the writing of such a book justified by the current needs of clinical practice? We think the answer is yes, because of the rapid and steady increase in the use of allogeneic donor tissues in a diverse field of orthopaedic reconstruction procedures. This situation has evolved dramatically in recent years and represents a general acceptance of the concept of using transplants for the biological reconstruction of skeletal defects, an idea that goes a long way back in history.

The scholars of orthopaedic transplantation know that their discipline began in 1668 when Job van Meekeren grafted a defect in a soldier's cranium with bone from a dog's skull. The idea of bone grafting was advanced by scientists like Van Leeuwenhoek, Duhamel, De Heyde, and Ollier, who described the structure of bone, callus formation, and osteogenesis in the late 17th and early 18th century. However, the most important contribution setting the stage for clinical bone transplantation was the description of "creeping substitution" by Barth, Curtis, and Phemister at the turn of the 19th century. The first clinical autograft was performed by Phillips von Walter in 1820 who reconstructed parts of a skull after trepanotomy. The first allograft in the practice of orthopaedics was performed in 1880 by W. Macewen from Scotland who reconstructed an infected humerus in a 4-year old boy with a tibial graft from a child with rickets. The practice of autogenous bone grafting in orthopaedic surgery became widely used after Albee's work published in 1915; this set the stage for the similar employment of allograft tissue.

Over the last century, the knowledge related to the allotransplantation of musculoskeletal tissues has progressed steadily, leading to a better understanding of the biology and immunology of these grafts, to safer methods of tissue banking, and to increased clinical experience related to graft use in surgical reconstruction. The end result of this increasing knowledge is that, today, the use of allograft bone and soft tissue has become an integral part of the technology utilized in the practice of orthopaedic surgery. Allograft bone is used in routine orthopaedic procedures, such as the filling of bone cysts and buttressing depressed fractures of the tibial plateau and os calcis. Bone and cartilage allografts play a major role in limb salvage surgery after the excision of bone tumors. The role of allograft bone in reconstructive surgery is increasing rapidly because of the need to restore bone stock in the multiply revised hip and knee implant. Recently, sports medicine has been the newest branch of orthopaedics to adopt the use of allograft tissue to replace torn knee ligaments and menisci.

We planned this book to cover all aspects of clinical orthopaedic allotransplantation that are in use today. It is hoped that the orthopaedic surgeon or resident in training will receive enough theory and, more importantly, enough practical information to understand the indications and the techniques for using allograft tissue. The sections on biology, immunology, and tissue banking cover basic knowledge with which we believe clinicians who perform allograft surgery should be acquainted. We kept the number of contributors to the minimum and tried to focus the text to the theoretical and practical aspects of allograft surgery that are reasonably well established. The brief discussion of allograft surgery in the spine in the chapter on general orthopaedics is intentional, because we hold the view that the indications and results of allograft fusions in the spine are currently too controversial to merit a separate chapter on spine surgery. Our goal was to convey knowledge that establishes a firm base for the practicing orthopaedist who is faced with using a new technology that is still evolving. This is the mission of a textbook that, by necessity, has to have a more limited and focused viewpoint than those books that summarize proceedings of meetings and give a variety of approaches as pioneered by multiple authors.

This is the first true textbook on allograft surgery in orthopaedics and, therefore, its publication represents an experiment itself. We undertook this project because of our long-term experience and scholarship as "ortho-paedic transplanters." We are indebted to all of the other contributors who are experts in their field, to our colleague surgeons who allowed us to use their cases, and to the residents and fellows whose work over the years has advanced knowledge in this field. We also thank Mary-Anne Williams for skillfully illustrating the surgical tech-niques shown in this book. It is our hope that this text will truly help orthopaedic surgeons in their routine practice, which, in 1992, will include the need to use transplanted tissues.

Andrei A. Czitrom
Allan E. Gross

CONTRIBUTORS

ROBERT S. BELL, MD
Assistant Professor
Division of Orthopaedic Surgery
University of Toronto
Mount Sinai Hospital
Toronto, Ontario, Canada

ANDREI A. CZITROM, MD, FRCS(C), PhD
Clinical Associate Professor
Department of Orthopaedic Surgery
University of Texas Southwestern Medical Center
Humana Advanced Surgical Institutes
Dallas, Texas

VICTOR M. GOLDBERG, MD
Professor and Chairman
Department of Orthopaedics
Case Western Reserve University
Cleveland, Ohio

ALLAN E. GROSS, MD, FRCS(C)
A. J. Latner Professor and Chairman
Division of Orthopaedic Surgery
University of Toronto
Mount Sinai Hospital
Toronto, Ontario, Canada

CAMERON B. GUEST
Research Fellow
Division of Orthopaedic Surgery
University of Toronto
Mount Sinai Hospital
Toronto, Ontario, Canada

DOUGLAS W. JACKSON, MD
Medical Director
Southern California Center for Sports Medicine
Long Beach, California

C. ELIZABETH MUSCLOW, MD, FRCP(C)
Associate Professor
Department of Pathology
University of Toronto
Director, Bone and Tissue Bank
Mount Sinai Hospital
Toronto, Ontario, Canada

MARK ROSEN, MD
Private Practice
Murray, Utah
(formerly) Sports Medicine Fellow
Southern California Center for Sports Medicine
Long Beach, California

TIMOTHY M. SIMON, MS
Research Director
Southern California Center for Sports Medicine
Long Beach, California

SHARON STEVENSON, DVM, PhD
Assistant Professor
Department of Orthopaedics
Case Western Reserve University
Cleveland, Ohio

IAN STOCKLEY, FRCS
Consultant Orthopaedic Surgeon
Northern General Hospital
Sheffield, United Kingdom
(formerly) Clinical Fellow
Division of Orthopaedic Surgery
University of Toronto
Mount Sinai Hospital
Toronto, Ontario, Canada

CONTENTS

1

BIOLOGY OF BONE AND CARTILAGE ALLOGRAFTS

Victor M. Goldberg and Sharon Stevenson

BONE

Despite the widespread use of cortical bone grafts in reconstructive tumor, trauma, and total joint surgery, the physiological and biological events that are crucial to the process of incorporation and the mechanisms that control these events are only superficially understood. From a clinical standpoint, a bone graft successfully incorporates when the host/graft interface unites and the graft/host bone construct will tolerate physiological weight bearing without fracture or pain. From a basic science standpoint, the process of incorporation of a cortical autograft has been defined as the gold standard: rapid revascularization and substitution of graft bone with new host bone. We propose that successful bone graft incorporation may be defined as concurrent revascularization and substitution with host bone without significant loss of strength. The resulting composite can bear physiological loads and repair and remodel itself in response to fatigue damage or to changes in load.

Bone grafts have two major functions: enhancing os-

teogenesis and providing mechanical support. Osteogenesis, the process of bone formation, may originate from the graft or from the host. One way that the graft can contribute to osteogenesis is by direct bone formation by surviving graft cells. Surface cells of the graft can survive transplantation, divide, and produce new bone as well as cytokines relevant to bone formation (1–3). This process is most important in cancellous autografts, but also plays a role in fresh cortical grafts. Another process whereby bone grafts enhance osteogenesis is known as osteoinduction. Osteoinduction is the recruitment from the surrounding host bed of pluripotential cells that differentiate into bone-forming cells. Osteoinduction is primarily mediated by graft matrix-derived soluble factors, one of which is bone morphogenic protein (BMP), a hydrophobic nonspecies-specific glycoprotein that has been extracted from bone matrices as well as from bone tumors (4, 5). BMP activity does not require viable graft cells since it is a property of graft bone matrix. BMP activity may be present not only in autografts, but also in fresh and preserved allografts. Processing bone grafts by freezing or freeze-drying does not seem to destroy its activity, but autoclaving does. Osteogenins are also mediators of osteoinduction and are particularly active in demineralized bone matrix (6). Osteogenins appear to be species specific and are destroyed by treatment with alkaliproteases and mercaptoethanol. There is, however, homology in purified osteoinductive proteins from diverse species of mammals.

Osteoinduction requires migration, proliferation, and differentiation by cells of the host bed (7). The early host inflammatory response, which occurs within hours of graft implantation, provides programmable cells that can differentiate into osteoblasts and capillary buds. The early interactions between the graft and cells of the host are

1

critical in determining the pattern of incorporation of a bone graft.

Under certain conditions, e.g., vascularized autografts, the osteogenic potential of a graft is independent of the host bed. Graft surface cells survive because the anastomosed vasculature provides an important avenue of graft nutrition. These vascularized bone grafts may incorporate in a nonsupportive host bed. However, incorporation of nonvascularized or processed allografts is dependent on the host bed. The control of revascularization of bone grafts is central in the ultimate outcome of the incorporation. Optimal revascularization depends upon a relatively healthy host bed, the presence of a stable graft/host interface, and an ordered sequence of mediators and cellular responders. The balance between functional revascularization and concomitant mineralization is paramount in determining the ultimate success or failure of a bone graft.

The clinical success of a graft depends upon its ability to provide mechanical support for the skeleton. Cortical grafts and cortical cancellous grafts may act as mechanical struts immediately after grafting. However, the continued structural integrity of a graft depends on the interaction between the mechanical environment and the biological response. Mechanical strain of the graft will stimulate remodeling and substitution of a graft. In cortical grafts, this process occurs by osteoconduction. In osteoconduction, the bone graft serves as a trellis or scaffold for the ingrowth of new host bone (8). This three-dimensional process includes the ingrowth of new capillaries, perivascular tissue, and osteoprogenitor cells from the recipient bed (Fig. 1.1). Osteoconduction is an ordered, predictable spatial process that is critical in the remodeling of cortical and cortical cancellous bone. The process of osteoconduction leads to gradual, partial resorption of the graft and its replacement by new host bone, a process previously called creeping substitution. Remodeling to a mechanically efficient supporting structure is influenced by the mechanical loads to which the grafts are subjected and may take years. Bone graft incorporation is a sequential process that begins with inflammation and proceeds through stages of revascularization and osteogenesis, remodeling, and finally, under the influence of Wolff's law, to the establishment of a mechanically sound structure.

Cancellous Bone Grafts

The biological events in bone-graft incorporation may be studied by different techniques. These experimental methods include radiology, histology, bone scintigraphy, single- and dual-photon absorptiometry, and biomechanical testing.

EARLY PHASE

Inflammation is the hallmark of the early period after transplantation. However, surface osteocytes survive, are nourished by diffusion, and are capable of producing early new bone (9). Vascularization of cancellous grafts occurs quickly, primarily because the open structure of the graft provides an effective, porous, three-dimensional scaffold (10). Cells with osteoclastic activity rapidly migrate into the graft and are quickly followed by osteoblast precursors. Osteoinductive factors enhance migration of host mesenchymal cells into the graft. Osteoblasts line the edges of cancellous trabeculae and secrete seams of osteoid that are deposited around the central core of necrotic bone (11).

LATER PHASE

Osteoconduction continues. Active resorption and formation proceed. The graft subsequently is remodeled and complete replacement of the necrotic graft with viable host bone occurs. New bone marrow is formed during the first 3 months. The final phase of cancellous autograft incorporation is usually completed by 1 year after surgery. At this point, the graft is completely resorbed and replaced by viable host new bone and a mechanically sound structure is present. Peripheral callus is being consolidated into the cortex and is remodeling in response to Wolff's law (12).

Nonvascularized Cortical Autografts

Incorporation proceeds in a similar pattern in cortical autografts as in cancellous autografts. However, because the rate of revascularization is markedly slower due to the structure of cortical bone, the entire process of incorporation is prolonged (9). Vascular penetration of the graft is primarily the result of peripheral osteoclastic resorption and vascular invasion of Volkman's and Haversian canals (11). Cortical autografts initially become significantly osteoporotic because of the invasion of vessels from the surrounding host bed. During this period of time, the graft is significantly weaker than normal bone and this weakness persists for months to years depending upon the size of the grafts (8, 11). Since osteoclasts are capable of resorbing bone at a rate of 50 μm/day, while osteoblasts form bone at a rate of approximately 1 μm/day, even under optimum circumstances, resorption dominates over formation in the early phases of cortical bone-graft incorporation (Fig. 1.2).

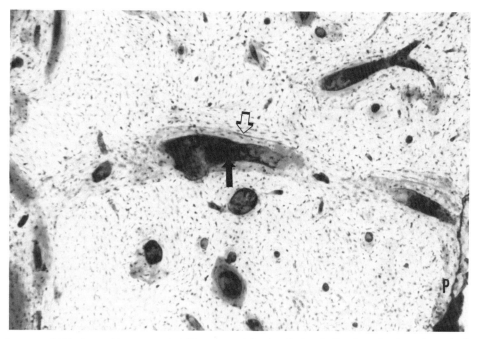

Figure 1.1. A large vessel (*black arrow*) has penetrated this nonvascularized cortical graft. New bone has been formed adjacent to the vessel (*open arrow*). This particular vessel has penetrated from the periosteal border (*P*) of the graft.

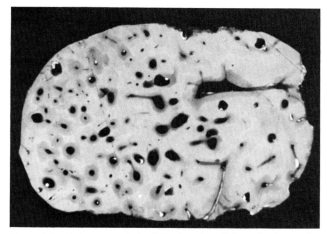

Figure 1.2. This nonvascularized fibular autograft is markedly porotic and has numerous vascular channels at 3 months after surgery. (Reprinted with permission from Goldberg VM, et al. Biologic and physical properties of vascularized fibular autografts in dogs. J Bone Joint Surg 72A:801–810, 1990.)

Appositional new bone formation is under way by 3 weeks, but, even at 1 year, cortical autografts remain an admixture of necrotic old bone and viable new bone. Although well fixed, weight-bearing cortical autografts remodel both spatially and temporally like a normal bone segment and the remodeling process remains active for a prolonged period of time; only rarely is all the graft bone removed and replaced by new host bone in a cortical autograft (Fig. 1.3).

Vascularized Cortical Autografts

The incorporation of vascularized cortical autografts is markedly different from that of nonvascularized cortical autografts because of the maintenance of a functional blood supply (13). Only transient intraoperative ischemia occurs and over 90% of the transplanted osteocytes survive (14). When the osteosynthesis site is well fixed, graft/host union occurs rapidly and little bone resorption is seen (Fig. 1.4). Vascularized cortical autografts incorporate independently of the host bed. There is little dependence on a bed-derived source of bone-forming cells and the turnover of the vascularized cortical autograft is similar to normal bone (Fig. 1.5). These grafts are especially useful in compromised host beds (14–16). Additionally, these grafts are clinically useful when segments of 6 cm or more are required for repair of a segmental defect (17, 18).

Cortical Allografts

In general, the bone incorporation of bone allografts and processed bone is inferior to autografts. It is almost invariably slower and less complete (19–21) (Fig. 1.6). Fresh allografts evoke an immune response that may result in aggressive resorption of the transplanted tissue or reduction of biological activity (22, 23). The inflammatory phase is exaggerated and the osteoinduction phase of bone-graft incorporation is reduced or destroyed. As de-

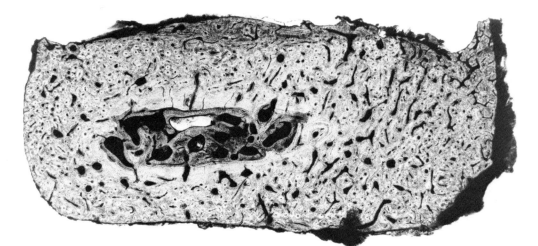

Figure 1.3. Approximately 35–55% of this cortical autograft had been replaced with new bone at 11 months after the surgery. There is a homogeneous admixture of old and new bone. (Reprinted with permission from Goldberg VM, et al. Natural history of autografts and allografts. Clin Orthop Relat Res 225:7–16, 1987.)

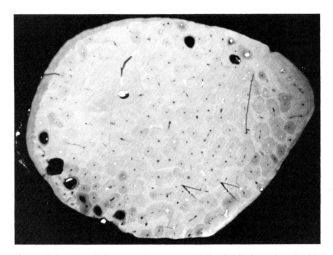

Figure 1.4. Very little resorption or remodeling had taken place in this vascularized fibular autograft at 3 months after the surgery. Vascularized grafts were significantly stronger and stiffer than nonvascularized grafts at 3 months (13). (Reprinted with permission from Goldberg VM, et al. Biologic and physical properties of vascularized fibular autografts in dogs. J Bone Joint Surg 72A:801–810, 1990.)

scribed in the following chapter, the immune response is usually directed toward the cells and vasculature of transplanted tissues. The immune response may be delayed because the host encounters graft-derived cellular antigens and becomes sensitized to those antigens only after partial revascularization of the graft. Under certain circumstances, such as appropriate weight bearing and a stable fixed construct, a segmental fresh cortical allograft may eventually incorporate and resemble autografts biomechanically and histologically. However, because of the variability in rate and patterns of incorporation of fresh

allografts, preserved cortical allografts are preferred. Ideally, preservation techniques would maintain the graft's mechanical properties and its ability to stimulate osteogenesis while reducing or eliminating its antigenicity. However, many of the processing methods, such as freeze-drying, although they may reduce immunogenicity, they may impair the mechanical properties of the bone graft (24, 25).

Freezing and freeze-drying are the most common processes of preservation. Processed cancellous allografts are clinically useful although revascularization and remodeling are delayed in comparison with fresh autografts. Osteoinduction, osteoconduction, and remodeling occur sequentially, but processed cancellous allografts may never be completely replaced by host-viable bone. Other preservation techniques, such as chemoextraction have also been shown to be clinically satisfactory. However, decalcification with deproteinization does not result in a bone graft that is as effective as frozen or freeze-dried grafts (24, 25). Cancellous allografts are clinically useful to provide filler material for cavitary skeletal defects. Frozen allografts are still immunogenic so revascularization is delayed when compared with fresh autografts. However, remodeling, osteoinduction, and osteoconduction occur over a period of time and these grafts, when rigidly fixed, are incorporated well and perform satisfactorily in clinical situations (26–28) (Fig. 1.7). It is important to realize that frozen allografts do remain in a mixture of necrotic graft bone and viable host tissue for a prolonged period of time. Although freeze-drying significantly reduces immunogenicity, it also alters the mechanical properties of the graft and results in signifi-

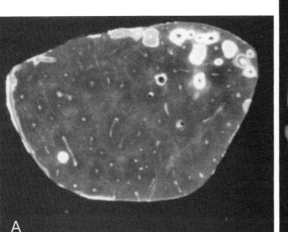
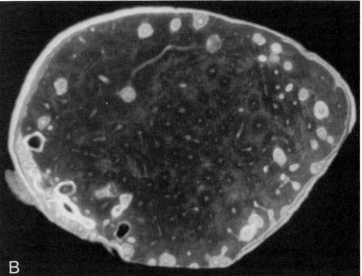

Figure 1.5. Only a few osteons had active bone formation and matrix mineralization in this sham-operated fibula (A) and vascularized fibular autograft (B) at 3 months after the surgery. (Reprinted with permission from Goldberg VM, et al. Biologic and physical properties of vascularized fibular autografts in dogs. J Bone Joint Surg 72A:801–810, 1990.)

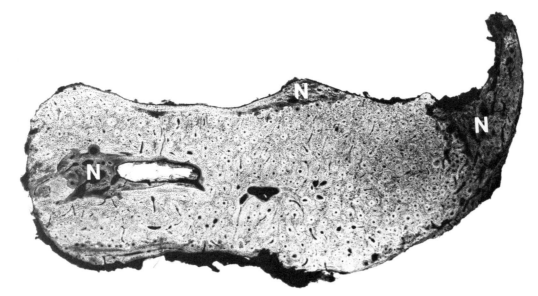

Figure 1.6. Some new bone (N) had formed around the plate and endosteally in this stably fixed fresh radial allograft. Even at 11 months, almost none of the original graft had been revascularized or substituted. (Reprinted with permission from Stevenson S, et al. The fate of cancellous and cortical bone after transplantation of fresh and cryopreserved tissue-antigen-matched and mismatched osteochondral allografts in dogs. J Bone Joint Surg 73A:1143–1156, 1991.)

cantly weaker grafts (24, 25). Complications such as fatigue fractures and graft/host nonunion or delayed union are possible (Fig. 1.8). Occasionally, freeze-dried grafts are completely resorbed. Other methods of preservation appear to preserve the osteoinductiveness of the allograft while reducing the immunogenicity. These preservation methods include irradiation and the use of chemical agents that produce a graft material known as chemosterilized

autolysed antigen-extracted allogenic bone (AAA). The sterilization of bone by irradiation of less than 3 megarads seems not to affect the material properties of bone significantly, but doses this high have been shown, in some studies, to destroy the bone inductive factors, such as BMP (6). Also, experimental studies have shown that irradiated bone appears to be incorporated more slowly then frozen or freeze-dried allogeneic bone (29). The

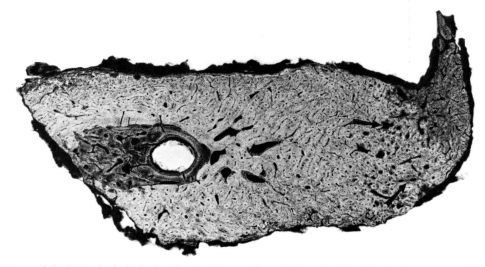

Figure 1.7. Some revascularization and substitution had occurred medially (*arrows*) in this frozen, stably fixed allograft. Marked resorption had occurred laterally with concomitant endosteal bone formation. (Reprinted with permission from Stevenson S, et al. The fate of cancellous and cortical bone after transplantation of fresh and cryopreserved tissue-antigen-matched and mismatched osteochondral allografts in dogs. J Bone Joint Surg 73A:1143–1156, 1991.)

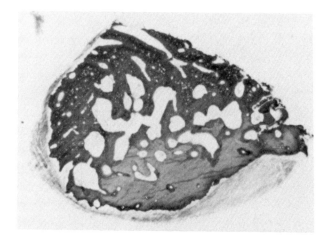

Figure 1.8. Very little of the original substance of this nonvascularized cortical allograft remains at 3 months after surgery. The construct is markedly porotic, composed of woven bone, and weak.

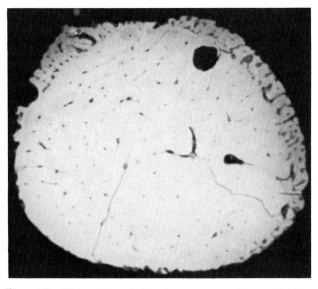

Figure 1.9. When cyclosporin A, an immunosuppressive agent, is given, vascularized allografts remodel similarly to vascularized autografts. At 3 months after surgery, this vascularized allograft had a normal structure.

AAA bone provides an implant that has preserved BMP and other inductive factors while dramatically reducing the immunogenicity of the graft (4, 5). Because of its demineralization, however, it has little strength and it is a poor weight-bearing construct.

Experimental studies have indicated that vascularized fresh allografts may become clinically useful. Several studies have shown that the immunosuppressive agents, such as cyclosporin A, can successfully maintain a vascularized cortical allograft in a canine model (30). The vascularized allograft appears to incorporate rapidly and bone union occurs quickly at the graft host junction. The bone segment remodels in a similar fashion to vascularized autografts (Fig. 1.9).

Xenografts

Xenografts, usually processed bovine bone, may be used in special circumstances. These grafts may provide a reasonable mechanical construct; however, they do incite a marked inflammatory response and are incorporated slowly, if at all (8, 31). These grafts may, however, preserve some of their osteoinductive capacity since BMP is thought to be nonspecies specific (5). All preserved allografts are superior to processed xenografts.

Successful bone-graft incorporation is a sequential event that proceeds from initial inflammatory response to an exquisitely balanced mechanical structure. The sum of the interactions between the cells of the host inflammatory/wound healing response and the net biological activity of a graft (cells, capacity for osteoinduction, ability to support osteoconduction) determines the process of bone-graft incorporation. The optimum revascularization and substitution, i.e., incorporation, occur when a normal inflammatory response is invoked in the absence of a specific immune response and the cells of that response interact with living cells of the bone graft. Monocyte/macrophages, lymphocytes, and bone cells all synthesize, release, and respond to interleukin-1, transforming growth factor β, tumor necrosis factor α, and prostaglandin E_2 (32–39). We believe that bidirectional actions of these and other mediators modulate healing, revascularization, immune response, and bone physiology.

CARTILAGE

Articular cartilage is transplanted in one of two forms: as a fresh shell osteochondral allograft or as a preserved massive (hemijoint) osteochondral allograft. The cartilaginous component of these grafts is critical in their successful function. Normal articular cartilage distributes load, minimizing peak forces on subchondral bone; it can be deformed and regain its original shape; it has remarkable durability and provides an unequaled low friction-bearing surface (40). Articular cartilage is an avascular tissue, composed of approximately 10% collagen, 10% proteoglycan, and 80% water (41). The collagen comprises mainly type II collagen with small amounts of at least two other collagens, types IX and XI, and forms a dense network of fibers. The proteoglycans, principally the large aggregating type, are enmeshed within and constrained by the collagen network. Noncollagenous proteins, such as anchorin, decorin, chondronectin, and link protein help stabilize the matrix (42). The collagen component of articular cartilage resists tension and the proteoglycan component, because of its high viscosity, resists compression. Chondrocytes synthesize all matrix components. Their chief energy source is anaerobic glycolysis; more than 90% of the glucose metabolized ends up as lactic acid. Chondrocytes rely on diffusion of nutrients and metabolites through the matrix rather than on a blood supply. Movement of fluid through the matrix is facilitated by the intermittent compression and release (pumping action) of cartilage during weight bearing and motion (42). Cel-

lular activity in the articular cartilage depends upon the maturity of the tissue. Immature cartilage is the most active metabolically, but even immature cartilage has a low mitotic rate (43). No mitoses are present in adult articular cartilage under normal conditions. However, chondrocytes remain metabolically active throughout life. In normal articular cartilage, the matrix components are slowly but continually being turned over and the production of proteoglycans increases markedly in osteoarthritic conditions (44).

Functional articular cartilage comprises both an intact macrostructure of articular cartilage and intact underlying subchondral bone (Fig. 1.10). The underlying subchondral bone is important biomechanically in acting as a load-

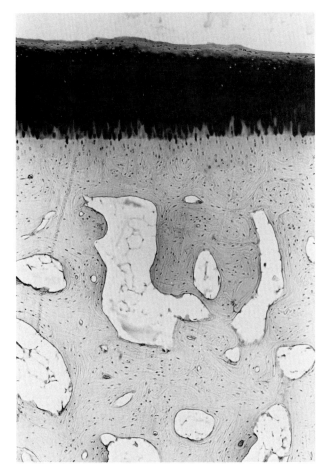

Figure 1.10. Normal subchondral bone is important for the health of transplanted articular cartilage. Most of the necrotic trabeculae in this nonvascularized osteochondral autograft has been replaced with new, host bone. The subchondral bone has retained its normal architecture during the process and the articular cartilage is healthy at 11 months after surgery. (Reprinted with permission from Stevenson S, et al. The fate of articular cartilage after transplantation of fresh and cryopreserved tissue-antigen-matched and mismatched osteochondral allografts in dogs. J Bone Joint Surg 71A:1297–1307, 1989.)

carrying mechanism and as a relatively stiff backing of the articular cartilage, which facilitates the pumping action responsible for diffusion to the chondrocytes. Thus, when articular cartilage is transplanted, consideration must be given to the articular cartilage/subchondral bone unit and not merely to the cartilage alone.

Shell Osteochondral Allografts

Fresh shell allografts (articular cartilage with a thin shell of underlying bone) have been used clinically with some success (45–48). Because of their unique method of nutrition, chondrocytes can survive the transplantation procedure and receive nutrients by diffusion from the synovial fluid. Living chondrocytes are required to maintain the matrix, particularly the proteoglycan component. The subchondral bone, however, is resorbed and replaced by host bone (49). It is during this process of vascular invasion and replacement by new bone that the host becomes sensitized to cellular antigens of the graft (*see* Chapter 2). Experimentally, the cartilage of shell allografts undergoes fibrillation, fragmentation, and erosion (50–52). An inflammatory synovial pannus may be present and immune response to donor-tissue antigens and cartilage-matrix antigens has been described (50–52). Additionally, inflammatory mediators may play a role in immune-mediated cartilage destruction. Although erosions of cartilage are contiguous with proliferating synovial pannus, proteoglycan loss from the matrix is widespread. It has been hypothesized that destructive enzymes may have diffused into the matrix or that chondrocytes may have been induced actively to degrade their own matrix (53). Inflammatory cells within proliferating synovial pannus produce collagenase and proteases and, in addition, produce factors (mononuclear cell factor, macrophage-activating factors, interleukin-1) that induce other cells. These inducing factors stimulate fibroblasts of the synovial membrane and chondrocytes to produce collagenase, prostaglandin E_2, and other proteases (54–56).

Massive (Hemijoint) Osteochondral Allografts

Massive osteochondral allografts consist of cortical bone, cancellous metaphyseal bone, and articular cartilage with underlying subchondral bone (Fig. 1.11). These grafts are almost always preserved prior to implantation and usually have been treated with a cryoprotectant, such as dimethylsulfoxide (DMSO) or glycerol, to help maintain viability of chondrocytes during the process of freezing and thawing. These cryopreservants are not effective for intact cartilage and, at best, 40–50% of chondrocytes survive (57, 58). When a conventional freezer is used, fewer then 10%

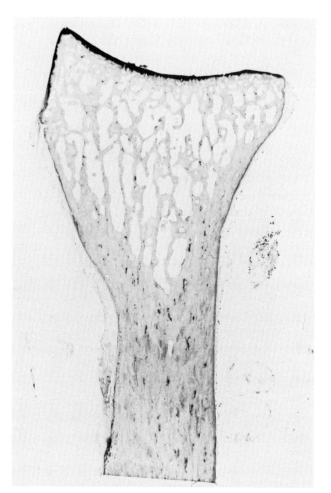

Figure 1.11. The large proportion of metaphyseal cancellous bone, which comprises a massive osteochondral graft, is evident in this photo. Note the delicate trabeculae and subchondral plate that can only be partially protected from weight bearing during graft incorporation.

of chondrocytes survive freezing and thawing. Thus, almost immediately, the articular cartilage is at risk for degeneration and replacement by fibrocartilage. Transplanted hyaline articular cartilage has been noted both clinically and experimentally to degenerate and to be replaced with fibrocartilage (59–63). In addition, these massive grafts do sensitize the host; 15–100% of the patients develop a measurable humoral antibody response to donor tissue antigens following massive allografting (25, 64, 65). Experimentally, both a local (intra-articular) response and a systemic humoral response have been documented as well as antibody-dependent cell-mediated cytotoxicity and cell-mediated immunity directed toward cell surface antigens at the graft (22). In a study of massive osteochondral allografts in dogs, all allografts, whether histocompatibility antigen-matched or -mismatched or whether fresh or frozen, did poorly compared with autogenous grafts. However, a differential response was consistently seen. Histocompatibility antigen-matched fresh grafts were the most successful, histocompatibility antigen-mismatched fresh allografts and histocompatibility-matched frozen allografts were intermediately successful, and histocompatibility antigen-mismatched frozen allografts were the least successful (66). Certain effects seemed to be attributable to freezing of the grafts; whereas others appeared to be attributable to the response of the host to histoincompatible tissue. All grafts that had been frozen had significantly less glycosaminoglycan per milligram of dry weight, more hydroxyproline per milligram of dry weight, and a lower galactosamine-glucosamine ratio than the grafts that had been implanted without cryopreservation. The host response to histoincompatible tissue manifested itself mainly in a loss of cartilage substance or mass. After 11 months in vivo, the dry weight of cartilage of the antigen-mismatched grafts, as a group, was significantly less of that of histocompatibility antigen-matched grafts (66). Degenerative changes that were observed in the articular cartilage were similar to those of osteoarthrosis—that is, formation of osteophytes, loss of proteoglycans, decrease in galactosamine-glucosamine ratio, little change in collagen content (as measured by

the concentration of hydroxyproline), and variable synovitis (44, 67, 68). Abnormal biomechanical forces secondary to postoperative instability will result in degeneration of cartilage, even that of autogenous grafts (69, 70). However, in this animal model, degenerative changes were not seen in autografts and it was believed that the degenerative changes resulted from the host response to the allografts rather than from abnormal biomechanical forces. The histological appearance of synovial membranes, (accumulation of plasma cells and large and small lymphocytes) paralleled the immunogenicity of the grafts. Additionally, titers of antibody in joints that received fresh histocompatibility antigen-mismatched grafts were four or five times higher then systemic titers in the same dogs. Others have documented in vivo, intra-articular synthesis of IgM and IgG (71). This immune response and the ensuing inflammatory changes may be responsible for the loss of cartilage mass seen. For instance, interleukin-1 has been found in synovial fluid of rheumatoid joints and dendritic cells from rheumatoid inflammatory synovial tissue can be stimulated to produce interleukin-1 in vitro (72). This immune-inflammatory response may well trigger the cascade that was described under shell osteochondral grafts (Fig. 1.12).

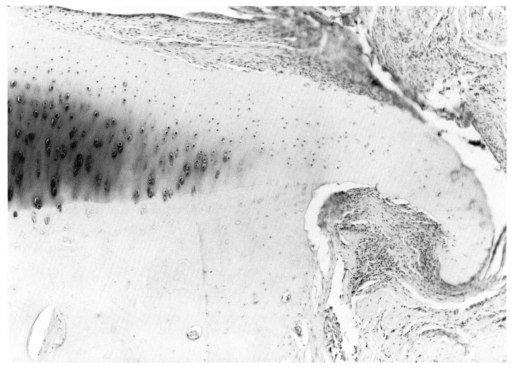

Figure 1.12. Inflammatory pannus covers the surface of this fresh osteochondral allograft and is invading and destroying the joint margin 11 months postoperatively. Note the loss of safranin-o staining in the cartilage that is covered with pannus. (Reprinted with permission from Stevenson S, et al. The fate of articular cartilage after transplantation of fresh and cryopreserved tissue-antigen-matched and mismatched osteochondral allografts in dogs. J Bone Joint Surg 71A:1297–1307, 1989.)

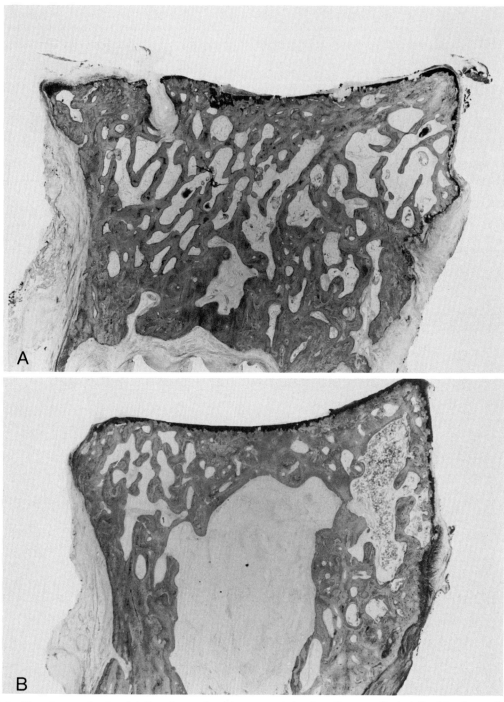

Figure 1.13. Both of these frozen osteochondral allografts are vulnerable to subchondral collapse at 11 months after surgery. There has already been a disruption of the subchondral plate with maintenance of trabecular architecture in one graft (*A*) and a large cyst surrounded by sclerotic bone has formed in the subchondral area of the other (*B*). (Reprinted with permission from Stevenson S, et al. The fate of cancellous and cortical bone after transplantation of fresh and cryopreserved tissue-antigen matched and mismatched osteochondral allografts in dogs. J Bone Joint Surg 73A:1143–1156, 1991.)

After implantation, massive osteochondral allografts cannot be completely protected from weight bearing and are susceptible to collapse during incorporation, revascularization, and substitution. In addition, a massive osteochondral allograft comprises not only cortical bone, but also cancellous bone within the metaphyseal area. In the canine model described previously, the repair process of cortical bone was similar for all grafted segments. New periosteal and endosteal bone were formed and the cortical bone became porotic as vessels penetrated it. Autografts were the most actively remodeled and fresh histocompatibility antigen-mismatched grafts were the least actively remodeled. The major differences between the bone of massive osteochondral allografts and massive osteochondral autografts occurred in the metaphyseal cancellous bone. All allografts had significantly more cancellous bone volume and thicker trabeculae than sham-operated bones and autografts (73). Intertrabecular fibrous connective tissue was directly proportional to the immunogenicity of the allograft and the bone-forming surface tended to be inversely proportional to the immunogenicity of the allograft. The metaphyseal area had been revascularized by the ingrowth of vessels into intratrabecular spaces without necrotic trabeculae being penetrated by vessels. This pattern was particularly pronounced in histocompatibility antigen-mismatched grafts. The metaphyseal portion of a massive osteochondral graft is subjected to weight bearing in the postoperative period and the persistence of necrotic bone, which cannot repair fatigue damage, may contribute to the subchondral collapse and degenerative joint disease noted clinically (74) (Fig. 1.13).

In summary, the biology of a bone or cartilage graft is a summation of complex processes, structures, and interactions. The inherent properties of the graft are important as is the ability of the host bed to respond to the graft and to the mechanical environment into which the graft is placed. An understanding of these processes is important in clinical decision-making when implanting bone or cartilage grafts.

REFERENCES

1. Bassett CAL. Clinical implications of cell function in bone grafting. Clin Orthop 1972; 87:49.
2. Bonfiglio M. Repair of bone-transplant fractures. J Bone Joint Surg 1958; 40A:446.
3. Gray JC, Elves MW. Early osteogenesis in compact bone isografts: a quantitative study of the contributions of the different graft cells. Calcif Tissue Int 1979; 29:225.
4. Mitzutani H, Urist MR. The nature of bone morphogenetic protein (BMP) fractions derived from bovine bone matrix gelatin. Clin Orthop 1982; 171:213.
5. Urist MR. Bone transplantation. In Urist MR (ed): Fundamental and Clinical Bone Physiology. JB Lippincott, Philadelphia, 1980.
6. Reddi AH, Weintrub S, Muthurumaran N. Biologic principles of bone induction. Orthop Clin North Am 1987; 18:207.
7. Reddi AH, Cunningham NS. Bone induction by osteogenin and bone morphogenetic proteins. Biomaterials 1990; 11:33.
8. Burwell RG. The fate of bone grafts. In Apley AG (ed). Recent advances in orthopaedics. Serological studies. J Bone Joint Surg 1961; 43B:814.
9. Burchardt H, Jones H, Glowczewskie F, et al. Freeze-dried allogeneic segmental cortical-bone grafts in dogs. J Bone Joint Surg 1978; 60A:1082.
10. Ray RD. Vascularization of bone grafts and implants. Clin Orthop 1972; 87:43.
11. Enneking WF, Burchardt H, Puhl JJ, et al. Physical and biological aspect of repair in dog cortical transplant. J Bone Joint Surg 1975; 57A:232.
12. Kushner A. Evaluation of Wolff's law of bone formation. J Bone Joint Surg 1940; 22A:589.
13. Goldberg VM, Stevenson S, Shaffer JW, et al. Biologic and physical properties of vascularized fibular autografts in dogs. J Bone Joint Surg 1990; 72A:801.
14. Doi K, Tominaga S, Shibata T. Bone grafts with microvascular anastomoses of vascular pedicles. J Bone Joint Surg 1977; 59A:809.
15. Goldberg VM, Porter BB, Lance EM. Transplantation of the canine knee joint on a vascular pedicle. J Bone Joint Surg 1980; 62A:414.
16. Goldberg VM, Shaffer JW, Field G, Davy DT. Biology of vascularized bone grafts. Orthop Clin North Am 1987; 18:197.
17. Taylor GI, Miller GDH, Ham FJ. The free vascularized bone graft: a clinical extension of microvascular techniques. Plast Reconstr Surg 1979; 64:745.
18. Weiland AJ, Kleinert HE, Kutz JE, et al. Free vascularized bone grafts in surgery of the upper extremity. J Hand Surg 1979; 4:129.
19. Elves MW, Gray JC, Thorogood PV. The cellular changes occurring with allografts of marrow containing cortical bone. J Anat 1976; 122:253.
20. Goldberg VM, Lance EM. Revascularization and accretion in transplantation. J Bone Joint Surg 1972; 54A:807.
21. Heiple KG, Chase SW, Herndon CH. A comparative study of the healing process following different types of bone transplantation. J Bone Joint Surg 1963; 45A:1593.
22. Stevenson S. The immune response to osteochondral allografts in dogs. J Bone Joint Surg 1987; 69A:573.
23. Kliman M, Halloran PF, Lee E, et al. Orthotopic bone transplantation in mice. III. Methods of reducing the immune response and their effect on healing. Transplantation 1981; 31:34.
24. Friedlaender GE, Strong DM, Sell KW. Studies on the antigenicity of bone. I. Freeze-dried and deep frozen allografts in rabbits. J Bone Joint Surg 1976; 58A:854.
25. Friedlaender GE, Strong DM, Sell KW. Studies of the antigenicity of bone. II. Donor-specific anti-HLA antibodies in human recipients of freeze-dried allografts. J Bone Joint Surg 1984; 66A:107.

26. Spence KF, Bright PW, Fitzgerald SP, et al. Solitary unicameral bone cyst: treatment with freeze-dried crushed cortical bone allograft. A review of one hundred forty-four cases. J Bone Joint Surg 1976; 58A:636.

27. Spence KF, Sell KW, Brown RH. Solitary bone cyst: treatment with freeze-dried cancellous bone allograft. J Bone Joint Surg 1969; 51A:87.

28. Tomford WW, Ploetz JP, Mankin HJ. Bone allografts of femoral heads: procurement and storage. J Bone Joint Surg 1986; 68A:534.

29. Pelker RR, Friedlaender GE, Panjabi JJ, et al. Chemotherapy-induced alterations in the biomechanics of rat bone. J Orthop Res 1985; 3:91.

30. Davy D, Bensusan J, Klein L, et al. Physical and biological properties of vascularized and nonvascularized fibular allografts in dogs. Trans Orthop Res Soc 1988; 13:61.

31. Lance EM. Bone and cartilage. In Najarian JS, Simmons RL (eds). Transplantation. Lea & Febiger, Philadelphia, 1984.

32. Bertolini DR, Nedwin GE, Bringmann TS, et al. Stimulation of bone resorption and inhibition of bone formation in vitro by human tumour necrosis factor. Nature (London) 1986; 319:516.

33. Centrella E, McCarthy TL, Canalis E. Transforming growth factors B is a bifunctional regulator of replications and collagen synthesis in osteoblast-enriched cell cultures from fetal rat bone. J Biol Chem 1987; 262:2869.

34. Dewhurst FE, Stashenko PP, Mole JE, et al. Purification and partial sequence of human osteoblast activating factor: Identify with interleukin 1B. J Immunol 1985; 135:2563.

35. Gowen M, Mundy GR. Actions of recombinant interleukin 1, interleukin 2, and interferon-γ on bone resorption in vitro. J Immunol 1986; 136:2478.

36. Tashjian AH, Hohmann EL, Antoniades HN, et al. PDGF stimulates bone resorption via a PG-mediated mechanism. Endocrinology 1982; 111:118.

37. Triffitt JT. Initiation and enhancement of bone formation: a review. Acta Orthop Scand 1987; 58:673.

38. Harvey W, Bennett A. Prostaglandins in Bone Resorption. CRC Press, Inc., Boca Raton, 1988.

39. Chensue SW, Shnyr-Forsch C, Weng A, et al. Biologic and immunohistochemical analysis of macrophage interleukin-1 α, -1 β, and tumor necrosis factor production during the peritoneal exudative response. J Leukocyte Biol 1989; 46:529.

40. Buckwalter J, Hunziker E, Rosenberg L, et al. Articular cartilage: Composition and Structure. In: Woo SL-Y, Buckwalter JA (eds). Injury and Repair of the Musculoskeletal Soft Tissues. Amer Acad Orthop Surg 1988; p. 405.

41. Muir IHM. The chemistry of the ground substance of joint cartilage. In: Joints and Synovial Fluid. New York, Academic Press, 1980; 2:27.

42. Ratcliffe A, Mow VC. The structure, function, and biologic repair of articular cartilage. In: Friedlaender G, Goldberg V (eds). Bone and Cartilage Allografts. Amer Acad Orthop Surg 1990; p. 123.

43. Mankin HJ. Mitosis in articular cartilage of immature rabbits: a histologic, stathokinetic (colchicinic) and autoradiographic study. Clin Orthop 1964; 34:170.

44. Mankin HJ, Lilliello L. Biochemical and metabolic abnormalities in articular cartilage from osteoarthritis human hips. J Bone Joint Surg 1970; 52A:424.

45. Gross AE, Silverstein EA, Falk J, et al. The allo-transplantation of partial joints in the treatment of osteoarthritis of the knee. Clin Orthop 1975; 108:7.

46. Locht RC, Gross AE, Langer F. Late osteochondral allograft resurfacing for tibial plateau fractures. J Bone Joint Surg 1984; 66A:328.

47. Meyers MH, Chatterjee SN. Osteochondral transplantation. Surg Clin North Am 1978; 58:429.

48. Outerbridge RE. Joint surface transplants—a preliminary report. J West Pacif Orthop Assoc 1971; 8:1.

49. Lane JM, Brighton CT, Ottens HR, Lipton M. Joint resurfacing in the rabbit using an autologous osteochondral graft. J Bone Joint Surg 1977; 59A:218.

50. Campbell CJ, Ishida H, Takahaski H, Kelly F. The transplantation of articular cartilage. J Bone Joint Surg 1963; 45A:1579.

51. Rodrigo JJ, Sakovich L, Travis L, Smith G. Osteocartilaginous allografts as compared with autografts in the treatment of knee joint osteocartilaginous defects in dogs. Clin Orthop 1978; 134:342.

52. Yablon IG, Brandt KD, DeLellis R, Covall D. Destruction of joint homografts. Arthritis Rheum 1977; 20:1526.

53. Krane SM, Amento EP. Cellular interactions and control of collagenase secretion in the synovium. J Rheumatol 10 (Suppl. 11): 7, 1983.

54. Pettipher ER, Higgs GA, Henderson B. Interleukin 1 induces leukocyte infiltration and cartilage prosteoglycan degradation in the synovial joint. Proc Natl Acad Sci USA 1986; 83:8749.

55. Sin YM, Sedgwick AD, Willoughby DA. Studies on the mechanism of cartilage degradation. J Pathol 1984; 142:23.

56. Ziff M. Factors involved in cartilage injury. J Rheumatol 10 (suppl. 11): 13, 1983.

57. Schachar NS, McGann LE. Cryopreservation of Articular Cartilage. In: Friedlaender GE, Goldberg VM, (eds). Bone and Cartilage Allografts. Amer Acad Orthop Surg 1991; p. 211.

58. Tomford WW, Mankin HJ. Investigational approaches to articular cartilage preservation. Clin Orthop 1983; 174:22.

59. Ahlo AJ. Allogenic joint transplantation in the dog. Ann Chir Gynaecol 1973; 62:226.

60. Campbell CJ. Homotransplantation of a half or whole joint. Clin Orthop 1972; 87:146.

61. Herndon CH, Chase SW. Experimental studies in the transplantation of whole joints. J Bone Joint Surg 1952; 34A:564.

62. Kandel RA, Pritzker KPH, Langer F, et al. The pathologic features of massive osseous grafts. Hum Pathol 1984; 15:141.

63. Salenious P, Holmstrom E, Koskinen E, Alho A. Histological changes in clinical half-joint allograft replacements. Acta Orthop Scand 1982; 53:295.

64. Langer F, Gross AE, West M, Urovitz EP: The immunogenicity of allograft knee joint transplants. Clin Orthop 1978; 132:155.

65. Rodrigo JJ, Travis CR, Thompson EC. Improvement of dog total

knee joint allografts with preadministration of sensitized T-cells from rabbits. Trans Orthop Res Soc 1979; 4:62.

66. Stevenson S, Dannucci GA, Sharkey NA, Poole RR. The fate of articular cartilage after transplantation of fresh and cryopreserved tissue-antigen-matched and mismatched osteochondral allografts in dogs. J Bone Joint Surg 1989; 71A:1297.

67. Mankin HJ. The reaction of articular catilage to injury and osteoarthritis (first of two parts). New Engl J Med 1974; 291:1285.

68. Mankin HJ. The reaction of articular cartilage to injury and osteoarthritis (second of two parts). N Engl J Med 1974; 291:1335.

69. Entin MA, Daniel G, Kahn D. Transplantation of autogenous half-joints. Arch Surg 1968; 96:359.

70. Kettlekamp DB. Experimental autologous joint transplantation. Clin Orthop 1972; 87:138.

71. Mims CA, Stokes A, Grahame R. Synthesis of antibodies, including antiviral antibodies, in the knee joints of patients with arthritis. Ann Rheumat Dis 1985; 44:734.

72. Nouri AME, Panayi GS, Goodman SM. Cytokines and the chronic inflammation of rheumatic disease. II. The presence of interleukin-2 in synovial fluids. Clin Exper Immunol 1984; 58:402.

73. Stevenson S, Li XQ, Martin B. The fate of cancellous and cortical bone after transplantation of fresh and cryopreserved tissue—antigen matched and mismatched osteochondral allografts in dogs. J Bone Joint Surg 1991; 73A:1143–1156.

74. Mankin HJ. Complications of allograft surgery. In: Friedlaender G, Mankin H, Sell K (eds). Osteochondral Allografts. Little Brown and Co., Boston, 1983; p. 259.

2

IMMUNOLOGY OF BONE AND CARTILAGE ALLOGRAFTS

Andrei A. Czitrom

A discussion of the immunology of musculoskeletal tissue transplantation must start, by necessity, with reasoning how one would explain the different biological behavior of autografts and allografts. Although the topic of biology is covered extensively in Chapter 1, it seems reasonable to re-emphasize that there is a profound difference in the outcome of autologous (or syngeneic) as compared with allogeneic bone transplants when grafted to either heterotopic or orthotopic sites. This can be demonstrated readily in a system where mouse calvaria-derived bone cells are transplanted heterotopically under the kidney capsule of syngeneic or allogeneic recipients. At 6 weeks after transplantation, the syngeneic transplant forms an ossicle containing marrow cells while the allogeneic transplant is destroyed by a strong inflammatory response dominated by small lymphocytes (Fig. 2.1 *A–D*). A similar but more subtle difference is noted after orthotopic transplantation of diaphyseal cortical bone grafts where the delay in remodeling serves as an indicator of immunological recognition. This is shown in Figure 2.2 (*A–D*), representing the remodeling of orthotopic cortical bone grafts in dogs at 20 weeks after transplantation. The remodeling seen on both longitudinal and transverse sections is significantly more advanced in autografts over allografts as measured by sequential fluorochrome labeling. The difference in the biological behavior of autologous (or syngeneic) versus that of allogeneic bone grafts in both situations must be attributed to the genetic differences in the respective donor-recipient combinations and is, therefore, by necessity, a manifestation of the host's ability to discriminate between self and nonself. This feature, by definition, represents immune recognition and tells us that the rules of transplantation immunology govern the outcome of bone allografts as they do that of other transplanted tissues or organs.

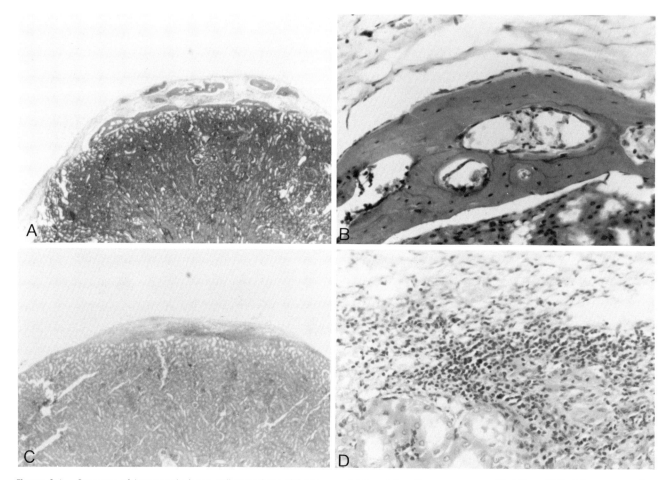

Figure 2.1. Outcome of heterotopic bone cell transplants. Calvaria-derived bone cells from DBA/2 (H-2^d) mice were transplanted under the kidney capsule of syngeneic DBA/2 (H-2^d) (A, B) or allogeneic CBA (H-2^k) (C, D) recipients and assessed by histology at 6 weeks after grafting. A. Low-power photomicrograph of syngeneic transplant showing bone formation (*top*) next to the normal kidney parenchyma (H & E, × 63). B. High-power view from area of bone formation shown in A demonstrating viable ossicle with marrow spaces (H & E, × 325). C. Low-power photomicrograph of allogeneic transplant showing fibrous tissue with no bone formation under the kidney capsule (H & E, × 63). D. High-power view from area of fibrous tissue shown in C demonstrating inflammatory response with lymphocytic infiltrate indicative of immune rejection (H & E, × 325).

BASIC CONCEPTS OF TRANSPLANTATION IMMUNOLOGY
Induction of Transplantation Responses

Organ or tissue grafts transplanted across genetic differences in animals or humans are generally rejected by the immune system. The response of the immune system is triggered by two separate signals derived from the graft: (*a*) alloantigen, and (*b*) a "second signal" provided by specialized antigen-presenting cells (APC) (1). The principal alloantigens are glycoproteins on the cell surface encoded by the major histocompatibility complex (MHC) (human lymphocyte antigen [HLA] in man, H-2 in the mouse). There are two classes of such antigens: (*a*) 45 K MHC molecules, which associate with β-2 microglobulin (class I: HLA A,B,C in man), and (*b*) 28–32 K molecules (class II: HLA D in man). Class I antigens are recognized preferentially by CD8$^+$ cytotoxic T cells while class II molecules trigger preferentially CD4$^+$ helper T cells (2, 3). Class I antigens are present on most nucleated cells while class II molecules have a more restricted expression on marrow-derived cells but can be induced by products of T cells (γ-interferon) on a variety of cell types (4). As class I antigens are ubiquitous on organs and tissues, they generally serve as the first signal to trigger the allograft response but are, by themselves, poor immunogens (1, 5). Effective activation of T cells requires stimulation by specialized APC which, in general, express class II antigens. These APC are equipped to provide the so-called second signal for T-cell activation in the form of either accessory molecules or soluble mediators, such as inter-

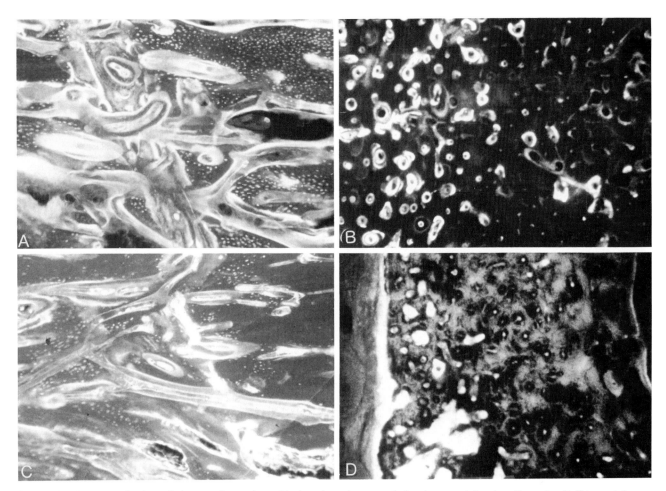

Figure 2.2. Outcome of orthotopic bone cell transplants. Diaphyseal autograft and allograft bone segments were transplanted in a dog model and assessed at 20 weeks by examining longitudinal and transverse sections labeled by sequential fluorochromes. *A.* Longitudinal section of autologous transplant at host/graft junction (*graft on the right*) showing early and extensive remodeling indicated by the abundance of fluorochromes administered during the first 2–4 weeks after transplantation (bright-staining areas). *B.* Transverse section through midportion of auto- logous graft showing remodeling from the cortex (*left*) toward the medullary canal (*right*) and spanning two-thirds of the diameter (bright-stained osteons). *C.* Longitudinal section of allograft at host/graft junction (*graft on the right*) showing late and limited remodeling indicated by less abundant early fluorochrome label. *D.* Transverse section through middle of allograft showing limited remodeling (bright-staining osteons) confined to the outer periphery of the cortex. (Courtesy of Dr. O. Schwarzenbach and Dr. M. Aebi, University of Bern, Switzerland.) (91, 96).

leukin-1 (3, 6). They include a heterogeneous group of cells of marrow origin, such as dendritic cells, macrophages, B lymphocytes, and other cell types (3, 6–9).

Effector Mechanism of Transplantation Responses

The effector arm of the immune system in transplantation responses is a cellular response mediated by CD4$^+$ helper and CD8$^+$ cytotoxic T cells and modulated by suppressor T cells (10–12). Acute rejection is mediated by similar mechanisms as the delayed-type hypersensitivity reaction and occurs within days to weeks after transplantation. This complex event involves T cells (primarily CD4$^+$ cells), soluble mediators or cytokines (interleukin-2, -3, -4, -5; γ-interferon, tumor necrosis factor), arachidonic acid and its metabolites (thromboxane A2 and B2), macrophages, and endothelial cells; all of which, in concert, produce parenchymal injury and occlusion of graft vessels (11). Although antibody responses generally do not mediate the transplantation responses to tissue or organ grafts, transplants do sensitize recipients to donor alloantigens by inducing specific alloantibodies. Donor-specific lymphocytotoxic HLA antibodies produce hyperacute rejection, although uncommonly, this type of immunological rejection can be mediated by cellular mechanisms (10). Chronic rejection occurs by similar cellular mechanisms as acute rejection but occurs months or years later (10, 13).

Recognition of Alloantigen

The intensity of allograft rejection depends on the degree of antigen mismatch between graft and host. It is strongest with mismatch at all MHC loci but is still present if all the MHC antigens are matched because of multiple minor, non-MHC antigenic differences. MHC antigens are not equally immunogenic and their immunogenicity is determined by the mode of their presentation to the immune system and by the genetic control of the response. When donor and recipient are MHC-identical but different at minor, non-MHC loci, the triggering of the host's cellular immune system can be a result of direct stimulation via donor APC or a result of indirect stimulation by reprocessing of donor alloantigen onto host APC (14, 15). This latter indirect route can also occur in MHC class I-different, class II-compatible combinations, while in MHC class I- and class II-incompatible transplants, stimulation is more likely to occur directly via donor APC (16, 17). Direct recognition of donor MHC alloantigen is most likely to occur by a mechanism that mimics recognition of self-MHC plus peptide as in conventional immune responses (10, 18).

Induction of Unresponsiveness

The two-signal model of alloreactivity predicts that the selective removal of APC from tissue or organ grafts will result in allograft survival (1, 19, 20). Transplantation experiments of cultured or ultraviolet light-treated endocrine tissues or of anti-class II monoclonal antibody-treated organs provide support for this notion (21–24). Thus, the selective manipulation of grafts prior to transplantation is one way to prevent allograft rejection without inducing a generalized suppression of the immune system. Specific immunosuppression of the host response against graft antigens can be readily induced in newborn animals by the perinatal injection of graft-derived lymphoid cells (neonatal tolerance) (25–27). An analogous tolerant state is present in radiation chimeras where the repopulating bone marrow stem cells become tolerant of host tissues (28). Specific tolerance cannot be induced readily in adult animals but convincing evidence showing a remarkable immunosuppressive effect of pretransplant blood transfusions (which most likely operates by inhibiting interleukin-2 production by T cells) suggests that specific perturbations of the immune system resulting in reduced responsiveness can be induced to the advantage of transplanters (29, 30). Finally, nonresponsiveness of the immune system can be induced by generalized immunosuppression of the host, an approach that has been revolutionized by the use of cyclosporin A for clinical organ transplantation (31).

IMMUNE RESPONSES TO BONE ALLOGRAFTS

The role of transplantation immunity with relationship to the outcome of bone allografts was recognized over three decades ago (32), concomitant with the development of knowledge of the events involved in the rejection of foreign tissues in general (33, 34). Studies that relate to host immunity to bone allografts have used a variety of methods including (a) histological assessments, (b) in vivo assays of cellular immunity, (c) measurements of humoral immunity and, (d) in vitro assays of cell-mediated immunity.

Histological Assessments

Histology invariably demonstrates a difference in the biological behavior of allografts and autografts. This issue is discussed extensively in Chapter 1. From the viewpoint of transplantation immunology, the histological evidence presented by Chalmers (32), Hutchinson (36), Burwell (37), and numerous subsequent investigators (35, 38–43) indicate, without doubt, that bone allografts are immunogenic and are rejected by the host. This is shown by the lack or delay in bone formation in heterotopic transplantation models or by the slow healing and remodeling after orthotopic grafting in association with the detection of inflammatory immune infiltrates.

Immunologic rejection interferes with graft function by abrogating bone formation by donor-derived osteogenic cells that are destroyed by the allogeneic response (32, 35). Histological techniques alone are subject to sampling errors and offer only limited information with regard to immune mechanisms and effector or target cells and tissues involved, although some degree of immune specificity can be determined by using inbred strains of animals.

In Vivo Assays of Cellular Immunity

The assessment of cellular immunity in vivo allows the measurement, to some extent, of the quantity and specificity of the immune response. The measurement of the weight of regional lymph nodes draining subcutaneously implanted allogeneic bone grafts has been used by Burwell and Gowland (44, 45) to show the different immunogenicity of allografts and autografts. Skin grafting is another method to measure cellular immunity in vivo and was used by Chalmers (32) and others (46–49) to investigate the immunogenicity of bone allografts and the specificity of the response. The results of these investigations are somewhat contradictory; some found that, after allogeneic bone grafting, there was a significant acceleration of the rejection of skin grafts (second-set reaction) derived from the same donor strain (32, 46), yet in other studies, there was only a minimal acceleration (47, 48) or a prolongation of skin graft survival (49). These results suggest that bone allografts can stimulate or suppress the immune system in specific ways that are not completely understood.

Measurements of Humoral Immunity

Humoral immunity to allogeneic bone grafts has been demonstrated in numerous experimental studies using a variety of assay systems, the most common being the detection of cytotoxic antibodies (47, 49–53). Similar observations have been made when studying sera from patients receiving bone and cartilage transplants (54, 55). These results indicate that bone allografts can sensitize recipients to donor cell surface alloantigens. They are not directly relevant to the rejection process, which is mediated by immune T cells rather than by antibody (10–12). However, the quantitation of humoral immunity to bone allografts is useful, similarly to the way skin grafts are, for the assessment of the relative immunogenicity of various types of grafts and for determining the specificity of the response that they induce.

In Vitro Assays of Cell-mediated Immunity

Cell-mediated immunity assayed in vitro, using a number of different methods, has allowed the detection of responses to allograft bone in experimental animals (49, 51, 53) and in humans (56). These in vitro tests, like antibody assays, indicate specific immunity to cell surface alloantigens of allogeneic bone grafts. Although they measure cellular responses, these tests do not necessarily correlate with the in vivo events of transplant rejection. However, T-cell assays, such as the mixed lymphocyte reaction, T-cell cytotoxicity, and interleukin-2 production, measure the function of specific T-lymphocyte subsets that are known to be involved in allogeneic responses and, thus, reflect best the specific immunity to allografts.

IMMUNOGENIC COMPONENTS OF BONE AND CARTILAGE GRAFTS
Importance of MHC Class II Antigens

The relative antigenicity of allografts is related to the presence of bone marrow-derived immunogenic cells (referred to earlier as APC) that reside within them and are capable of delivering the second signal required to activate fully the T-lymphocyte system, which cannot respond to alloantigen alone (1, 5, 19–24). These cells are known to express class II MHC molecules, which play a role in their ability to trigger allogeneic responses (6–9). The importance of class II MHC antigens for the immunogenicity of bone allografts is supported by evidence indicating that, in certain situations, fetal bone grafts that are blocked by anti-class II antibody do not elicit allograft rejection (57). In addition, data showing that bone allografts elicit anti-class II alloantibody responses and that treatment with anti-class II serum decreases their immunogenicity indicate that a population of class II-positive cells are responsible for triggering allogeneic responses against these transplants (52, 58, 59). These living immunogenic cells have been shown to survive for several weeks after retransplantation to a second recipient (52).

Role of Bone Marrow

The immunogenic cells of bone allografts would be expected logically to reside in bone marrow. The notion that the marrow is the immunogenic compartment of allogeneic bone grafts is supported by two different lines of experimental evidence. First, it has been shown early that bone allografts that are washed free of marrow prior to transplantation elicit lower measurable immune responses than grafts containing marrow (44, 47, 53, 60). Second, experiments that examined the outcome of bone allografts derived from radiation chimeras have demonstrated that genetic matching for marrow but not for nonmarrow elements results in decreased humoral immunity and improved healing (61). This latter finding has been confirmed for vascularized limb allografts (62) and makes a strong argument for attributing the immunogenicity of allogeneic bone to its marrow component.

Immunogenic Cells in Bone Marrow

The nature of the immunogenic cell within the bone marrow component of bone allografts has been the subject of studies in my laboratory. The approach taken was to fractionate bone marrow cells sequentially and to enrich for functional activity as stimulators of allospecific T-lymphocyte responses in vitro, concomitant with examining the morphology of the cells that were enriched at each step. It was shown that the most potent immunogenic cells within bone marrow share many of the physical properties of dendritic cells, express class II MHC antigens, and stimulate both helper (interleukin-2-producing) and cytotoxic T cells strongly in vitro, albeit with less efficiency than splenic dendritic cells (Table 2.1) (63). These cells were identified as myeloid cells of the granulocyte lineage (Fig. 2.3). They are the most likely candidates of the various cell types present in bone allografts to represent the relevant "passenger cells" that initiate transplantation immunity (64, 65).

Immunogenicity of Other Compartments

The contribution of components other than living bone marrow cells to the immunogenicity of bone allografts is likely to be of minimal importance. There is evidence that bone cells (osteocytes and osteoblasts) are not immunogenic because they express class I but not class II MHC antigens and they do not stimulate lymphocytes in mixed cultures (66). The immunogenic property of osteoclasts, which are marrow-derived cells, is unclear. Elements other than cells, such as matrix components (proteoglycan subunits and collagen), although antigenic in experimental systems of autoimmunity (67, 68), are not relevant in alloreactivity and transplantation where immunity is triggered by and directed at alloantigens on the cell surface.

Immunogenicity of Cartilage

Cartilage allografts differ fundamentally from bone allografts in terms of immunogenicity because they do not contain a large load of marrow-derived cells. However, allogeneic cartilage or chondrocytes have been shown to stimulate both humoral and cellular immunity after transplantation in vivo (69–71). Moreover, chondrocytes bear both class I and class II MHC antigens and can stimulate allogeneic lymphocytes in mixed cultures (72–74). De-

spite this, ample experimental evidence indicates that cartilage or chondrocyte grafts remain viable after allotransplantation (75–80). This ability of cartilage allografts to escape rejection has been attributed to the pericellular cartilage matrix, which exerts afferent and efferent blocks that interfere with effective immunological stimulation and effector function (70, 71, 80–82). Composite osteochondral allografts follow the rules described for both bone and cartilage grafts with the bone component undergoing rejection and the cartilage component generally surviving transplantation (83–85).

Vascularized Transplants

Vascularized bone and limb allografts are composed of multiple types of tissues and cell types that can act as stimulators and targets of the transplantation response. These transplants are far too complex to allow a systematic analysis of relative immunogenicities of the individual components. However, histological data indicate that an early target of the rejection response in these composite allografts is the bone marrow while the endothelium of the vascular pedicle is attacked at a later stage of graft rejection (86, 87).

APPROACHES FOR DECREASING THE IMMUNOGENICITY OF BONE ALLOGRAFTS

The aim of decreasing the immunogenicity of bone allografts is to obtain better healing and mechanical strength. Assessments that deal directly with these parameters are more relevant than immunological assays because they reflect the ultimate function and effectiveness of allografts when compared to autografts. The principal methods that

Table 2.1.
Allostimulatory Potential of Bone Marrow APC and Spleen Dendritic Cells[a]

Stimulator Cell Type[b]	Cell No.[b]	Supernatant Dilution[b]	IL-2 Production (cpm ± SD)[b]	CTL Activity (LU/culture)[b]
Bone marrow APC	2 × 10⁴	1 : 2	110,498 ± 3,096	31.2
		1 : 4	69,724 ± 2,247	
	5 × 10³	1 : 2	22,814 ± 2,102	16.6
		1 : 4	9,190 ± 1,000	
Dendritic cells	2 × 10⁴	1 : 2	198,399 ± 21,326	81.0
		1 : 4	161,977 ± 16,604	
	5 × 10³	1 : 2	210,039 ± 5,332	80.0
		1 : 4	147,654 ± 11,579	

[a]Reproduced with permission from Czitrom AA, et al. Granulocyte precursors are the principal cells in bone marrow that stimulate all specific cytolytic T-lymphocyte responses. Immunology 1988; 64:655.
[b]T cells from C57 BL/6 mice were cultured with allogeneic DBA/2 stimulator cells (irradiated 2000 rads) for 72 hours for interleukin-2 (IL-2) production and for 5 days for cytotoxic T-lymphocyte (CTL) activity. IL-2 production is expressed as proliferative responses of an indicator cell line in counts per minute (cpm) ± SD (³H-thymidine incorporation). CTL activity is expressed in lytic units (LU) per culture calculated from individual dose-response curves of ⁵¹Cr release from a fixed number of target cells.

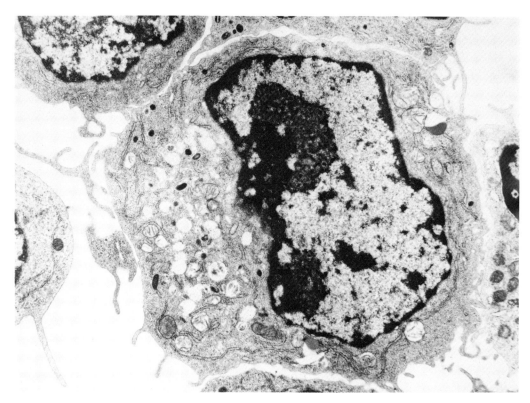

Figure 2.3. The immunogenic cell in bone marrow. Electron micrograph of low-density, nonadherent, Fc-receptor-negative cell that was purified for the most potent stimulatory activity of cytotoxic T cells in vitro (63, 64). The cell has a few surface projections, an indented nucleus, a small nucleolus, a prominent Golgi, numerous mitochondria, scanty lysosomes, and many intracytoplasmic granules (× 9940). The features are those of a myeloid cell of the granulocyte lineage.

have been used to evaluate these parameters include histological or radiotracer techniques to assess osteogenesis (32, 36, 37, 39–41, 43, 88), measurement of blood flow (89, 90), quantitation of remodeling after sequential fluorochrome labeling (91, 92), and biomechanical testing (48, 59, 61, 92, 93). No single technique is uniquely reliable to measure the ultimate outcome of success of bone grafting and therefore, ideally, a combination of techniques should be used. The main approaches used to reduce the immunogenicity of bone allografts aiming to increase their success are: (*a*) immunosuppression of the host, (*b*) histocompatibility matching of host and graft, and (*c*) altering the graft.

Immunosuppression of the Host

The effect of immunosuppression in experimental bone transplantation has been studied extensively. Early studies examined the effect of agents such as azathioprine, prednisolone, antilymphocyte serum, or sublethal whole body irradiation (41, 47, 59, 94–96). The results of these experiments showed that osteogenesis and revascularization of nonvascularized bone allografts were significantly improved in immunosuppressed animals and were al-

most identical to autografts. However, similar immunosuppression did not prevent chronic rejection of vascularized joint transplants (97). Another agent, methotrexate, was found to depress antibody responses but interfered with the healing of nonvascularized bone allografts (59). Cyclosporin A has been investigated in numerous, more recent studies and found to be effective in improving the incorporation of nonvascularized bone allografts (91, 96, 98). Moreover, cyclosporin A has been effective in preventing the rejection of vascularized bone and joint allografts in several experimental models (91, 96, 99–101). Immunosuppression has no current application in clinical bone transplantation because of the potential side effects of chronic treatment, which are not sufficiently justified for the purpose of limb salvage.

Histocompatibility Matching

Experiments of bone transplantation carried out in inbred animals controlling the genetic differences between host and recipient have provided evidence supporting the notion that the outcome of bone allografts correlates with the degree of histocompatibility. Thus, the immune response to allogeneic bone grafts was found to be greater than the response generated by semiallogeneic grafts (53). The analysis of defined histocompatibility differences showed that the healing and mechanical strength of MHC-incompatible bone grafts are significantly reduced compared with that of MHC-compatible but minor alloantigen-incompatible grafts (48, 92). Such results suggest that histocompatibility matching would reduce the immunogenicity of and improve the outcome of bone allografts. This has been shown to be the case in experiments examining the immunogenicity and healing of MHC-matched and MHC-mismatched bone and osteochondral allografts (102–104). The possible role of histocompatibility matching in human bone transplantation has been examined in a retrospective review (105) but its potential benefit in clinical practice is currently unresolved.

Altering the Graft

This approach has been investigated extensively not only because of efforts to decrease the immunogenicity of bone allografts but also for the purpose of developing storage methods of grafts for use in clinical practice. The principal methods used for these purposes have been deep-freezing and freeze-drying of allogeneic bone grafts. Numerous studies in both heterotopic and orthotopic transplantation models using a variety of immunological assay systems of humoral and/or cellular responsiveness have demonstrated decreased or absent immunity to deep-frozen and freeze-dried bone allografts (32, 45–47, 49–52, 59). The logical explanation of these results is that these treatment methods kill all living cells and, thus, there is no direct immunogenic signal to stimulate the host transplantation response. Theoretically, these dead tissues still contain cell-surface glycoprotein fragments of histocompatibility antigens that can stimulate antibody responses and can be picked up, processed, and presented indirectly by host-APC to the T-lymphocyte system (14–16). As this indirect route for stimulating transplantation immunity is much less efficient than the direct route (16, 17), for practical purposes, frozen and freeze-dried bone allografts can be considered as being nonimmunogenic biological implants. The same holds true for allogeneic bone grafts treated by other methods that kill living cells, such as autoclaving, deproteinizing, decalcifying, and high doses of radiation (46).

The major disadvantage of deep-freezing and freeze-drying of bone grafts is the absence of live osteogenic cells. Graft-derived osteogenesis is an important event in the early phases of graft repair and is readily demonstrated in fresh autografts but is deficient in allografts because of destruction of osteogenic cells by the immune system (32, 35, 39, 40, 88). The lack of graft-derived osteogenic potential in deep-frozen and freeze-dried bone allografts (and also in frozen syngeneic or autologous grafts) results in slower healing and remodeling as well as in decreased mechanical strength when compared with fresh autologous grafts (59, 93). Ideally, one would like to use an allograft that has been altered in such a way as to be nonimmunogenic but it still contains live osteogenic cells. This may be possible by selectively eliminating immunogenic APC by methods such as treatment with anti-class II reagents, low doses of irradiation, or organ culture (59, 106, 107). At the present time, these approaches are experimental and they do not resolve the concomitant need for long-term preservation of the tissues involved. Deep-frozen and freeze-dried allografts remain the most used tissues in orthopaedic practice and the clinical demand for these biological materials is increasing at a constant rate.

REFERENCES

1. Lafferty KJ, Andrus L, Prowse SJ. Role of lymphokine and antigen in the control of specific T cell responses. Immunol Rev 1980; 51:279.
2. Mitchison NA. The major histocompatibility complex: the modern synthesis. Immunology Today 1980; 1:91.
3. Sprent J, Schaefer M. Antigen presenting cells for unprimed T cells. Immunology Today 1989; 10:17.
4. Pober JS, Collins T, Gimbrone Jr MA, Cotran RS, Gitlin JD, Fiers W, Clayberger C, Krensky AM, Burakoff SJ, Reiss CS. Lymphocytes recognize human vascular endothelial and dermal fibroblast Ia antigens induced by recombinant immune interferon. Nature 1983; 305:726.
5. Batchelor JR, Welsh KI, Burgos H. Transplantation antigens per se are poor immunogens within a species. Nature 1978; 273:54.
6. Weaver CT, Unanue ER. The costimulatory function of antigen presenting cells. Immunology Today 1990; 11:49.
7. Sunshine GH, Katz DR, Czitrom AA. Heterogeneity of stimulator cells in the murine mixed leukocyte response. Eur J Immunol 1982; 12:9.
8. Czitrom AA, Katz DR, Sunshine GH. Alloreactive cytotoxic T lymphocyte responses to H-2 products on purified accessory cells. Immunology 1982; 45:553.
9. Czitrom AA, Sunshine GH, Reme T, Ceredig R, Glasebrook AL, Kelso A, MacDonald HR. Stimulator cell requirements for allospecific T cell subsets: specialized accessory cells are required to activate helper but not cytolytic T lymphocyte precursors. J Immunol 1983; 130:546.
10. Morris PJ. Rejection—unanswered questions. Hum Immunol 1990; 28:104.
11. Tilney NL, Kupiec-Weglinski JW. Advances in the understanding of rejection mechanisms. Transplant Proc 1989; 21:10.
12. Bach FH. Reconsideration of the mechanism of first-set vas-

cularized allograft rejection: some concluding remarks. Hum Immunol 1990; 28:263.

13. Harder F, Landman J. General aspects of organ transplantation surgery. In: Aebi M, Regazzoni P (eds). Bone Transplantation. Springer-Verlag, Berlin, Heidelberg, 1989; p. 98.

14. Czitrom AA, Gascoigne NRJ, Edwards S, Waterfield DJ. Induction of minor alloantigen-specific T cell subsets in vivo: recognition of processed antigen by helper but not by cytotoxic T cell precursors. J Immunol 1984; 133:33.

15. Owens T, Czitrom AA, Gascoigne NRJ, Crispe IN, Ratcliffe MJH, Lai PK, Mitchison NA. The presentation of cell surface alloantigens to T cells. Immunobiology 1984; 168:189.

16. Sherwood RS, Brent L, Rayfield LS. Presentation of alloantigens by host cells. Eur J Immunol 1986; 16:569.

17. Lechler RI, Batchelor JR. Restoration of immunogenicity to passenger cell-depleted kidney allografts by the addition of donor strain dendritic cells. J Exp Med 1982; 155:31.

18. Batchelor JR, Kaminski E, Lombardi G, Goldman JM, Lechler RI. Individual variation in alloresponsiveness and the molecular basis of allorecognition. Hum Immunol 1990; 28:96.

19. Lafferty KJ, Prowse SJ, Simeonovic CJ. Immunobiology of tissue transplantation: a return to the passenger leukocyte concept. Ann Rev Immunol 1983; 1:143.

20. Silvers WK, Kimura H, Desquenne-Clark L, Miyamoto M. Some new perspectives on transplantation immunity and tolerance. Immunol Today 1987; 8:117.

21. Lafferty KJ, Prowse DJ. Theory and practice of immunoregulation by tissue treatment prior to transplantation. World J Surg 1984; 8:187.

22. Silvers WK, Flemming HK, Naji A, Barker L. Influence of removing passenger cells on the fate of skin and parathyroid allografts. Diabetes 1982; 31(Suppl. 4):60.

23. Lau H, Reemtzma K, Hardy MA. Prolongation of rat islet allograft by direct UV irradiation of the graft. Science 1984; 223:607.

24. Lloyd DM, Weiser MR, Kang RH, Buckingham M, Stuart FP, Thistlethwaite JR. Does depletion of donor dendritic cells in an organ allograft lead to prolongation of graft survival on transplantation? Transplant Proc 1989; 21:482.

25. Brent L, Brooks CG, Medawar PB, Simpson E. Transplantation tolerance. Br Med Bull 1976; 32:101.

26. Streilein JW. Neonatal tolerance: towards an immunogenetic definition of self. Immunol Rev 1979; 46:125.

27. Holan V. Absolute specificity of neonatally induced transplantation tolerance. Transplantation 1990; 50:1072.

28. Sykes M, Sachs DH. Mixed allogeneic chimerism as an approach to transplantation tolerance. Immunol Today 1988; 9:23.

29. Opelz G, Senger DPS, Mickey MR, Terasaki PT. Effect of blood transfusion on subsequent kidney transplants. Transplant Proc 1973; 5:253.

30. Hadley GA, Kenyon N, Anderson CB, Mohanakumar T. Downregulation of antidonor cytotoxic lymphocyte responses in recipients of donor-specific transfusions. Transplantation 1990; 50:1064.

31. Cockfield SM, Halloran PF. Cyclosporin: a new decade. Ann Roy College of Phys Surg Canada 1991; 24:25.

32. Chalmers J. Transplantation immunity in bone homografting. J Bone Joint Surg 1959; 41B:160.

33. Billingham RE, Brent L, Medawar PB. The antigenic stimulus in transplantation immunity. Nature 1956; 178:514.

34. Medawar PB. The homograft reaction. Proc Roy Soc 1958; 145:145.

35. Chalmers J. Bone transplantation. Symp Tissue Org Transplant. (Suppl) J Clin Pathol 1967; 20:540.

36. Hutchinson J. The fate of experimental bone autografts and homografts. Br J Surg 1952; 39:552.

37. Burwell RG. The fate of bone grafts. In: Apley AG (ed). Recent Advances in Orthopaedics. Williams & Wilkins, Baltimore, 1969.

38. Chase SW, Herndon CH. The fate of autogenous and homogeneous bone grafts. A historical review. J Bone Joint Surg 1955; 37A:809.

39. Hammack BL, Enneking WF. Comparative vascularization of autogenous and homogenous bone transplants. J Bone Joint Surg 1960; 42A:822.

40. Sabet TY, Hidvegy EB, Ray RD. Bone Immunology. II. Comparison of embryonic mouse isografts and homografts. J Bone Joint Surg 1961; 43A:1007.

41. Goldberg VM, Lance EM. Revascularization and accretion in transplantation. Quantitative studies of the role of the allograft barrier. J Bone Joint Surg 1972; 54A:807.

42. Bonfiglio M, Jeter WS. Immunological responses to bone. Clin Orthop 1972; 87:19.

43. Goldberg VM, Stevenson S. Natural history of autografts and allografts. Clin Orthop 1987; 225:7.

44. Burwell RG, Gowland G. Studies in the transplantation of bone. II. The changes occurring in the lymphoid tissue after homografts and autografts of fresh cancellous bone. J Bone Joint Surg 1961; 43B:820.

45. Burwell RG, Gowland G. Studies in the transplantation of bone. III. The immune responses of lymph nodes draining components of fresh homologous cancellous bone and homologous bone treated by different methods. J Bone Joint Surg 1962; 44B:131.

46. Brooks DB, Heiple KG, Herndon AH, Powell AE. Immunological factors in homogeneous bone transplantation. IV. The effect of various methods of preparation and irradiation on antigenicity. J Bone Joint Surg 1963; 45-A:1617.

47. Elves MW. Newer knowledge of the immunology of bone and cartilage. Clin Orthop 1976; 120:232.

48. Halloran PF, Ziv I, Lee EH, Langer F, Pritzker KPH, Gross AE. Orthotopic bone transplantation in mice. I. Technique and assessment of healing. Transplantation 1979; 27:414.

49. Langer F, Czitrom A, Pritzker KP, Gross AE. The immunogenicity of fresh and frozen allogeneic bone. J Bone Joint Surg 1975; 57A:216.

50. Elves NW. Humoral immune response to allografts of bone. Int Arch Allergy 1974; 47:708.

51. Friedlaender GE, Strong DM, Sell KW. Studies on the antigen-

icity of bone. I. Freeze-dried and deep-frozen bone allografts in rabbits. J Bone Joint Surg 1976; 58A:854.

52. Halloran PF, Lee HE, Ziv I, Langer F, Gross AE. Orthotopic bone transplantation in mice. II. Studies of the alloantibody response. Transplantation 1979; 27:420.

53. Muscolo DL, Kawai S, Ray RD. Cellular and humoral immune response analysis of bone-allografted rats. J Bone Joint Surg 1976; 58A:826.

54. Rodrigo JJ, Fuller TC, Mankin HJ. Cytotoxic HLA antibodies in patients with bone and cartilage allografts. Trans Orthop Res Soc 1976; 1:131.

55. Friedlaender GE, Strong DM, Sell KW. Donor graft specific anti-HLA antibodies following freeze-dried bone allografts. Trans Orthop Res Soc 1977; 2:87.

56. Langer F, Gross AE, West M, Urovitz EP. The immunogenicity of allograft knee joint transplants. Clin Orthop 1977; 132:155.

57. Segal S, Siegal T, Altaraz H, Lev-El A, Nevo Z, Nebel L, Katzenelson A, Feldman M. Fetal bone grafts do not elicit allograft rejection because of protecting anti-Ia alloantibodies. Transplantation 1979; 28:88.

58. Halloran PF, Lee E, Ziv I, Langer F. Bone grafting in inbred mice: evidence for H-2K, H-2D, and non-H-2 antigens in bone. Transplant Proc 1979; 11:1507.

59. Kliman M, Halloran PF, Lee E, Esses S, Fortner P, Langer F. Orthotopic bone transplantation in mice. III. Methods of reducing the immune response and their effect on healing. Transplantation 1981; 31:34.

60. Burwell RG, Gowland G, Dexter F. Studies in transplantation of bone. VI. Further observations concerning the antigenicity of homologous cortical and cancellous bone. J Bone Joint Surg 1963; 45B:597.

61. Esses SI, Halloran PF. Donor marrow-derived cells as immunogens and targets for the immune response to bone and skin allografts. Transplantation 1983; 35:169.

62. Lee WPA, Yaremchuk M, Manfrini M, Pan YC, Randolph MA, Weiland AJ. Prolonged survival of vascularized limb allografts from chimera donors. Trans Orthop Res Soc 1989; 14:468.

63. Czitrom AA, Axelrod TS, Fernandes B. Granulocyte precursors are the principal cells in bone marrow that stimulate allospecific cytolytic T-lymphocyte responses. Immunology 1988; 64:655.

64. Czitrom AA, Axelrod T, Fernandes B. Antigen presenting cells and bone allotransplantation. Clin Orthop 1985; 197:27.

65. Czitrom AA. Bone transplantation, passenger cells and the major histocompatibility complex. In: Aebi M, Regazzoni P (eds). Bone Transplantation. Springer-Verlag, Berlin, Heidelberg, 1989; p. 103.

66. Muscolo DL, Kawai S, Ray RD. In vitro studies of transplantation antigens present on bone cells in the rat. J Bone Joint Surg 1977; 59B:342.

67. Champion BR, Sell S, Poole AR. Immunity to homologous collagen and cartilage proteoglycans in rabbits. Immunology 1983; 48:605.

68. Terato K, Hasty KA, Cremer MA, Stuart JM, Townes AS, Kang AH. Collagen induced arthritis in mice. Localization of arthritogenic determinant to a fragment of type II collagen molecule. J Exp Med 1985; 162:637.

69. Stjernsward J. Studies in the transplantation of allogeneic cartilage across known histocompatibility barriers. Proc 10th Congr Int Soc Blood Transf, Stockholm, 1965; p. 197.

70. Langer F, Gross AE, Greaves MF. The immunogenicity of articular cartilage. Clin Exp Immunol 1972; 12:1.

71. Langer F, Gross AE. Immunogenicity of allograft articular cartilage. J Bone Joint Surg 1974; 56A:297.

72. Malseed ZM, Heyner S. Antigenic profile of the rat chondrocyte. Arthritis Rheum 1976; 19:223.

73. Tiku ML, Liu S, Weaver CW, Teodorescu M, Skoskey JL. Class II histocompatibility antigen-mediated immunologic function of normal articular chondrocytes. J Immunol 1985; 135:2923.

74. Gertzbein SD, Tait JD, Devlin SR, Argue S. The antigenicity of chondrocytes. Immunology 1977; 33:141.

75. Craigmyle MBL. An autoradiographic and histochemical study of long-term cartilage grafts in the rabbit. J Anat London 1958; 92:467.

76. Gibson T, Davis WB, Curran RC. The long-term survival of cartilage homografts in man. Br J Plast Surg 1958; 11:177.

77. Schatten WE, Bergenstal DB, Kramer WM, Swarm RL, Siegel S. Biological survival and growth of cartilage grafts. Plast Reconstr Surg 1958; 22:11.

78. Depalma AF, Tsaltas TT, Mauler GG. Viability of osteochondral grafts as determined by uptake of S^{35}. J Bone Joint Surg 1963; 45A:1565.

79. Chesterman PJ, Smith AU. Homotransplantation of articular cartilage and isolated chondrocytes. An experimental study in the rabbit. J Bone Joint Surg 1968; 50B:184.

80. McKibbin B, Ralis ZA. The site dependence of the articular cartilage transplant reaction. J Bone Joint Surg 1978; 60B:561.

81. Heyner S. The significance of the intercellular matrix in the survival of cartilage allografts. Transplantation 1969; 8:666.

82. Heyner S. The antigenicity of cartilage grafts. Surg Gynecol Obstet 1973; 136:298.

83. Kandel RA, Gross AE, Ganel A, McDermott AGP, Langer F, Pritzker KPH. Histopathology of failed osteoarticular shell allografts. Clin Orthop 1984; 197:103.

84. Oakeshott RD, Farine I, Pritzker KPH, Langer F, Gross AE. A clinical and histologic analysis of failed fresh osteochondral allografts. Clin Orthop 1988; 233:283.

85. Czitrom AA, Keating S, Gross AE. The viability of articular cartilage in fresh osteochondral allografts after clinical transplantation. J Bone Joint Surg 1990; 72A:574.

86. Gotfried Y, Yaremchuk MJ, Randolph MA, Weiland AJ. Histological characteristics of acute rejection in vascularized allografts of bone. J Bone Joint Surg 1987; 69A:409.

87. Gotfried Y, Yaremchuk MJ, Randolph MA, Weiland AJ. The target cells in vascularized bone allografts. In: Aebi M, Regazzoni P (eds). Bone Transplantation. Springer-Verlag, Berlin, Heidelberg, 1989; p. 111.

88. Elves MW. Studies of the behaviour of allogeneic cancellous bone grafts in inbred rats. Transplantation 1975; 19: 416.

89. Ogata K, Kuroki T, Sugioka Y. Measurement of blood flow in rabbit bone transplants. Int Orthop (SICOT) 1990; 14: 75.

90. Kirkeby OJ. Revascularization of bone grafts. J Bone Joint Surg 1991; 73B:501.

91. Schwarzenbach O, Regazzoni P, Aebi M. Segmental vascularized and non-vascularized bone allografts. In: Aebi M, Regazzoni P (eds). Bone Transplantation. Springer-Verlag, Berlin, Heidelberg, 1989; p. 78.

92. Goldberg VM, Powell A, Shaffer JW, Zika J, Stevenson S, Davy D, Heiple K. The role of histocompatibility in bone allografting. In: Aebi M, Regazzoni P (eds). Bone Transplantation. Springer-Verlag, Berlin, Heidelberg, 1989; p. 126.

93. Pelker RR, McKay J, Troiano N, Panjabi MM, Friedlaender GE. Allograft incorporation: a biomechanical evaluation in a rat model. J Orthop Res 1989; 7:585.

94. Burchard H, Glowczewskie FP, Enneking WF. Allogeneic segmental fibular transplants in azathioprine immunosuppressed dogs. J Bone Joint Surg 1977; 59A:881.

95. Burchard H. Short-term immunosuppression and dog cortical allografts. In: Aebi M, Regazzoni P (eds). Bone Transplantation. Springer-Verlag, Berlin, Heidelberg, 1989; p. 135.

96. Aebi M, Schwarzenbach O, Regazzoni P. Long-term versus short term immunosuppression in experimental bone allotransplantation. Trans Orthop Res Soc 1987; 12:89.

97. Goldberg VM, Porter BB, Lance EM. Transplantation of the canine knee joint on vascular pedicles. J Bone Joint Surg 1973; 55A:1314.

98. Kraay MJ, Davy DT, Goldberg VM, Shaffer JM, Klein L, Powell A. Influence of cyclosporin-A treatment and sham surgery on mechanical properties in a canine fibular graft model. Trans Orthop Res Soc 1986; 11:275.

99. Stewart J, Kiuchi T, Langer F, Halloran P, Gross AE. The effect of immunosuppression on vascularized bone grafts. Orthop Trans 1983; 6:492.

100. Aebi M, Regazzoni P, Perren SM, Harder F. Microsurgically revascularized bone allografts with immunosuppression with cyclosporine: preliminary report of the effect in an animal model. Transplantation 1986; 42:564.

101. Paskert JP, Yaremchuk MJ, Randolph MA, Weiland AJ. The role of cyclosporin in prolonging survival in vascularized bone allografts. Plast Reconstr Surg 1987; 80:240.

102. Stevenson S. The immune response to osteochondral allografts in dogs. J Bone Joint Surg 1987; 69A:573.

103. Stevenson S, Sharkey N, Dannucci G, Martin R. The incorporation and function of DLA-matched and mismatched, fresh and cryopreserved massive allografts in dogs. In: Aebi M, Regazzoni P (eds). Bone Transplantation. Springer-Verlag, Berlin, Heidelberg, 1989; p. 76.

104. Stevenson S, Dannucci GA, Sharkey NA, Pool RR. The fate of articular cartilage after transplantation of fresh and cryopreserved tissue-antigen-matched and mismatched osteochondral allografts in dogs. J Bone Joint Surg 1989; 71A:1297.

105. Muscolo DL, Caletti E, Schajowicz F, Araugo ES, Makino A. Tissue typing in human massive allografts of frozen bone. J Bone Joint Surg 1987; 58A:826.

106. Gonzales del Pino J, Benito M, Randolph MA, Weiland AJ. The effects of different schedules of total body irradiation in heterotopic vascularized bone transplantation. Transplantation 1990; 50:920.

107. Schwarzenbach O, Czitrom AA, Aebi M, Payne U. In vitro culture to enhance allogeneic bone grafts. A rat model. Orthop Trans 1989; 13:340.

3

BONE AND TISSUE BANKING

C. Elizabeth Musclow

Bone is a frequently transplanted tissue (1, 2). Bone banks developed as a response to the need for an adequate, readily available stock of quality and efficacious bone allografts to meet the various and increasing requirements of recipients. The scope of this enterprise ranges from identifying the donor to medical screening for donor acceptability; from recovering and processing the bone to testing for tissue safety; from preserving the bone biomechanical integrity to documenting and distributing it to qualified institutions; all of this must be accomplished while adhering to accepted standards and practices of operation. The duty placed upon the modern bone bank is to supply bone allografts for replacement or repair of bone lost due to trauma, for failed joint arthroplasty, and for limb-sparing procedures following bone tumor excision (3).

Autologous bone is recognized as superior to and is preferred over allograft bone (4–6). However, autologous bone is not always available in sufficient quantities, or is it feasible to obtain if morbidity at the donor site is expected to be high (7) or if a joint surface is needed. Banked donor bone allows for an unlimited quantity of bone, no donor site morbidity, and the advantages of having long bones or large pelvic bones available for transplantation.

Large bone transplants are becoming increasingly effective as innovative reconstructive orthopaedic procedures are developed to manage tumors of the pelvis and extremities. Use of banked bone allografts for a variety of orthopaedic applications is escalating and is gaining acceptance as a worthwhile procedure (8–34).

Early attempts at bone transplantation by placing human autografts or animal xenografts into human subjects make for interesting reading (35–37). Transplanted bovine bone, Kiel bone, has received both positive and negative reviews (38–40). Coral implants and synthetics, composed mainly of hydroxyapatite, have received some praise (41–45). In looking to the future, one envisions the possibility of using materials that will induce host bone formation to fill skeletal defects autogenously. The concept of biodegradable materials, molded to the exact shape and size of the bony defect, and then, polymerized to maintain that configuration may replace human bone as graft substitutes for orthopaedic surgery, oral surgery, and neurosurgery (46). The ultimate, of course, is to prevent the occurrence of the events that allow or precipitate the pathology treated with bone transplantation.

For the present, however, banked human bone remains a valued resource for relieving suffering, for providing mechanical support, and for providing a better quality of life for many patients requiring reparative and reconstructive orthopaedic surgery. This chapter will review bone banking strategies to meet these challenges.

CONTROLS ON BONE DONATION

Legislation

In the United States, the Uniform Anatomical Gift Act (47–50) is the basic legal framework that defines the terms of reference for and contains the conditions pertaining to the altruistic donation of all or part of a human body for therapeutic transplantation into another person, for teaching, or for research endeavors. The Act is adapted by state legislatures in principle, but may differ in detail across the country because it is a state rather than a federal legislation. The National Conference of Commissioners for Uniform State Laws (NCCUSL) drafted an updated version of the Act hoping for general and consistent acceptance by all state governments.

Many states have adopted the Required Request Law (51). This legislation requires that the next of kin of a deceased person be given the option of donating the loved one's tissues and/or organs for transplantation use. The offer may be accepted or rejected without fear of incurring prejudice. The decision is recorded in the medical record of the deceased. It is also required by American National Legislation (PL99–509, Section 9318) that

hospitals have written protocols for the identification of potential donors.

The Joint Commission on the Accreditation of Healthcare Organizations publishes a standards manual that requires inpatient charts to contain documentation defending the failure to retrieve tissues and/or organs from a deceased patient. It requires that policies and procedures be in place for identification and referral of potential donors to procurement agencies or tissue banks (52). These legal considerations were recently summarized (8).

Similarly, in Canada, the federally developed Human Tissue Gift Act is modified and interpreted at the provincial level for establishing standards of organ and tissue donation practices (53). Health and Welfare Canada guidelines for organ and tissue donation in hospitals were published in 1986 (54). This document provides a consistent definition of recommended requirements for health care institutions relative to organ and tissue donation services within the institution. The provincial health authorities, however, are at liberty to modify these guidelines; the ethics are not always clear-cut (55, 56). In June of 1990, Canada instituted a directive to all hospitals to prepare policy for identifying potential donors and for making potential donors and their families aware of the options of organ and tissue donations (57).

Personal Wish and Next of Kin

Mentally competent persons having attained the age of majority may make free and informed consent for their surgically discarded bone to be donated to the bone bank and used for allograft. Such a person will undergo surgery, during which time bone is removed that will not be reimplanted, e.g., total hip or knee replacements, other joint surgery, or thoracotomy. On preoperative office examination, the orthopaedic surgeon can predict with some certainty which patients may be potential bone donors of this type. This is an opportune time to present to the patient the option of donating the surgical discard bone to the bone bank. Such donation is the legal right of the individual and the human tissue gift act does not apply (47, 49).

Others may indicate their wish to be organ and/or tissue donors should they die by signing their driver's license, signing a donor card, indicating it in their will, or voicing their opinion during life in the presence of witnesses. In practice, consent is sought also from the potential donor's family, in addition to these evidences left by the deceased. Consents from the legal next of kin obtained in writing, by telegram, by telephone, or orally, in the presence of witnesses, are acceptable.

Religious and Ethical Considerations

Major religious groups allow tissue and organ donation as an act of charity for the betterment of one's fellow man (58–66). Families of the deceased find the act of donation a comfort, realizing that their tragedy may help others attain a better quality of life. The wishes of those whose faiths oppose donation, however, must be respected with sensitivity and understanding. The moral, ethical, and social aspects of transplantation challenge thought and the benefits of utilizing this technology must not be blind to the potential sinister nonmedical concerns that may lie hidden within it (55, 56, 67, 68).

TYPES OF BONE BANKS

In general, there are two types of bone banks: (*a*) the surgical and (*b*) the regional cadaver bone bank. The former is almost always associated with a community hospital. The latter may be based at a large medical center, may be operated by the blood transfusion service, or may exist as an independent facility (1–6, 8, 69–73).

Surgical

A surgical or community hospital bone bank need not be complex to be safe, highly valued, and cost effective. It involves collecting surgical discard bone, processing, storing, and distributing this bone. Such bone is used as allograft replacement of bone stock during reconstructive orthopaedic surgeries. Generally, bone collected during surgery would be discarded if not directed to a bone bank of this type. Femoral heads excised during hip arthroplasty, femoral condyles, tibial plateaus removed at total knee replacement, wedges removed at knee osteotomy, excised radial heads, ribs resected during thoracotomy, and selected cases of traumatic amputation when replantation is not possible represent the types of surgical discard bone that proves useful as allografts (6, 8, 74–82). Community bone banks may store and distribute larger allografts obtained from regional centers. This would be a convenience to the surgeon of the local area.

Regional

The more expensive, labor-intensive proposition of supplying large amounts and a large variety of bone and tissue allografts for a wide constituency of physician users is both challenging and rewarding. Regional banks are usually diverse, variously supplying bone, cornea, skin,

fascia lata, tendon, ligaments, dura mater, pericardium, heart valves, saphenous veins, and pancreatic islet cells.

The American Association of Tissue Banks (McLean, Virginia 22101) publishes a technical procedures manual that details the policies and procedures of practice for operating a bone and tissue bank (83). Others have produced guidelines gleaned from extensive personal experience for establishing, staffing, and operating a bone and tissue bank of this sophistication (1–5, 13, 69, 84–93).

BONE BANK ORGANIZATION

To be effective and responsible, the bone bank must have a functional identity enhanced by professional staff. It may be either an independent or an institutionally based organization; for example, part of a hospital complex (Fig. 3.1). Dedication to meticulous record keeping and careful adherence to a protocol promoting high standards of tissue banking practice are essential ingredients for a respected and reliable bone bank (73, 77, 88).

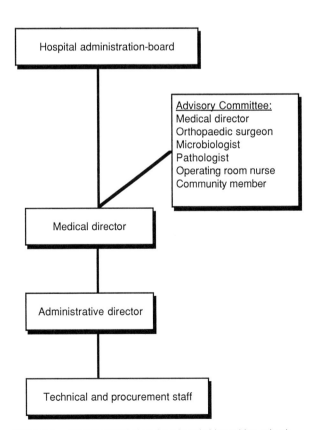

Figure 3.1. Organizational chart for a hospital-based bone bank.

Director

Day-to-day operations of the bone bank, whether it is a small and community hospital-based one or a regional one, that serves a large constituency of surgeons, are the responsibility of the on-site administrative director. Although this person need not be medically licensed, a licensed physician must be available to evaluate tissue safety and overall direction so that the bank is in compliance with medicolegal requirements. The medical director reviews all donor records for suitability and signs the final release allowing acceptable donor bone to enter the distribution pool. In a small bank, one physician may assume both administrative and medical duties. In a larger establishment, diversification of responsibility is imperative, with a business manager, technical director, and others reporting to a medical director and board of management or advisory committee. Dedication to staff training, quality control, high standards of performance, and progressive action advancing the science and safety of bone transplantation are inherent in a respected bone bank. A knowledgeable deputy medical director must be formally identified; this is someone who will assume the responsibilities of the bank in the medical director's absence.

Technical Staff

The coordinator or senior technical assistant to the medical director may be an operating room nurse, a medical laboratory technologist, a certified tissue bank specialist, or another medically oriented professional. Many duties may be delegated to this person by the medical director. He or she should be an able manager and supervisor, devoting special attention to the technical side of the bone bank's operation. The American Association of Tissue Banks offers excellent workshops and other educational programs that train individuals in all aspects of bone banking from retrieval through record keeping. This not only keeps technical staff current but also provides for certification of tissue bank specialists.

Advisory Committee

The bone bank interacts with the laboratory, the operating room, infection control and organ procurement agencies, and with the community. Therefore, an advisory committee composed of experts representing these groups plus surgeons, pathologists, microbiologists, and lay advisors will greatly enhance the bone bank's image.

The advisory body, along with the medical director, governs the bone bank's activities, revises policies and procedures, reviews liability concerns, advances public education, and, in general, affords a broad perspective on the performance, scope, and quality of the program.

Policy and Procedure Manuals

Written policies and procedures covering the full operation of the bone bank are essential resources to staff. They ensure uniformity and standardization of practice and are required for accreditation. They must be current and readily available to all staff and inspection teams.

Physical Plant

Equipment needs vary with the size and scope of the bone bank program. A surgical bone bank need not be an expensive or complicated enterprise to be efficient and effective. Security of tissue and confidentiality of records require a limited access area for storing donor and recipient files and for housing locked freezers. Freezers capable of maintaining $-70°C$ or colder are equipped with a constant temperature monitor and alarm system. Ideally, two freezers are available so that quarantined bone awaiting test results is stored separately from the bone ready for distribution.

When bone recovery is from living donors as part of an operative procedure, only sterile packaging materials are used; these are needed in addition to the usual surgical set-up. Prompt wrapping of the bone while still in the sterile field is essential. Cadaver bone collection requires specially prepared sterile instrument trays, which go with the procurement team to the donor's location. Collection is performed ideally in a sterile operating room environment. In the absence of sterile recovery and sterile processing facilities, it is necessary to have sterile drapes to cover all surfaces in the morgue or clean dissection area where the "clean" procurement will occur.

Donor reconstruction materials, such as wooden dowels or plaster rolls, must also be available. The bone bank should impose upon the host institution in which the retrieval occurs as little as possible. All supplies should be the responsibility of the procurement team. If the bank processes bone into frozen or freeze-dried iliac crest wedges, dowels, cancellous wedges, struts, or others, a sterile, class 100 room, surgical saws, orthopaedic instruments, bone grinders, freeze-driers, and surgical scrub facilities are among the requirements (79, 88).

DONOR SELECTION

The main goal of bone banks, either small and local or large and regional, is to provide safe bone allografts. Careful review of the medical record, thorough physical examination of the donor, autopsy, and prudent use of laboratory screening tests are tools to evaluate a bone donor's acceptability. Such strict criteria may reject some potential donors, but will provide a safer bone supply in keeping with the expectations of both the surgeon and the recipient (4, 13, 69, 70, 76, 78, 79, 85, 87, 88, 93–98). The living donor and family members of the deceased donor must cooperate with this process. When medical history is incomplete or the circumstances of death are questionable or unknown, a potential donor may be refused in the interest of safety to the recipients (Table 3.1). The Standards and the Technical Manual of the American Association of Tissue Banks details the credentials of an acceptable bone donor (77, 83).

Age

The young, healthy adult, 18–55 years old, is the best bone donor candidate for long bones intended to function in weight bearing after transplantation (94). Weightbearing allografts must be of optimal biomechanical strength. However, depending upon the intended use of the bone, age is not always a major factor. Those younger than 16–18 years may not have fused epiphyses. Individuals older than 50 years are more prone to osteoporosis, osteopenia, malignancy, or other diseases that may directly or indirectly affect the quality of the bone. Bone chips used for packing a cystic defect or stabilizing a prosthesis may be prepared from a donor of any age. The ideal donor of fresh osteochondral allografts is over 18 years and less than 30 years of age. Such donors have small risk for osteoporosis and/or arthritic changes of the joint surfaces, which are the source of cartilage required by the recipient.

History

Bone banks require a comprehensive medical and social history as part of the donor screening process. The history form will become part of the bone bank's permanent record. The aim is to detect potentially harmful diseases, infectious processes, toxic substances or high risk factors for these possible complications. Diseases and/or toxins that might be transmitted from the donor to the recipient through a bone allograft would contraindicate the acceptance of the donor tissue. It has been reported that Creutzfeld-Jakob disease was transmitted to a bone allograft recipient from a donor who had received human pituitary-derived growth hormone produced between 1963 and 1985. Donors treated with such growth hormone must be rejected (82, 99, 100). In one documented case, acquired immune deficiency syndrome (AIDS) was transmitted via a bone allograft from a donor not tested for human immunodeficiency virus (HIV) antibody (101). The risk of a donor found HIV antibody negative on screening and having a negative history and histology report but still carrying the AIDS virus has been estimated to be less than one in a million (102). Some bone banks reject donors who have received blood transfusions within the preceding 6 months because of the AIDS risk (82, 94). However, for the blood donor and the bone donor who received that blood transfusion both to elicit a false-negative HIV test must be extremely rare. HIV positivity has appeared in recipients of a blood transfusion that tested negative for HIV antibody at the time of its collection (103). Bone retrieval is contraindicated if the donor has a history of intravenous drug abuse; if the donor has a high risk for hepatitis and/or HIV exposure; if the donor

Table 3.1.
When To Decline a Bone Donation[a]

1. Presence of acute or chronic infection
2. Period of respirator-assisted breathing exceeds 72 hours
3. Presence of malignancy (other than basal cell carcinoma of skin)
4. Presence of autoimmune disease
5. Presence of inflammatory disease (including rheumatoid arthritis)
6. Presence of debilitating, degenerative neurological disease
7. Practice of intravenous drug abuse
8. Presence of high risk factors for AIDS and/or hepatitis
9. Presence of disease of unknown etiology
10. Prolonged corticosteroid therapy
11. Previous toxic exposures (industrial hazards)
12. Previous treatment with human pituitary-derived growth hormone
13. Presence of bone disease (osteoporosis, osteopenia, steroid-induced osteonecrosis)
14. Major surgical procedure more than 72 hours before death
15. Precise cause of death unknown

[a]Data from references 77–79, 85, 87, 88, 94.

has had respirator-assisted breathing for more than 3 days, with its risks of sepsis; or if the donor has antecedent disease of unknown etiology, such as rheumatoid arthritis, neurological disease, or cancer (92, 94). Prolonged corticosteroid use or other long-term medication may render bones to be of less than optimal strength (94). The American Association of Tissue Banks also endorses the exclusion of donors who have emigrated from a high-risk HIV area since 1977 or who have engaged in sexual practices that are high risk for HIV transmission (77) (Table 3.2).

Physical Examination

The careful physical examination is a revealing means of evaluating potential bone donors. In traumatic deaths, obvious tissue trauma, with bone fracture underlying or compounding it, usually rules that bone unacceptable. Tattoos, decubitus ulcers, skin lesions, needle tracks, or oral abscesses suggesting drug abuse negate bone donation (94). The physical examination confirms the general age, state of well-being, and nutritional status of the donor. Careful history from the family and thorough physical examination may fail to reveal an illness in deceased patients. This may be related to many factors, including sex and age of the patient, the type and size of the hospital involved, and the particular nature of the disease (98). Whenever possible, therefore, it is encouraged strongly to obtain a postmortem examination of bone donors. This not only elucidates disease processes but also affords increased protection of the allograft recipient from transmissible disease and from receiving a bone with a previously undiagnosed metabolic bone disorder. Study at autopsy and excision biopsy of lymph nodes are other ways of screening for AIDS (102).

Laboratory Screening

The question is: "How much testing is enough?" A definite answer is elusive. The advent of more sensitive and diverse diagnostic laboratory assays enables more thorough objective screening of donors. The American Association of Tissue Banks Standards require testing for hepatitis B surface antigen, hepatitis C antibody, and HIV antibody. Many banks also test for human T-cell lymphotropic virus, (HTLV-1), syphilis, rheumatoid factor, antinuclear antibody, antithyroglobulin antibody, serum tumor markers, prostatic acid phosphatase, and other indicators of inflammatory, autoimmune, or malignant disease. Such an approach to bone donor assessment has been termed the "serological autopsy" (88). A profile of such diagnostic tests may be more acceptable to some donor families than a traditional tissue autopsy. This option may salvage an otherwise refused bone donation. HTLV-1 has become more of an issue for bone bankers since the virus is thought to be transmissible by blood transfusion and since the Red Cross began to test donor blood for the antibody to HTLV-1 on a routine basis beginning in June 1990 (104–106).

Three instances of Rh sensitization attributed to bone grafting have been reported (107–110). Personal (unpublished) experience showed the development of anti-D and anti-E in an Rh-negative woman who received a fresh osteochondral allograft. Documenting the Rh status of donors, attempting to release Rh-negative allografts for Rh-negative recipients at risk, and recommending prophylactic anti-D immune γ-globulin for Rh-negative recipients who must use an Rh-positive allograft, are important considerations for the medical director of the bone bank.

Bone banks prefer a pretransfusion sample of blood for HIV and other serological testing of potential donors (100). This becomes imperative if the patient's blood is diluted by several blood transfusions and/or much intra-

Table 3.2.
Recommendations For The Prevention of Human Immunodeficiency Virus (HIV) Transmission By Blood and Blood Products[a]

1. Clinical or laboratory evidence of HIV infection
2. Men who have had sex with another man, even once, since 1977
3. Intravenous drug abuse
4. Persons born in or emigrating from countries where heterosexual activity may play a major role in transmission of HIV infection
5. Persons with hemophilia or other blood clotting disorders who have received clotting factor concentrates
6. Sexual partners of any of the above high risk persons
7. Men or women engaged in sex for money or drugs since 1977, or their sexual partners within the past 12 months
8. Persons who have had/been treated for syphilis or gonorrhea during the past 12 months
9. Persons who have received a blood transfusion within the past 12 months

[a]High Risk Criteria adapted from United States Public Health Services, Department of Health and Human Services, revised December 5, 1990.

venous fluid replacement given within the 24 hours preceding death (111).

Testing deceased bone donors for HIV antibody or antigen is an accepted mandatory practice, but testing living donors for HIV has met with controversy. Generally, the testing at the time of surgical donation is endorsed, but retesting at 6 months postoperation is resisted by busy surgeons from both philosophical and pragmatic points of view. However, both the American Association of Tissue Banks and the Canadian guidelines have adopted the required 6 month-retest protocol for both HIV and hepatitis C (77, 112–115). Six-month retesting is required also for semen donors (116, 117). It might be argued successfully that bone and tissue should be quarantined until both the serological and Western blot assays for HIV on donor blood are negative (113).

HIV antigen testing by p24 and/or polymerase chain reaction are attempts to narrow the window between infection and positive detection.

Blood cultures are recommended on both living and deceased bone donors to rule out sepsis. The best source of blood for culture in the deceased is cardiac blood or blood from a surgically exposed leg vessel. Of the blood volume, 5% is sequestered in bone; therefore, blood-borne disease transmission by bone allografts is possible (97). It has been proposed, as a further check against disease transmission, that residual bladder urine obtained by catheterization and pleural fluid obtained by thoracentesis from cadaver donors be obtained for culture just as bone recovery commences (92).

Vascularized perfusable organ tissue transplants may be rejected by the recipient due to histoincompatibility between the donor and the recipient. For bone allografts, however, the degree of immunogenic response is not well documented. In the clinical situation, a bone rejection response cannot be measured as directly as it can be in vascularized organ grafts. The best indication for possible incompatibility is delayed rate of bone union and incorporation. Animal studies have shown better graft incorporation if there is close histocompatibility matching between donor and recipient (118). Similarly, fresh autografts incorporate and heal more quickly than allograft counterparts. In humans, one study showed a better outcome for grafts matched for human lymphocyte antigen (HLA) (119). However, HLA typing is not performed routinely pretransplant of allogeneic bone. Similarly, post-transplant immunosuppressive therapy is not instituted routinely. Ultraviolet light has been demonstrated to decrease rejection of HLA-incompatible soft tissue grafts. Its penetration is probably too shallow to make it applicable to bone (46). Preservation of allografts by deep freezing or freeze-drying and the secondary sterilization of the bone by γ radiation may play a role also in reducing immunogenicity (46, 120–128).

In summary, the donor selection process requires both objective laboratory testing and careful medical judgment to ensure the supply of safe, quality bone for use in transplantation (4, 5, 8, 13, 69, 76, 79, 85, 87–90).

INFORMED CONSENT

The Uniform Anatomical Gift Act and Rules of Informed Consent attempt to balance patient risk-taking with rights of autonomy and self-determination (49, 129). The living donor who voluntarily consents to bone donation must understand the implications and the risks involved. A clear description of the donation procedure and explanation of the blood tests required to protect the interests of the recipient must be presented. An opportunity for the potential donor to ask questions and receive answers is essential. A copy of the signed consent form becomes part of the permanent bone bank record (78) (Fig. 3.2).

Informed consent for bone recovery from a deceased person may be given by the legal next of kin. This is sought even when there is evidence that tissue donation was the wish of the deceased, e.g., a signed donor card found on the person. The order of precedence for consent from the next of kin is the spouse, an adult son or daughter, either parent, an adult sibling, legal guardian, or a public trustee authorized to make the final arrangements for the body (54). Reluctance to donate on the part of the family and/or evidence that the deceased opposed donation must be respected.

A written consent reduces misunderstanding and is a legal document. It not only itemizes the exact tissues to be donated, but also states limitations, if any, on the use of the collected tissue.

BONE RECOVERY

Bone recovery may be performed either in a sterile operating theater or in a nonsterile, but clean, environment. Obligate sterile recovery is required for collection of both fresh (not to be frozen) osteochondral joint allografts and bone eventually transplanted without undergoing secondary sterilization.

Living Donor

Bone donation occurring as part of a surgical procedure is sterile (73, 78). Femoral heads, femoral condyles, tibial plateau removed during hip and knee arthroplasty, excised radial heads, rib portions, and skull flaps are do-

CONSENT TO BONE DONATION AND BLOOD TESTING

I understand that bone tissue may be taken from me at my upcoming surgery. I consent to such removal. I also consent to the removed bone being sent to the Bone Bank for whatever use may be made of it.

I understand one possible use for this bone may be for transplantation into other patients. Therefore, the bone must be free from infections or other potentially harmful processes. I consent to having my blood tested now as the bone bank deems appropriate. I understand that the blood tests will include screening for hepatitis and AIDS virus. I understand that an additional blood sample will be required from me six months after the surgery. I consent to this blood test also.

I understand that I or my doctor will be informed of any test result which is abnormal and that an abnormal result may be reported to the Medical Officer of Health.

I understand that my confidentiality will be respected and that no identifying information about me will be released to doctors or patients receiving my bone for transplant use.

I understand that I can refuse to donate my bone to the Bone Bank and that this decision will not affect the quality of medical care for me at this hospital.

I have had my questions about the bone donation process answered to my satisfaction.

_____   _____
            Date   Signature of Donor

_____   _____
Signature of Witness   Name of Donor (Please Print)

Figure 3.2.   Sample consent form for living donors.

nated commonly to the bone bank when reimplantation into the donor is not an option (76). The surgeon inspects the quality of the removed bone not only relative to its potential as an allograft, but also relative to the donor's medical condition. The bone is cultured, sampled for histological assessment, and packaged while still within the sterile operative field. The wrapped bone is labeled, documented for exposure to antibiotics during collection, and then promptly cooled or frozen. Bone should be on ice within 1 hour of collection, frozen at least to $-20°C$ within 4 hours of collection, and in the $-70°C$ freezer within 24 hours of collection (73, 74, 76, 79–82).

Deceased Donor

Cadaver bone collection performed in the operating room is an aseptic procedure. At times, an operating room may not be available and bone recovery occurs in a nonsterile environment. Although the body is surgically scrubbed and all surfaces in a nonsterile room are appropriately draped with sterile sheets, the bone procurement is termed "clean." Secondary sterilization becomes obligatory for all tissue recovered in a clean environment. Bone collection should be completed either within 12 hours of death if the body is kept at room temperature or within 24 hours if the body is kept at $4°C$ (1, 8, 77, 87). A standard orthopaedic instrument tray, including osteotomes, power saw, or Gigli saws is required. Sterile drapes, stockinette, clamps, sterile wrappings or specimen storage jars, labels,

culture tubes, and donor reconstruction materials are needed.

Personnel

The recovery team must be trained in bone retrieval and may be either technicians and/or surgeons. Each side of the donor is the responsibility of one member of the team to reduce cross-contamination (94). The assistance of scrub and circulating nurses is valued. As for any surgical procedure, the team must put on masks, scrub, and put on gowns. The donor is draped and the skin is surgically prepared. No incision should be made over an area of trauma or abrasion; even a needle puncture site must be avoided. Gowns and gloves should be changed as procurement proceeds from region to region of the body and between bone removal and bone wrapping. This reduces cross-contamination of bone by bacteria (94).

Procedure

Tissue donation to enhance the quality of life or ease the pain of another human being is a most unselfish gift. Although the tissue banker is focused on the safety of the tissue for the recipient and on maintaining an adequate inventory to meet the need, one must not forget that, of equal importance, is the procurement of the tissue. Tissue removal must be done in a professional, dignified manner, reflecting respect and concern for the deceased, the bereaved, and the funeral director charged with embalming and presenting the deceased in an acceptable manner for an open casket funeral. Special attention must be paid to preserving blood vessels necessary for embalming. Nicked or cut vessels leak fluid, disturbed tissues swell, and improperly placed ligatures thwart proper circulation of the embalming chemicals. Reconstruction materials must allow for a natural positioning of a limb. These very important aspects of tissue collection not only impact on the family who are concerned if their loved one does not look natural, but also place the funeral professional in an undeservedly awkward position. The funeral director should be viewed as a vital member of the tissue donation procedure for his/her role in dealing with the grieving family and performing postmortem services to the deceased.

The order of bone removal from the body is somewhat arbitrary. For the lower limb, a skin incision is made running from the antero-superior iliac spine, over the greater trochanter, down the lateral thigh to the knee, then directed medially to the midanterior aspect over the patellar tendon, and then, down the crest of the tibia to the ankle (4, 13, 17, 92, 94). Fascia lata is salvaged as the incision is enlarged. The femur is disarticulated at the knee with the posterior capsule of the knee and the collateral ligaments left attached to the femur. Sharp dissection and scraping away of muscle using an osteotome proceeds proximally. A scalpel is used to cut the abductor tendons about 1 inch proximal to their insertion into the greater trochanter. The capsule is removed from the neck of the femur and the head is dislocated anteriorly. The intact femur is lifted from the body with the insertions of iliopsoas, gluteus medius, and gluteus minimus muscles attached. Removal of the femur in two stages may be desirable. A power saw or Gigli saw can easily bisect the femur, yielding a distal and a proximal portion.

The tibia is similarly disarticulated and removed either as a full-length bone or bisected. Often, only the proximal tibia is removed from the body. Menisci may be procured separately or left in situ by slicing off the tibial plateaus. Documenting meniscal measurements, anteroposterior and mediolateral lengths, is an important aid when matching to a prospective recipient.

Patellar tendons with a large block of tibial tubercle attached distally and the patellar block attached proximally are useful for reconstruction of anterior cruciate ligaments (33). Procurement of an entire hemipelvis or the iliac crests only is performed by extending an incision from anterior to posterior along the iliac crest. The soft tissue is removed. The sacroiliac joint is separated and the symphysis pubis is cut to allow removal of the hemi-

pelvis. This procedure is technically difficult. Should bowel perforation occur, the procurement should be terminated in this area. The operator changes gown and gloves and proceeds with bone removal from another site.

Bone in the upper extremities is exposed using an incision through the deltoid-pectoral groove, extending distally along the biceps muscle to the elbow. A generous portion of capsule and rotator cuff is left on the humerus. The cuff is cut at its insertion into the glenoid and the anterior deltoid origin is severed to facilitate disarticulation of the humeral head. The collateral ligaments of radius and ulna and the triceps insertion into the olecranon are cut to free the distal end of the humerus, which may now be disarticulated. Removal of the radius and ulna must be done carefully to avoid visible incisions showing at the wrist. Consideration might be given to procuring only one upper limb so that the other is left for natural positioning in the casket. Rib segments may be removed in an alternative fashion so that the chest contour is maintained. Collection of the Achilles tendon should be in association with a generous attached bone block from the os calcis. Mandibular bone procurement should be done only when special consent is obtained and the body is to be cremated with no open casket viewing. Special requests for fresh intact knee, hip, or elbow joints may be received by the bone bank for selected recipients. Such fresh osteochondral allografts are never frozen or secondarily sterilized. In our institution, these are obtained under obligate sterile conditions and the allograft is immediately submerged into the following antibiotic solution held at 4°C: 3 L of Ringer's lactate (Abbott Laboratories) 50,000 U/L of Bacitracin (Upjohn), and 1 g/L Ancef (cefazolin sodium, Smith, Kline and French). The sterile container is sealed with a sterile, leak-proof lid, wrapped in sterile drapes, and labeled. It is stored at 4°C for not more than 24–36 hours, allowing time for the recipient to be readied for surgery (96).

Some bone banks advocate that all bone collected for allograft use should soak in antibiotic solution before wrapping and transport to the bone bank (94). If used, the name of the antibiotics must be documented on the tissue package label to protect the sensitized recipient.

Cultures

Whether it is surgical discard bone or cadaveric bone and whether it is collected aseptically or "clean," all bone must be cultured at the time of recovery. Swab cultures, covering a large surface area of the collected bone, bone chips from the cortical surface, and/or marrow from the medullary canal are sent for culture (Fig. 3.3). All cultures

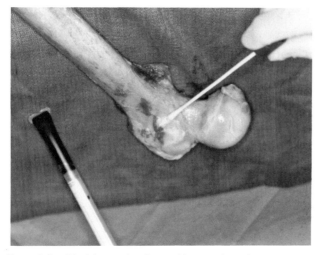

Figure 3.3. Obtaining swab cultures of bone at time of procurement.

must be obtained before placing bone in antibiotic soaks. Cultures are incubated both aerobically and anaerobically for 7–14 days. This allows for even a few slow-growing bacteria to be detected. Contaminated bone must be secondarily sterilized or discarded if resistant pathogens or endotoxin producers are identified. Certain banks will consider all bones to be contaminated if more than 25% (4) or 50% (94) of the cultures from one donor grow the same organism. Viral contamination of bones may go undetected because no practical screening method for pathogenic viruses is available at present; the exceptions are blood serology tests for hepatitis, AIDS, HTLV-1, and cytomegalovirus. The medical director must exercise discriminating clinical judgment in evaluating the laboratory reports from the screening tests before deciding donor acceptability.

Histology

Visual inspection plus either representative rongeurs-bitten-out chips or a sawed slice of donor bone for histological assessment are important recommended aspects of allograft bone quality control. The problem of sampling error, however, cannot be avoided. Some would argue that histological sampling damages the bone and is not necessary for assessing the safety of surgical discard femoral heads (81). Most of such bone is obtained from older donors, however, and the risk of malignancy rises in the elderly. Histology reports evaluating pathological and/or metabolic bone disease are entered into the bone bank records. A positive finding may result in bone being discarded. Histology may also prove important to the living donor if occult, but treatable, disease is detected.

Wrapping and Labeling

Wrappings provide a water-proof vapor barrier between the freezer environment and the sterile bone. Packaging must tolerate the extremes of temperature, must not leach toxins onto the bone, must prevent sharp bony surfaces from violating the wrappings, and must be suitable for the secondary sterilization process. Double polystyrene or glass wide-mouth jars, with the smaller jar nesting inside the larger jar, serve well for storing surgical discard bone. The double-jar type of packaging facilitates re-entry of the sterile inner jar containing the bone to the operative field at time of transplantation. Polyethylene plastic bags alternated with sterile towels are suitable for any bone, especially the larger allografts. Three to five layers of wrappings have been found satisfactory (72) (Fig. 3.4). Peelable, hermetically sealed, plastic pouches are also suitable.

Accurate tracking of allografts is important. Labels in indelible ink with the minimum of donor name, date of collection, which antibiotics were used, name of donor hospital, and which bone (right or left) will identify the donation. For reasons of confidentiality, this label will be removed later and a coded identifier label will be attached by the bone bank staff. Some banks will use the procurement date as a donor number because it is unique and also because it serves as a quick check of the length of time that the bone has been in storage. A final sterile plastic bag is placed over the labeled bag to protect the label from loss. Allograft bone should be refrigerated or frozen within 4 hours of collection (78, 83, 90). If this is not possible, packing the bone in insulated boxes with

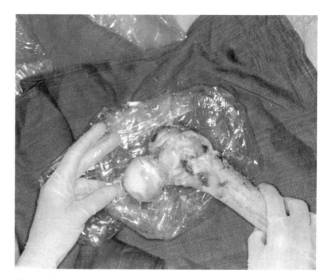

Figure 3.4. Wrapping bone in alternate layers of sterile plastic bags and sterile towels.

either dry ice, freezer packs, or bags of wet ice during the journey to the bank is important.

Reconstruction

Careful attention to donor reconstruction following bone removal is an imperative act of dignity for every donor even if a closed casket funeral or cremation is anticipated after bone recovery. Reconstruction allows for open casket funerals. Wooden dowels, plaster rolls, cotton padding, or commercially available supports may be used for reconstruction. Knee and pelvic areas may be padded to restore natural contours. Incisions are neatly stitched closed over these implants. Special mandibular implants are commercially available and should be used by the bone procurement team even if the body is destined for cremation and/or a closed casket funeral service.

BONE STORAGE AND PROCESSING

A separate, controlled access freezer room is best for bone storage. Separate freezers are allocated for quarantined bone awaiting screening tests and for fully screened bone ready for distribution (88). Bone kept at $-20°C$ is suitable for transplant use for up to 6 months (83). Autolytic enzyme action (collagenase) is abolished essentially after prolonged deep freezing at $-70°C$ to $-80°C$; (121, 130); therefore, storage of bone for at least 5 years is possible at these temperatures (83). Frozen rabbit femora were compared with femora that had never been frozen. No significant differences were seen in either histological appearance or shear fractures of the capital femoral growth plate (131). Others have found biomechanical properties to be similar in human tibia and femora, whether fresh or frozen (17). Repeated freeze-thaw and irradiation of patellar tendons have been reported not to have serious deleterious effects on the characteristics of the grafts (132). Freezing appears to affect adversely the ability of the host to incorporate the allograft and, therefore, directly influences the outcome of a bone transplant (133).

Lyophilization (freeze-drying) has the advantage of permitting long-term storage at room temperature, obviating the expenses associated with maintaining ultracold freezers; however, a lyophilizer increases set-up costs and technique is important. Tissue is taken to ultra-low temperatures and then dehydrated under high vacuum. Residual water content in freeze-dried tissue must be less than 8% by nuclear magnetic resonance (NMR) analysis or 5% by gravimetric analysis (13, 83, 134). Cryopreservatives, such as dimethyl sulfoxide (DMSO), glycerol, or 70% alcohol, may increase survival of resident cells, such as chondrocytes in cartilage or menisci during freezing and thawing (4, 135, 136). Ligaments, tendons, and fascia lata are being cryopreserved in these agents with some success. Costly, but effective liquid nitrogen storage has resulted in viable osteochondral cell cultures up to 4 months after tissue procurement (17). Good conservation of bone in commercial Cialit, [2-(ethyl 1-mercuro-mercaptol)- 5-benzoxazole-carbonate-sodium] has been reported (137).

Bone banks may choose never to unwrap or to violate a bone package between time of collection and time of transplant. Larger banks, however, under strict sterile conditions, will open bone packages and will both customize bone blocks to specific sizes and prepare bone chips or bone powder. This not only maximizes the number of bone allografts possible from each donor but also assists the surgeon. Consequently, the number of recipients who may benefit from each donor is enhanced and time in surgery may be shortened. Donor bone cut into optimal sizes or chips, fashioned into dowels, cubes, or wedges of certain sizes, is widely sought. Chemosterilized autolyzed antigen-extracted allogenic bone (AAA) has been prepared as an alternative to autologous bone for facilitating intertransverse process fusion and other arthrodeses and is a potent osteogenic influence (20, 28, 138).

Processing must be performed under sterile, level 100, conditions (139) by trained personnel who are surgically scrubbed, masked, gloved, and gowned. Cultures of randomly selected processed tissue at each step of the procedure are a vital part of the Quality Control and Quality Assurance programs.

Secondary Sterilization

There is lack of consensus on the extent and nature of adverse effects on bone by the various methods available for secondary sterilization (121, 140–149). Many banks rely heavily on careful donor selection, laboratory testing, and sterile procurement techniques so that they can bypass secondary sterilization entirely. This is especially true for surgical bone banks dealing mainly in surgical discard femoral heads and in programs using fresh allograft transplants. However, "clean" bone collections always require some form of secondary sterilization. It is observed, however, that even with sterile bone procurement practice, swab cultures taken from the recovered bone may be positive (150–152).

Data from the Bone Bank at the Naval Research Institute at Bethesda, Maryland found that the incidence of clinical infection in recipients of banked bone procured under sterile conditions compared favorably with the incidence of infection following autografts (153). Those patients at highest risk of postoperative infection also had some predisposing or comorbid factor. This suggests that complicating factors, rather than allograft contamination, were at fault (154). The onus is on the bone bank, however, to provide bone that is as safe as possible.

Various processes to sterilize bone are available. Boiling, steam sterilization, or autoclaving are not recommended even though they are effectively bacteriocidal (155–159). Ethylene oxide (ETO) is also an effective sterilizing agent, but it presents risks to personnel and is potentially deleterious to stored bone (46, 88, 156, 160, 161). Adequate airing is essential to allow toxic residues from ETO to dissipate. A study was performed placing vials containing HIV virus inside the medullary canal of human femoral shafts that were exposed to ETO for 250 minutes. The HIV was noninfectious after the ETO treatment (162). The uniform penetration of ETO into bone, however, is questioned (158). Chemicals, antibiotics, and antiseptics also have been tried to ensure bone graft sterility (20, 88, 156, 163–165). γ- and β-irradiation are effective sterilizers of bacteria (69, 79, 88, 121, 140, 144, 146, 149, 166, 167). Certain slow viruses, however, show a special resistance to both radiation and other disinfecting agents (168, 169). Potential transmission of AIDS from donor to recipient via bone transplantation poses a special problem. Since HIV was recognized and the first reported bone transplant-related transmission of it was published (101), a reliable sterilizing approach for HIV has been sought (88, 162, 170–175).

BONE DISTRIBUTION

Once bone is deemed safe for transplantation, it is ready for equitable distribution to user sites. Frozen bone cleared for use should be stored in a separate, limited access, ultra-cold freezer. It is efficient and convenient to store all bone of one type together. Freeze-dried bone can be stored at room temperature for easy access.

Long bones should be x-rayed. A radiopaque ruler or marker included on the x-ray with the bone serves as a size reference. Then, bone of specific anatomic size can be readily identified and dispatched (2, 4). Every bone leaving the bank must bear an information label and/or be accompanied by an information document. Instructions for proper storage, thawing, or rehydration/reconstitution procedures using sterile physiological solutions are included (73, 88). Suitable thawing procedures include exposing the wrapped bone to room temperature for several hours or submerging the unwrapped bone

into 37°C sterile saline baths with or without added antibiotics as the surgery is beginning. By the time the surgical site is prepared to receive the allograft, the bone will be thawed.

The package insert requests that a culture be obtained of the allograft bone in the operating room before it is exposed to antibiotics. An adverse reaction form also accompanies the bone. This allows for reporting to the bone bank of any untoward postoperative events believed attributable to the bone allograft. This is important for quality assurance.

Bone collected, but not suitable for allograft, is discarded by whatever method the local institution uses for discarding human tissue, e.g., incineration. The disposal date and the reason for discarding a bone or tissue are documented in the donor record (73).

During transit between the bone bank and hospital operating rooms, bone storage temperatures must be maintained and the mode of transport must not violate the sterile packaging (4). Dry ice packed around the bone in well-insulated styrofoam boxes has proven effective for maintaining frozen bone during transport to the user institution. For long journeys, bone could be shipped in liquid nitrogen in specially constructed canisters. Freeze-dried bone is packed to avoid breakage and is shipped at ambient temperatures.

DOCUMENTATION

Every step of the bone bank operation, from donor selection and consent to distribution and implantation, must be legibly and indelibly documented. Each bone allograft must have a complete audit trail to its source while maintaining donor and recipient confidentiality (88). Although this can be done adequately by manual record keeping, computer-assisted documentation is helpful and time saving (74). A detailed policy and procedures manual, reviewed and revised annually by the director, ensures standardized state-of-the-art practice. All records, reports, or other communications relative to a bone allograft should be retained indefinitely or for the period of time required by local legislation. Adverse reactions should be investigated with a written report entered into the donor records. The information obtained from the adverse event is utilized as appropriate in improving performance. Not to be forgotten is retention of all quality control and quality assurance documents of equipment function and maintenance, microbiological cultures, secondary sterilization certificates, and old copies when policy and procedure manuals are revised.

QUALITY CONTROL

Whether the facility is a small community hospital bone bank serving the patients of one transplant surgeon or a large regional bank serving a large patient/surgeon constituency, bone allografts must be of the highest quality possible. The reputation of the bone bank depends on the quality of its operation. Banks accredited by the American Association of Tissue Banks require an annual review of the tissue bank's records and performance by a professional knowledgeable of tissue banking practice but not affiliated with the bank under review.

Scrupulous attention to detail, protocol adherence, equipment maintenance, careful laboratory testing, and discerning medical and technical judgment are essential ingredients to realize this goal for recipient safety and bone utility (73, 88). An area of special concern is that of transmissible diseases. Histological and serological assessment of donor bone and blood in conjunction with an autopsy on the donor are especially helpful quality control practices. Utilization of radiosensitive bacterial spore strip (e.g., *B. pumilus*) as a quality control of radiation effectiveness is recommended. Similarly, radio sensitive color indicator labels on each bone package show, at a glance, that radiation sterilization has been done.

The American Association of Tissue Banks has established technical training courses and certification examination for tissue bank specialists in an effort to upgrade personnel and standardize bone retrieval and bone banking techniques.

LIABILITY

Not all state legislatures have designated tissue banking activities as a "service"; therefore, bone banks are not universally protected from certain "product" liability statutes. Bone is an anatomical gift. It is not to be bought or sold. The onus is on the bone bank to supply high-quality bone for allograft use by maintaining high standards of donor identification and tracking, bone bank operation, tissue storage, and quality control. Voluntary self-scrutiny and adherence to recognized standards of excellence safeguard the recipients, generate the respect and confidence of the surgeons, and stimulate community support for the bone bank.

The bone bank does not assume any responsibility or liability for the clinical use of the allograft tissue (72, 88). Hospital-based bone banks usually are under the legal advice and liability protection of the hospital. Independent facilities will require their own sources of insurance protection. These concerns may increase in importance if allograft bone is shipped interstate or across international boundaries. Insurance carriers must be knowledgeable of the existing dilemma. Two great legal contributions to the general field of tissue banking and allograft preparations have been the Uniform Anatomical Gift Act in the United States (48) and the Human Tissue Gift Act in Canada (53).

ACCREDITATION

In 1986, the American Association of Tissue Banks initiated an accreditation program. Involvement was voluntary. The aims of both the American Association of Tissue Banks and the participating institutions were both to standardize the operation of bone and tissue banks across the country and to achieve nationally recognized uniform levels of quality (77, 83). A detailed questionnaire prepared by the American Association of Tissue Banks and answered by the director of the bone and tissue bank and an on-site visit by a team of experienced tissue bankers are the main features of the inspection process. Accreditation is granted for a 3-year period, after which the facility requests a repeat inspection to regain accreditation. Accreditation status ensures that bone and tissue banking activities are being performed in a professional, consistent manner. Accreditation serves as an assurance to recipients and transplant surgeons that their source of bone allografts is creditable, peer reviewed, and complying with nationally accepted standards of operations. It is independent of government agencies (73). The American Association of Tissue Banks has extended its accreditation service into Canada. It is better to be proactive and volunteer to maintain standards than to be legislated toward excellence.

THE FUTURE

In spite of the risks, the most convincing argument in favor of allograft bone transplantation is its clinical success (75). Ultimately, however a substitute for human bone is desired that will lack the problems of rejection, disease transmission potential, and the biomechanical lesions induced by secondary sterilization procedures. Probably, factors that stimulate osteoblastic activity and bone regeneration will be isolated. Lymphocyte-stimulated rejection reactions may be preventable by improving penetration of ultraviolet irradiation or other manipulations to reduce immunogenicity (46, 158). Improved cryopreservation techniques may be found that reduce tissue damage by ice crystal formation and/or thawing and will allow for viable osteocyte and chondrocyte preservation over longer periods of time (46). Vascularized allografts may be realized in the future (176). Secondary sterilization procedures may be found that are less toxic, produce less tissue damage, and are fully reliable for killing viral agents. Many of these concerns were reviewed also by Friedlaender and Mankin in 1983 (177).

In the shorter term, the limiting factor for bone and tissue transplantation will continue to be the availability of suitable allograft donors. Consequently, a great challenge to those interested in bone and tissue banking is the education of the public and health professionals to the need for and the use of allograft musculoskeletal tissue—bone, ligaments, tendons, cartilaginous surfaces, and menisci. Education in the schools, to service organizations, of the clergy, and of the public will yield a heightened awareness of the need and the value of human allograft bone. It also may uncover sources of funding to support further research needed for understanding the scientific mysteries and clinical strengths of the endeavor.

Continued and accelerated cooperation among organ procurement agencies and bone and tissue banks, equally compulsive and dedicated to common high standards of operation, will contribute to meeting the needs of allograft recipients across the country (2, 5). Larger tissue banks will produce specialized or customized allografts that are beyond the capabilities of a community bone bank. Appropriately presized and/or preprocessed bone will complement innovative reconstructive orthopaedic surgeries as they emerge.

With increasing need for bone and increasing donor recruitment, there will be increasing demands on the clinical laboratory. Their support is vital to assess, interpret, and report results of donor screening (178). Bone banking is very much a team effort to provide a better quality of life for many patients.

REFERENCES

1. Cruz LD. A look inside a bone bank. AORN J 1988; 47:1196–1200.
2. Friedlaender GE. Tissue transplantation: Allocation and related issues. Trans Proceed 1988; 1:1017–1021.
3. Cruess RL. Bone banking, 1989: Challenges and opportunities. Can J Surg 1989; 32:227–228.
4. Friedlaender GE, Mankin HJ. Bone banking: current methods and suggested guidelines. (Parts A and B). In: Murray DG (ed). Am Acad Ortho Surg. Instr Course Lectures. CV Mosby Co, St. Louis, 1981; 36–55.
5. Friedlaender GE. Current concepts review—Bone banking. J Bone Joint Surg 1982; 64A:307–311.
6. Hart MM, Campbell ED, Kartub MG. Bone banking: a cost effective method for establishing a community hospital bone bank. Clin Orthop Relat Res 1986; 206:295–300.
7. Grob D. Autologous bone-grafts: problems at the donor site. In: Aebi M, Regazzoni P (eds). Bone Transplantation. Springer-Verlag, Berlin Heidelberg, 1989; p. 245.
8. Czitrom AA, Gross AE, Langer F, Sim FH. Bone banks and allografts in community practice. In: Bassett A III (ed). AAOS Instructional Course Lectures. CV Mosby Co, St. Louis, 1988; 13–24.
9. Dartée DA, Huij J, Tonino AJ. Bank bone grafts in revision hip arthroplasty for acetabular protrusion. Acta Orthop Scand 1988; 59:513–515.
10. Delloye C, de Nayer P, Coutelier L, Vincent A. Our experience with massive deep-frozen allografts in limb salvage surgery and with cryopreserved osteoarticular allografts in joint lesions. In: Aebi M, Regazzoni P (eds). Bone Transplantation. Springer-Verlag, Berlin, Heidelberg, 1989; pp. 323–324.
11. Mnaymneh W, Malinin T, Mnaymneh LG, Robinson D. Pelvic allograft–A case report with a follow-up evaluation of 5.5 years. Clin Orthop Relat Res 1990; 255:128–132.
12. Delloye C, Allington N, Munting E, Geulette B, Vincent A. Three-years' experience with small freeze-dried bone implants used in various conditions. In: Aebi M, Regazzoni P (eds). Bone Transplantation. Springer-Verlag, Berlin, Heidelberg, 1989; pp. 325–326.
13. Friedlaender GE. Bone banking: In support of reconstructive surgery of the hip. Clin Ortho Relat Res 1987; 225:17–21.
14. Gross AE, Lavoie MV, McDermott P, Marks P. The use of allograft bone in revision of total hip arthroplasty. Clin Orthop Relat Res 1985; 197:115–122.
15. Head WC, Berklacich FM, Malinin TI, Emerson RH. Proximal femoral allografts in revision total hip arthroplasty. Clin Orthop Relat Res 1987; 225:22–36.
16. Malinin TI, Brown MD. Bone allografts in spinal surgery. Clin Orthop Relat Res 1981; 154:68–73.
17. Malinin TI, Martinez OV, Brown MD. Banking of massive osteoarticular and intercalary bone allografts—12 years' experience. Clin Orthop Relat Res 1985; 197:44–57.
18. Marx RE, Kline SN, Johnson RP, et al. The use of freeze-dried allogeneic bone in oral and maxillofacial surgery. J Oral Surg 1981; 39:264–274.
19. Freeman E, Turnbull RS. Histologic evaluation of freeze-dried fine particle bone allografts. Preliminary observations. J Periodontol 1977; 48:288–289.
20. Urist MR. Chemosterilized antigen-extracted surface-demineralized autolysed allogeneic (AAA) bone for arthrodesis. In: Friedlaender GE, Mankin HJ, Sell KW (eds). Osteochondral Allografts: Biology, Banking and Clinical Applications. Little, Brown and Co., Boston, 1983; pp. 193–201.
21. Oakeshott RD, McAuley JP, Gross AE, et al. Allograft reconstruction in revision total hip surgery. In: Aebi M, Regazzoni P (eds). Bone Transplantation. Springer-Verlag, Berlin, Heidelberg, 1989; pp. 265–274.

22. Parrish FF. Total and partial half joint resection followed by allograft replacement in neoplasms involving ends of long bones. Transpl Proc 1976; 8(Suppl. 1):77–81.

23. Schneider JR, Bright RW. Anterior cervical fusion using pre-served bone allografts. Transpl Proc 1976; 8(Suppl. 1):73–76.

24. Sim FH, Bowman Jr WE, Wilkins RM, Chao EYS. Limb salvage in primary malignant bone tumours. Orthopedics 1985; 8:574–581.

25. Urist MR. Introduction to update on osteochondral allograft surgery. In: Aebi M, Regazzoni P (eds). Bone Transplantation. Springer-Verlag, Berlin, Heidelberg, 1989; pp. 1–6.

26. Brown KLB, Cruess RL. Bone and cartilage transplantation in orthopaedic surgery. J Bone Joint Surg 1982; 64A:270–279.

27. Burchardt H. Biology of bone transplantation. Orthop Clin North Am 1987; 18:187–196.

28. Reddi AH, Wientroub S, Muthukumaran N. Biological princi-ples of bone induction. Orthop Clin North Am 1987; 18:207–212.

29. Itoman M, Sasamoto N, Yamamoto M. Banked bone grafting for bone defect repair—Clinical evaluation of bone union and graft incorporation. J Jpn Orthop Assoc 1988; 62:461–469.

30. Moskowitz GW, Lukash F. Evaluation of bone graft viability. Sem Nucl Med 1988; 18:246–254.

31. Handelberg F, Yde P, de Boeck H, Casteleyn PP, Opdecam P. Our experience with frozen allografts: First short-term results. In: Aebi M, Regazzoni P (eds). Bone Transplantation. Springer-Verlag, Berlin, Heidelberg, 1989; pp. 321–322.

32. Harris WH. Allografting in total hip arthroplasty: in adults with severe acetabular deficiency including a surgical technique for bolting the graft to the ilium. Clin Orthop Relat Res 1982; 162:150–164.

33. Noyes FR, Barber SD, Magine RE. Bone-patellar ligament-bone and fascia lata allografts for reconstruction of the anterior cru-ciate ligament. J Bone Joint Surg 1990; 72A:1125–1136.

34. Malinin T, Carneiro R. Transplantation of vascularized bone allografts. Transact Orthop Res Soc 1990; 15:228.

35. de Boer H. Early research on bone transplantation. In: Aebi M, Regazzoni P (eds). Bone Transplantation. Springer-Verlag, Berlin, Heidelberg, 1989; p. 7–19.

36. de Boer HH. The history of bone grafts. Clin Orthop Relat Res 1988; 226:292–298.

37. Albee FH. Fundamentals in bone transplantation: Experiences in three thousand bone graft operations. JAMA 1923; 81:1429–1432.

38. Siqueira EB, Kranzler LI. Cervical interbody fusion using calf bone. Surg Neurol 1982; 18:37–39.

39. Goran A, Murthy KK. Fracture dislocation of the cervical spine. Value of anterior approach with bovine bone interbody fusion. Spine 1978; 3:95–102.

40. McMurray GN. The evaluation of Kiel bone in spinal fusions. J Bone Joint Surg 1982; 64B:101–104.

41. Council on Dental Materials, Instruments and Equipment; Council on Dental Research; Council on Dental Therapeutics. Hydroxylapatite, beta tricalcium phosphate and autogenous and allogeneic bone for filling periodontal defects, alveolar ridge augmentation and pulp capping. J Am Dent Assoc 1984; 108:822–831.

42. Shimazaki K, Mooney V. Comparative study of porous hy-droxyapatite and tricalcium phosphate as bone substitute. J Orthop Res 1985; 3:301–310.

43. White E, Shors EC. Biomaterial aspects of interpore-200 porous hydroxyapatite. Dent Clin North Am 1986; 30:49–67.

44. Holmes RE, Bucholz RW, Mooney V. Porous hydroxyapatite as a bone-graft substitute in metaphyseal defects. J Bone Joint Surg 1986; 68A:904–911.

45. Sartoris DJ, Gershuni DH, Akeson WH, Holmes RE, Resnick D. Coralline hydroxyapatite bone graft substitutes: preliminary report of radiographic evaluation. Radiology 1986; 159:133–137.

46. Meryman HT. Tissue banking: present status and future prom-ise. In: Fawcett KJ, Barr AR (eds). Tissue Banking. Am Assoc Blood Banks, Arlington, VA, 1987; pp. 1–15.

47. Nortell B. Legal aspects of transplantation: a solution in search of a problem? In: Freidlaender GE, Mankin HJ, Sell KW (eds). Osteochondral Allografts: Biology, Banking and Clinical Ap-plications. Little, Brown and Co, Boston, 1983; pp. 301–306.

48. National Conference of Commissioners on Uniform State Laws: The Uniform Anatomical Gift Act Proceedings, Section 7B, July 30, 1968.

49. Sadler AM, Sadler BL, Stason EB. The uniform anatomical gift act. A model for reform. JAMA 1968; 206:2501–2506.

50. Curran WJ. The uniform anatomical gift act. N Engl J Med 1969; 280:36–37.

51. Weedn VW, Leveque B. Routine inquiry for organ and tissue donations. Texas Med 1988; 84:30–37.

52. Francisco CJ, III, JD. Organ donation and transplantation—what every physician should know. Texas Med 1988; 84:92–95.

53. Ministry of the Solicitor General. Human Tissue Gift Act, Re-vised Statutes of Ontario, 1980, (October, 1982.) Chapter 210.

54. Minister of Supply and Services Canada—Health and Welfare Canada. Organ and Tissue Donation Services in Hospitals—Guidelines, 1986, Ottawa, Canada.

55. Keyserlingk EW. Human dignity and donor altruism—are they compatible with efficiency in cadaveric human organ pro-curement? Transpl Proc 1990; 22:1005–1006.

56. Scott R. The human body: belonging and control. Transpl Proc 1990; 22:1002–1004.

57. Public Hospitals Act (O. Reg. 34/90) Hospital Management, Regulation to amend Ontario Regulation 518/88 made under the Public Hospitals Act. January 18, 1990, Toronto, Canada.

58. Geiser F. Sharing body and blood is familiar to Christians. Transplants are solace to the grieving and hope for the des-perately ill. The Lutheran 1985; April:5–7.

59. Scorsone S. Christianity and the significance of the human body. Transpl Proc 1990; 22:943–944.

60. Bulka RP (Rabbi). Jewish perspective on organ transplantation. Transpl Proc 1990; 22:945–946.

61. Sahin AF. Islamic transplantation ethics. Transpl Proc 1990; 22:939.

62. Namihira E. Shinto concept concerning the dead human body. Transpl Proc 1990; 22:940–941.

63. Trivedi HL. Hindu religious view in context of transplantation of organs from cadavers. Transpl Proc 1990; 22:942.

64. Sugunasiri SHJ. The Buddhist view concerning the dead body. Transpl Proc 1990; 22:947–949.

65. Kalshoven PJ. A humanistic conception of the human body after death. Transpl Proc 1990; 22:950–951.

66. United Network for Organ Sharing and South Eastern Organ Procurement Foundation. VI. General religious beliefs concerning organ donation and transplantation. Richmond, VA, 1989.

67. Friedlaender GE. In defense of science and the soul. Transpl Proc 1985; 17(Suppl. 4):11–12.

68. Freedman B. The ethical continuity of transplantation. Transpl Proc 1985; 17(Suppl. 4):17–23.

69. Friedlaender GE. Bone banking and clinical applications. Transpl Proc 1985; 17(Suppl. 4):99–104.

70. Malinin TI, Brown MD, Mnaymneh W, Martinez O, Marx RE, Kline SN. Bone banking—Experience with 1175 donors. In: Aebi M, Regazzoni P (eds). Bone Transplantation. Springer-Verlag, Berlin, Heidelberg: 1989; pp. 170–171.

71. Kalbe P, Illgner A, Berner W. Organization of a bone bank: experience over 16 years. In: Aebi M, Regazzoni P (eds). Bone Transplantation. Springer-Verlag, Berlin, Heidelberg, 1989; pp. 172–173.

72. Tomford WW, Doppelt SH, Mankin HJ. Organization, legal aspects and problems of bone banking in a large orthopedic center. In: Aebi M, Regazzoni P (eds). Bone Transplantation. Springer-Verlag, Berlin, Heidelberg, 1989; pp. 145–150.

73. Buckham KR. Surgical bone banking—Recommendations for setting up a program. AORN J 1989; 50:765–783.

74. La Prairie AJP, Gross M. A simplified protocol for banking bone from surgical donors requiring a 90-day quarantine and an HIV-1 antibody test. Can J Surg 1991; 34:41–48.

75. Paterson MP, Du Toit G. The use of banked femoral head bone allograft in spinal surgery. S Afr J Surg 1989; 27:89–92.

76. Czitrom AA. Bone banking in community hospitals. In: Aebi M, Regazzoni P (eds). Bone Transplantation. Springer-Verlag, Berlin, Heidelberg, 1989; pp. 151–154.

77. Mowe JC (ed). Standards for tissue banking. American Association of Tissue Banks, Arlington, VA, 1984, revision 1985, 1987, 1988.

78. Jacobs NJ. Establishing a surgical bone bank. In: Fawcett KJ, Barr AR (eds). Tissue Banking. American Association of Blood Banks, Arlington, VA, 1987; pp. 67–96.

79. Jacobs NJ, Kline WE, McCullough JJ. Bone transplantation, bone banking, and establishing a surgical bone bank. In: Bradford DS, Lonstein JE, Moe JH, Ogilvie JW, Winter RB (eds). Moe's Textbook of Scoliosis and Other Spinal Deformities. WB Saunders, Philadelphia, 1987; pp. 592–607.

80. Hart MM, Campbell ED, Kartub MG. Establishing a bone bank—Experience at a community hospital. AORN J 1986; 43:808–819.

81. Tomford WW, Ploetz JE, Mankin HJ. Bone allografts of femoral heads: procurement and storage. J Bone Joint Surg 1986; 68A:534–537.

82. Steckler D. Issues confronting the surgical bone bank. In: Fawcett KJ, Barr AR (eds). Tissue Banking Updates. American Association of Blood Banks, Arlington, VA, 1989; pp. 7–9.

83. Mowe JC (ed). Technical Manual for Tissue Banking. American Association of Tissue Banks, Arlington, VA, 1987.

84. Practices Subcommittee of the Technical Practices Coordinating Committee, AORN. Proposed recommended practices for storing, preserving and maintaining skin, bone, cartilage and blood vessel tissue. AORN J 1982; 35:934–940.

85. Russell G, Hu R, Raso VJ. Bone banking in Canada: a review. Can J Surg 1989; 32:231–236.

86. Johnson GV. Bone banks in the 1980s (Editorial). Br J Hosp Med 1988; 39:15.

87. Jackson JB. Bone banking: An overview. Lab Med 1987; 18:830–833.

88. Kateley JR. Establishing a tissue bank. In: Fawcett KJ, Barr AR (eds). Tissue Banking. American Association of Blood Banks, Arlington, VA, 1987; pp. 17–27.

89. Chase GJ, Boral LI. Establishing a bone bank: thoughts for a pathologist to consider. ASCP Check Sample, Immunohematology 1986; I86–3:2–7.

90. Knappenberger KR, Bartal E, Romanos R. Cadaveric bone retrieval/banking techniques. Kansas Med 1986; Feb:42–43.

91. Panel discussion on tissue banking. Transpl Proc 1985; 17(Suppl. 4):121–126.

92. Doppelt SH, Tomford WW, Lucas AD, Mankin HJ. Operational and financial aspects of a hospital bone bank. J Bone Joint Surg 1981; 63A:1472–1481.

93. Freidlaender GE. Personnel and equipment required for a "complete" tissue bank. Transpl Proc 1976; 8(Suppl. 1):235–240.

94. Tomford WW, Mankin HJ. Cadaver bone procurement. In: Fawcett KJ, Barr AR (eds). Tissue Banking. American Association of Blood Banks, Arlington, VA, 1987; pp. 97–107.

95. Motzkin GW. Organ donation . . . a license to butcher? Canadian Funeral Director 1990; 66:32–33.

96. McDermott AGP, Langer F, Pritzker KPH, Gross AE. Fresh small-fragment osteochondral allografts—long term follow-up study on first 100 cases. Clin Orthop Relat Res 1985; 197:96–102.

97. Tomford WW. Cadaver bone procurement. In: Fawcett KJ, Barr AR (eds). Tissue Banking Updates. American Association of Blood Banks, Arlington, VA, 1989; pp. 11–13.

98. Battle RM, Pathak D, Humble CG, et al. Factors influencing discrepancies between premortem and postmortem diagnoses. JAMA 1987; 258:339–344.

99. Centers for Disease Control. Update: rapidly progressive dementia in a patient who received a cadaveric dura mater graft. MMWR 1987; 36:49–50, 55.

100. Standards Committee Continues Discussion. American Association of Tissue Banks. Newsletter 1989; 12:1, 3–4.

101. Centers for Disease Control. Leads from MMWR 1988; 37; 597–599. Transmission of HIV through bone transplantation: case report and public health recommendations. JAMA 1988; 260(17):2487–2488.

102. Buck BE, Malinin TI, Brown MD. Bone transplantation and human immunodeficiency virus: an estimate of risk of acquired immunodeficiency syndrome (AIDS). Clin Orthop Relat Res 1989; 240:129–136.

103. Ward JW, Holmberg SD, Allen JR, et al. Transmission of human immuno-deficiency virus (HIV) by blood transfusions screened as negative for HIV antibody. N Engl J Med 1988; 318:473–478.

104. The Canadian Red Cross Society. The Canadian Red Cross Blood Programme from 1974 to 1990-A report to the Canadian Hematology Society. Ottawa, December, 1990; pp. 13, 61.

105. Herst R. Testing of transfusion products to include Hepatitis C and HTLV-1 (letter) Toronto: The Canadian Red Cross Society, Toronto Centre. June, 1990.

106. Delamarter RB, Carr J, Saxton EH. HTLV-1 viral associated myelopathy after blood transfusion in a multiple trauma patient. Clin Orthop Relat Res 1990; 260:191–194.

107. Johnson CA, Brown BA, Lasky LC. Rh immunization caused by osseous allograft (letter). N Engl J Med 1985; 312:121–122.

108. Jensen TT. Rhesus immunization after bone allografting. Acta Orthop Scand 1987; 58:584.

109. Van Dijk BA, Stassen J, Kunst VAJM, Sloof TJJH, Van Horn JR. Rhesus immunization after bone allografting (letter). Acta Orthop Scand 1988; 59:482.

110. Hill Z, Vacl J, Kalasová E, Calábková M, Pintera J. Hemolytic disease of the newborn due to anti-D antibodies in a D^u positive mother. Vox Sang 1974; 27:92–94.

111. Bowen PA, Lobel SA, Caruana RJ, Leffell MS, House MA, Rissing JP, Humphries AL. Transmission of human immunodeficiency virus (HIV) by transplantation: clinical aspects and time course analysis of viral antigenemia and antibody production. Ann Intern Med 1988; 108:46–48.

112. Chateauvert M, Duffie A, Gilmore N. Human immunodeficiency virus antibody testing: Counseling guidelines from the Canadian Medical Association. Canadian Medical Association, Ottawa, Canada, 1990.

113. Health and Welfare Canada Working Group on HIV Infection in Organ and Tissue Transplantation: Guidelines for prevention of HIV infection in organ and tissue transplantation. Canada Disease Weekly Report 1989; 15(Suppl. 4):1–17.

114. Warren J (ed). Transplant News 1990(Nov 16); 1:7.

115. 180-day quarantine for HCV and HIV for living donors effective April 1, 1991. Newsletter, American Association of Tissue Banks 1990; 13:1.

116. Centers for Disease Control. Semen banking, organ and tissue transplantation, and HIV antibody testing. MMWR 1988; 37:57–58, 63.

117. Semen banking, organ and tissue transplantation and HIV antibody testing. Lab Med 1988; 19:509.

118. Goldberg VM, Powell A, Shaffer JW, Zika J, Bos GD, Heiple KG. Bone grafting: role of histocompatibility in transplantation. J Orthop Res 1985; 3:389–404.

119. Muscolo DL, Caletti E, Schajowicz F, Araujo ES, Makino A. Tissue-typing in human massive allografts of frozen bone. J Bone Joint Surg 1987; 69A:583–595.

120. Friedlaender GE. Immune responses to preserved bone allografts in humans. In: Friedlaender GE, Mankin HJ, Sell KW (eds). Osteochondral Allografts: Biology, Banking and Clinical Applications. Little, Brown and Co, Boston, 1983; pp. 159–164.

121. Friedlaender GE. Current concepts review: bone grafts: The basic science rationale for clinical applications. J Bone Joint Surg 1987; 69A:786–790.

122. Friedlaender GE, Mankin HJ, Langer F. Immunology of Osteochondral allografts: background and general considerations. In: Friedlaender GE, Mankin HJ, Sell KW (eds). Osteochondral Allografts: Biology, Banking and Clinical Applications. Little, Brown and Co, Boston, 1983; pp. 133–140.

123. Hosny M. Recent concepts in bone grafting and banking. J Craniomandib Pract 1987; 5:170–182 (Erratum 289).

124. Stevenson S. The immune response to osteochondral allografts in dogs. J Bone Joint Surg 1987; 69A:573–582.

125. Horowitz MC, Friedlaender GE. Immunologic aspects of bone transplantation. Orthop Clin North Am 1987; 18:227–233.

126. Czitrom AA, Axelrod T, Fernandes B. Antigen presenting cells and bone allotransplantation. Clin Orthop Relat Res 1985; 197:27–31.

127. Czitrom AA. Bone transplantation, passenger cells and the major histocompatibility complex. In: Aebi M, Regazzoni P (eds). Bone Transplantation. Springer-Verlag, Berlin, Heidelberg, 1989; pp. 104–110.

128. Goldberg VM, Stevenson S. Natural history of autografts and allografts. Clin Orthop Relat Res 1987; 225:7–16.

129. LeBlanc B. Informed consent and refusal: the medical-legal debate continues. Ont Med Rev 1990; 57:16–19.

130. Ehrlich MG, Lorenz J, Tomford WW, Mankin HJ. Collagenase activity in banked bone. Trans Orthop Res Soc 1983; 8:166.

131. Lee KE, Pelker RR. Effect of freezing on histologic and biomechanical failure patterns in the rabbit capital femoral growth plate. J Orthop Res 1985; 3:514–515.

132. Eastlund DT. Effect of repeated freeze-thaw or irradiation on patellar tendon mechanical properties. American Red Cross Tissue Services Newsletter 1990; 3:1–2.

133. Bos GD, Goldberg VM, Gordon NH, Dollinger BM, Zika JM, Powell AE, Heiple KG. The long-term fate of fresh and frozen orthotopic bone allografts in genetically defined rats. Clin Orthop Relat Res 1985; 197:245–254.

134. Malinin TI, Wu NM, Flores A. Freeze-drying of bone for allotransplantation. In: Friedlaender GE, Mankin HJ, Sell KW (eds). Osteochondral Allografts: Biology, Banking and Clinical Applications. Little, Brown and Co, Boston, 1983; pp. 181–192.

135. Tomford WW. Cryopreservation of articular cartilage. In: Frielaender GE, Mankin HJ, Sell KW (eds): Osteochondral Allografts: Biology, Banking and Clinical Applications. Little, Brown and Co, Boston, 1983; pp. 215–217.

136. Tomford WW, Mankin HJ, Friedlaender GE, Doppelt SH, Gebhardt MC. Methods of banking bone and cartilage for allograft transplantation. Orthop Clin North Am 1987; 18:241–247.

137. Ghisellini F, Palamini G, Brugo G. Conservation of bone homografts in cialit: 5 year clinical experience. In: Aebi M, Regazzoni P (eds). Bone Transplanation. Springer-Verlag, Berlin, Heidelberg, 1989; pp. 176–177.

138. Urist MR, Dawson E. Intertransverse process fusion with the aid of chemosterilized autolyzed antigen-extracted allogeneic (AAA) bone. Clin Orthop Relat Res 1981; 154:97–113.

139. Present DA, Anderson DW, Glowczewskie FA, Vanjonack WJ. Procedures and practices for aseptic processing of sterile bone for banking. In: Aebi M, Regazzoni P (eds). Bone Transplantation. Springer-Verlag, Berlin, Heidelberg, 1989; pp. 178–179.

140. Pelker RR, Friedlaender GE. Biomechanical aspects of bone autografts and allografts. Orthop Clin North Am 1987; 18:235–239.

141. Burwell RG. The fate of freeze-dried bone allografts. Transplant Proc 1976; 8(Suppl. 1):95–111.

142. Jackson DW, Windler GE, Simon TM, Intra-articular reaction associated with the use of freeze-dried, ethylene oxide-sterilized bone-patella tendon-bone allografts in the reconstruction of the anterior cruciate ligament. Am J Sports Med 1990; 18:1–10.

143. Bright RW, Burchardt H. The biomechanical properties of preserved bone grafts. In: Friedlaender GE, Mankin HJ, Sell KW (eds). Osteochondral Allografts: Biology, Banking and Clinical Applications. Little, Brown and Co, Boston, 1983; pp. 241–247.

144. Mukherjee JS, Cowling KM, Soutas-Little RW, Hubbard RP, Kateley J. Mechanical analysis and finite element modelling of bone allografts after different types of sterilization. In: Butler DL, Torzilli PA (eds). Biomechanics Symposium. American Society of Mechanical Engineers, New York, 1987; pp. 109–111.

145. Butler DL, Noyes FR, Walz KA, Gibbons MJ. Biomechanics of human knee ligament allograft treatment. Proceedings of the 33rd Annual Meeting, Orthopedic Research Society, San Francisco, California. January 19–22, 1987; p. 128.

146. Haut RC, Powlison AC, Rutherford GW, Kateley JR. Order of irradiation and lyophilization on the strength of patellar tendon allografts. 35th Annual Meeting, Orthopedic Research Society, Las Vegas, Nevada, February 6–9, 1989.

147. Duval P, Yahia H, Zukor D, Rubins I, Drouin G. Effects of irradiation on the mechanical properties of knee meniscal grafts. Transact Orthop Res Soc 1990; 15:218.

148. Zukor DJ, Rubins IM, Daigle MR, Rudan JF, Roy I, Duval P, Yahia H, Farine J, Gross AE. Allotransplantation of frozen irradiated menisci in rabbits. Transact Orthop Res Soc 1990; 15:219.

149. Haut RC, Powlison AC, Rutherford GW, Kateley JR. Some effects of donor age and sex on the mechanical properties of patellar tendon graft tissues (abstract). Annual Winter Meeting, American Society of Mechanical Engineers, Chicago, Illinois, November 26–December 2, 1988.

150. Kostiak PE, Bender TM, Connors JJ, Sebastianelli MJ, Burchardt H. The procurement environment and the incidence of contaminated tissue (abstract). Presented at 13th Annual Meeting of the Am Assoc of Tissue Banks. Baltimore, Maryland, Oct. 1-4, 1989.

151. de Vries P. Before freezing culture allograft for bacteria. The Medical Post, Maclean Hunter Ltd., Canada, August 11, 1981; p. 49.

152. McMahon CA, Lamberson HV. Comparison of bacterial contamination of cadaver bone donations collected under operating room and morgue conditions (abstract). 13th Annual Meeting, Am Assoc Tissue Banks, Baltimore, Maryland, October 1–4, 1989.

153. Tomford WW, Starkweather RJ, Goldman MH. A study of the clinical incidence of infection in the use of banked allograft bone. J Bone Joint Surg 1981; 63A:244–248.

154. Lord CF, Gebhardt MC, Tomford WW, Mankin HJ. Infection in bone allografts: Incidence, nature and treatment. J Bone Joint Surg 1988; 70A:369–376.

155. Kreicbergs A, Köhler P. Bone exposed to heat. In: Aebi M. Regazzoni P (eds). Bone Transplantation. Springer-Verlag, Berlin, Heidelberg, 1989; pp. 155–161.

156. Evanoff J. Sterilizing and preserving human bone. AORN J 1983; 37:972–980.

157. Köhler P, Kreicbergs A. Incorporation of autoclaved autogeneic bone supplemented with allogeneic demineralized bone matrix—an experimental study in the rabbit. Clin Orthop Relat Res 1987; 218:247–258.

158. Meryman HT. Transmission of viral disease and recent advances in transplantation immunology. In: Fawcett KJ, Barr AR (eds). Tissue Banking Updates. Amer Assoc Blood Banks, Arlington, VA, 1989; pp. 1–5.

159. Köhler P, Kreicbergs A, Strömberg L. Physical properties of autoclaved bone-Torsion test of rabbit diaphyseal bone. Acta Orthop Scand 1986; 57:141–145.

160. Occupational safety and health agency defines ethylene oxide excursion limit. Newsletter, American Association of Tissue Banks 1988; 11:5.

161. Johnson AL, Moutray M, Hoffmann WE. Effect of ethylene oxide sterilization and storage conditions on canine cortical bone harvested for banking. Vet Surg 1987; 16:418–422.

162. Eastlund T, Jackson B, Havrilla G, Sonnerud K. Preliminary study results using ethylene oxide (ETO) or heat to inactivate HIV in cortical bone (abstract). Thirteenth Annual Meeting, Am Assoc Tissue Banks, Baltimore, Maryland, Oct 1–4, 1989.

163. Prolo DJ, Oklund SA. Sterilizing of bone by chemicals. In: Friedlaender GE, Mankin HJ, Sell KW (eds). Osteochondral Allografts: Biology, Banking and Clinical Applications. Little, Brown and Co, Boston, 1983; pp. 233–238.

164. Gray JC, Elves MW. Osteogenesis in bone grafts after short-term storage and topical antibiotic treatment. J Bone Joint Surg 1981; 63B:441–445.

165. von Versen R, Starke R. The peracetic acid/low pressure cold

sterilization—A new method to sterilize corticocancellous bone and soft tissue. Z Exp Chir Transplant Künstl 1989; 22:18–21.

166. Bright RW, Smarsh JD, Gambill VM. Sterilization of human bone by irradiation. In: Friedlaender GE, Mankin HJ, Sell KW (eds). Osteochondral Allografts: Biology, Banking and Clinical Applications. Little, Brown and Co, Boston, 1983; pp. 223–232.

167. Hernigou P, Delepine G, Goutallier D. Control of sterility in bone banking with irradiation. In: Aebi M, Regazzoni P (eds). Bone Transplantation. Springer-Verlag, Berlin, Heidelberg, 1989; pp. 174–175.

168. Gibbs CJ Jr, Gajdusek DC, Latarjet R. Unusual resistance to ionizing radiation of the viruses of Kuru, Creutzfeldt-Jakob disease and Scrapie. Proc Natl Acad Sci USA 1978; 75:6268–6270.

169. CDC Indicts Dura Mater in Second CJD Transmission. Newsletter, Am Assoc of Tissue Banks, McLean, VA, 1989; 12:1–2.

170. Buck BE, Resnick L, Shah SM, Malinin TI. Human immunodeficiency virus cultured from bone: Implications for transplantation. Clin Orthop Relat Res 1990; 251:249–253.

171. Bigbee PD. Inactivation of human immunodeficiency virus (AIDS virus) by gamma and x-ray irradiation in body fluids and forensic evidence. FBI Law Enforcement Bulletin July, 1988; 8–9.

172. Spire B, Dormont D, Barré-Sinoussi F, Montagnier L, Chermann JC. Inactivation of lymphadenopathy-associated virus by heat, gamma rays, and ultraviolet light. Lancet 1985; 1:188–189.

173. Conway B, Tomford WW, Hirsch MS, Schooley RT, Mankin HJ. Effects of gamma irradiation on HIV-1 in a bone allograft model. Transact Orthop Res Soc 1990; 15:225.

174. Withrow SJ, Oulton SA, Suto TL, Wilkins RM, Straw RC, Rose BJ, Gasper PW. Evaluation of the antiretroviral effect of various methods of sterilizing/preserving corticocancellous bone. Transact Orthop Res Soc 1990; 15:226.

175. Conway B, Strick DA, Beghian LE, Montesalvo M, Jahngen E, Schooley RT, Tomford WW. Radiosensitivity of HIV-1: Demonstration of an inoculum effect. (Poster) American Assoc. Tissue Banks, 14 Annual Meeting, Sept. 23–26, 1990; M15.

176. Burwell RG, Friedlaender GE, Mankin HJ. Current perspectives and future directions: The 1983 invitational conference on osteochondral allografts. Clin Orthop Relat Res 1985; 197:141–157.

177. Friedlaender GE, Mankin HJ. Future goals in bone transplantation. In: Friedlaender GE, Mankin HJ, Sell KW (eds). Osteochondral Allografts: Biology, Banking and Clinical Applications. Little, Brown and Co, Boston, 1983; pp. 309–318.

178. Polesky HF, Lasky LC. Transplantation: its impact on the laboratory. Lab Med 1987; 18:829.

4

INDICATIONS AND USES OF MORSELLIZED AND SMALL-SEGMENT ALLOGRAFT BONE IN GENERAL ORTHOPAEDICS

Andrei A. Czitrom

A variety of orthopaedic procedures make use of bone graft in the form of morsellized material or small pieces of bone of particular shapes and sizes (small-segment bone grafts). In these circumstances, either autograft or banked allograft bone can be used. The recent rapid development of tissue banking techniques has made banked allograft bone readily available and this has contributed to an increased use of allogeneic bone in general orthopaedic practice. This chapter discusses the indications and techniques of using this type of allograft material.

BANKING AND SUPPLY OF MORSELLIZED AND SMALL-SEGMENT BONE GRAFTS

The technology of bone banking is discussed extensively in Chapter 3 and, therefore, only a few specific items relevant to the use of morsellized and small-segment allograft material will be mentioned here.

The author thanks Dr. Fred Langer for his assistance in providing some of the clinical examples presented in this chapter.

Types of Processing

Morsellized and small-segment bone is generally supplied in three different forms that result from different processing techniques: (*a*) deep-frozen; (*b*) freeze-dried; and (*c*) demineralized. Deep-frozen bone is stored at $-70°C$ while freeze-dried or demineralized material can be stored on the shelf at room temperature. For the purpose of morsellized and small-segment grafting, deep-frozen and freeze-dried bone are equivalent. Demineralized material obviously has less mechanical strength than deep-frozen or freeze-dried bone and its use at the present time is experimental for the purpose of bone induction. Morsellized and small-segment bone is sometimes treated by radiation or ethylene oxide for the purpose of additional sterilization.

Comparison of Bank Bone and Autograft Bone

Bank bone can be immunogenic and sensitize recipients to donor antigens while autografts can not. This is not an issue that is of relevance in common clinical practice except when bone is transplanted to Rh-negative females of child-bearing age where Rh-sensitization may be a problem. Osteogenesis is a property of autografts only as bank bone contains no living cells and is not osteogenic. Osteoconduction is the ability to allow bone ingrowth and is similar for bank bone and autografts. Osteoinduction is provided by autografts but not at all or only very poorly by bank bone that is not demineralized. As a result of the combination of absent osteogenic potential and decreased osteoinductive capacity, the healing of bank bone is slower than the healing of autografts. However, bank bone does heal and incorporate by allowing ingrowth of host bone because of its osteoconductive property. The possibility of disease transmission exists when bank bone is used but is not an issue with autografts. These factors constitute advantages of autografts over allografts. However, bank bone has certain advantages over autografts. It is unlimited in quantity (this is important in children where the availability of autogenous bone is limited) and is supplied ready in many sizes and shapes. Its use has the potential to decrease blood loss and anesthesia time and, therefore, may decrease patient morbidity. The use of bank bone avoids the donor site morbidity associated with harvesting the iliac crest, which includes potential problems such as infection, hematoma, nerve injury, muscle hernia, or chronic pain referable to the donor site, which can be as high as 37% (1). The use of bank bone versus autograft bone is a choice that has to balance the advantages and disadvantages of these grafting materials.

Supply

Morsellized or small-segment allografts can be obtained from either local surgical bone banks or from regional tissue banks. The major source of procurement for surgical bone banks is the operating room. The most frequent bone that is harvested is the femoral head, but other surgical discard, such as wedges removed at osteotomy, tibial plateaus and femoral condyles removed at knee arthroplasty, excised patellae or radial heads, ribs taken at thoracotomy, or bones from traumatic amputations can be stored in surgical banks. Current standards from the American Association of Tissue Banks require a 180-day quarantine of such live donor tissues with an HIV-negative test result prior to use. Many surgical bone banks store a small stock of large deep-frozen bone allografts used in revision arthroplasty of the hip and these grafts can also be a source of morsellized or small-segment material if large quantities of bone graft are required. Femoral heads and other large deep-frozen bones have to be cut, shaped, or morsellized in the operating room after thawing. Commercial bone mills are useful and necessary for morsellizing large amounts of deep-frozen allograft bone.

Regional tissue banks supply a great variety of shapes, sizes, and types of bone grafts that are processed and packaged under sterile conditions. They include cortical, cancellous, or cortical-cancellous bone preparations in the form of struts, dowels, strips, blocks, chips, or granules. Generally, these are available in both deep-frozen or freeze-dried varieties. Deep-frozen grafts are thawed in the operating suite prior to use and freeze-dried bone is generally reconstituted in sterile saline solution. The incorporation of morsellized banked bone grafts can be enhanced by the addition of host autogenous bone at a 1:3 ratio of autograft to allograft (2). Alternatively, they can be mixed with bone marrow cells obtained by aspiration of the iliac crest for the purpose of stimulating osteogenesis (3, 4).

INDICATIONS AND TECHNIQUES

The general indications for morsellized or small-segment allograft bank bone in orthopaedic reconstruction are: (*a*) to fill a cavity, (*b*) as a buttress, and (*c*) to augment the quantity of autograft bone. They are not indicated as bone grafts for the treatment of nonunions or in situations that require the stimulation of osteogenesis, such as enhancing primary union or arthrodesis (2). The third indication, that of augmenting the quantity of autograft bone, is applicable to various situations where autograft bone is insufficient in quantity, including the use of allograft bone as a filling or buttressing material in combination with autograft bone. In addition, it applies to spinal fusions for scoliosis where bank bone can serve as a vehicle to spread limited amounts of autograft bone over large areas providing osteoconductive material for osteogenesis derived from the autograft and the host bed. The contribution of the allograft bone to the efficacy of this method cannot be determined with precision and, therefore, this indication will not be discussed in more detail. The technique of reconstruction for the first two indications will be shown with appropriate case examples to illustrate their effectiveness.

Filling of a Bone Cavity

The need to fill a bone cavity (Figs. 4.1–4.10) arises most often after the excision of cysts or benign tumors. In these situations, control of the disease and preservation of function in the bone and neighboring joint is achieved by curettage or simple excision. The eradication and cure of the lesion requires the total removal of the lesion and the restoration of the osseous structure with bone graft material that will allow healing and remodeling. The technique of curettage and bone grafting of a benign bone lesion is shown in Figure 4.1. The most important single parameter for curettage to be effective is adequate exposure and visualization. This requires a large cortical window, which allows complete exteriorization of the cyst or tumor. Generally, one must remove half or more of the circumference of the bone to get adequate expo-

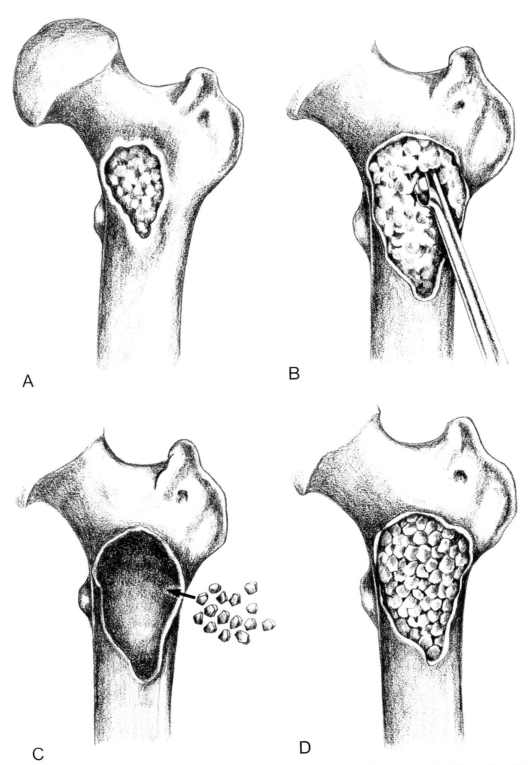

A

B

C

D

Figure 4.1. Technique of curettage and bone grafting of a benign bone lesion. *A.* Exposure of the lesion by creating a cortical window. *B.* Exteriorization of the tumor by enlarging the window and curettage (this is followed by extension of the margin with a motorized burr and, in some cases, by adjuvant treatment). *C.* The cavity is filled with morsellized allograft (deep-frozen or freeze-dried bone). *D.* Complete tight packing of the cavity with allograft bone.

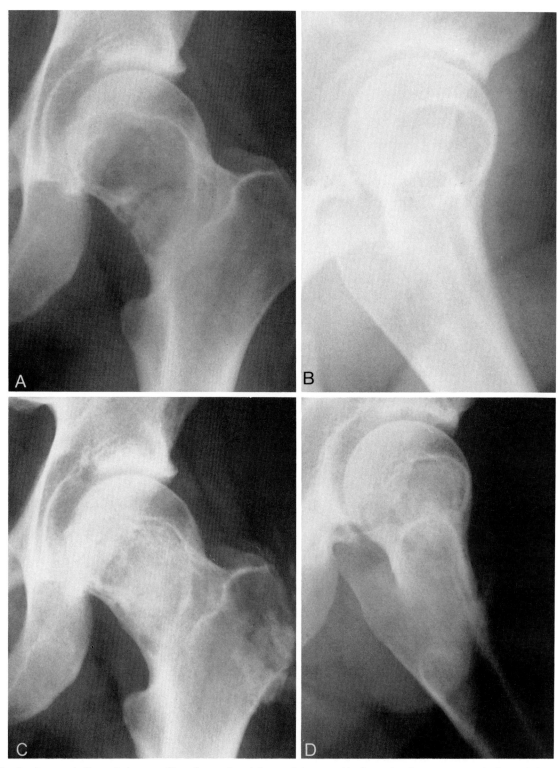

Figure 4.2. Curettage and allogeneic bone grafting of cyst. *A* and *B*. Anteroposterior and lateral radiographs of the hip in a 28-year-old man showing large cyst involving the femoral head and neck. *C* and *D*. Views of the same hip 3 months after curettage and allogeneic bone grafting showing incorporation of graft.

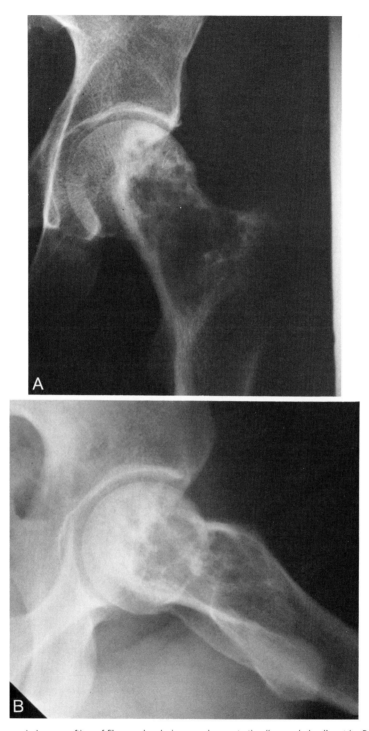

Figure 4.3. Curettage and allogeneic bone grafting of fibrous dysplasia. *A* and *B.* Anteroposterior and lateral hip radiographs showing fibrous dysplasia involving femoral head and neck. *C.* Anteroposterior tomogram demonstrating "ground glass" matrix. *D* and *E.* Postoperative views of the hip 5 months after curettage and grafting with morsellized allograft and autologous marrow showing incorporation and healing.

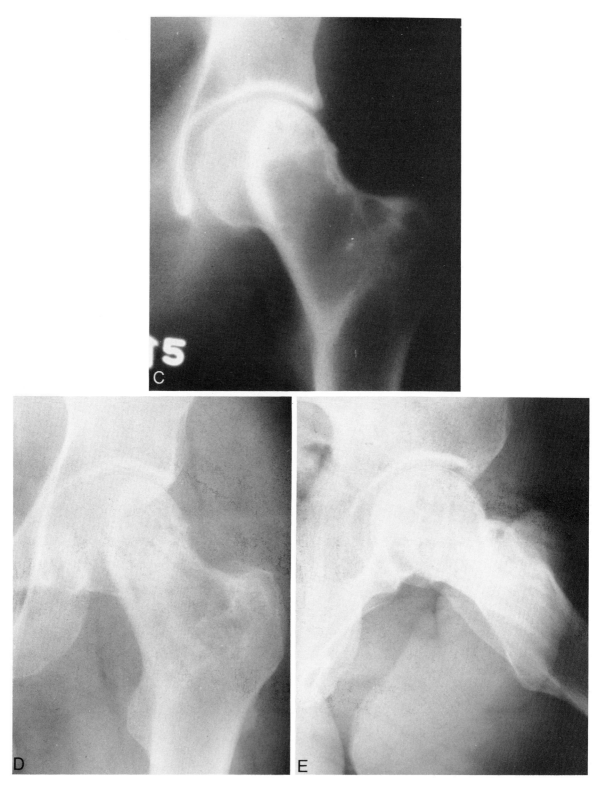

Figure 4.3. *C, D,* and *E.*

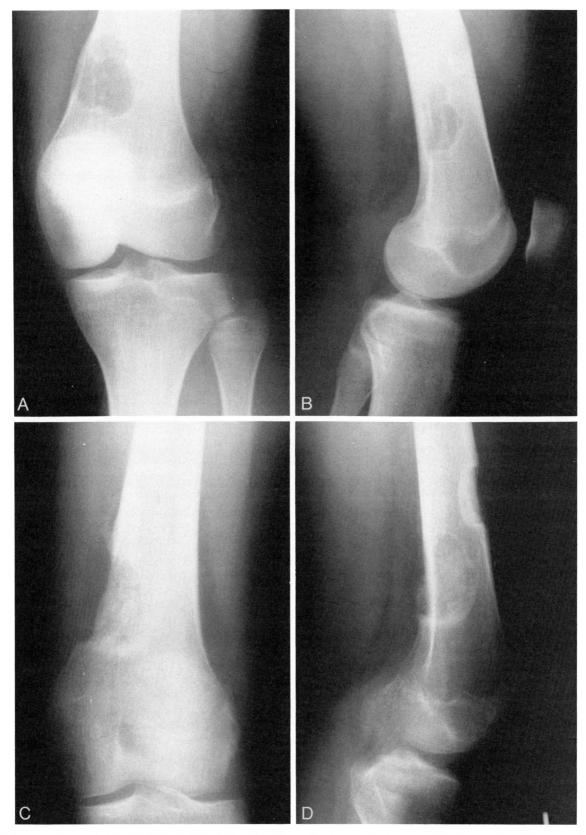

Figure 4.4. Curettage and allogeneic bone grafting of nonossifying fibroma. *A* and *B.* Anteroposterior and lateral radiographs of the distal femur of a 12-year-old girl showing two lesions that were symptomatic; they turned out to be nonossifying fibromas. *C* and *D.* Postoperative views at 3 months showing good healing and incorporation of the allograft used to pack the defects.

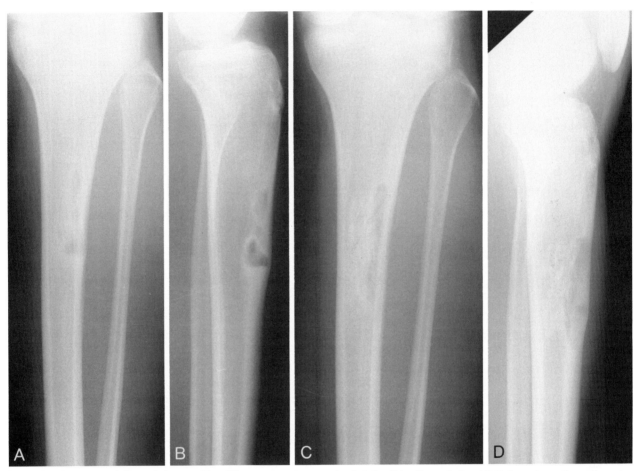

Figure 4.5. Curettage and allogeneic bone grafting of fibro-osseous dysplasia. *A* and *B*. Preoperative radiographs of the tibia of a 16-year-old female showing multiple cortical lesions characteristic of fibro-osseous dysplasia (ossifying fibroma). *C* and *D*. Early postoperative radiographs at 1 month showing the reconstruction with morsellized allograft after curettage.

sure. Following this, the cyst wall or the tumor is excised with a curette and the margin is extended with a motorized burr. This is generally sufficient to control cysts and most benign tumors but, in the case of locally aggressive lesions, such as giant cell tumors, it is necessary to extend the margins by adjuvant treatment. This is done by electrocauterizing the tumor walls or by filling the cavity with phenol or hydrogen peroxide followed by lavage with 95% acid alcohol and isotonic saline. The cavity is then packed tightly with morsellized deep-frozen or freeze-dried bank bone with or without supplemental autograft or autologous bone marrow cells. If there is a danger of collapse of the articular surface, cortical strut allografts are added to the reconstruction. The allografts perform as an osteoconductive scaffold placed in a well-vascularized bed of cancellous bone that has an abundance of osteogenic cells and osteoinductive factors. Therefore, the allograft material must not necessarily contribute to bone formation, which it cannot do in any case. Addi-

tion of autogenous bone or bone marrow can, however, at least theoretically, contribute to more rapid incorporation by bringing in a source of osteogenesis and osteoinduction. The outcome is predictably good with rapid healing and good incorporation. The clinical examples shown (Figs. 4.2–4.10) represent a range of lesions (cyst, fibrous tumors, cartilage tumors, and giant cell tumors) treated with this technique. Morsellized deep-frozen cortical-cancellous or cancellous allograft without additional autograft but with supplemental autologous bone marrow cells (at a ratio of 1:5 marrow versus allograft, volume per volume) was utilized in all cases. The use of a cortical strut allograft to support the joint surface is shown in Figure 4.9. The technique of salvage of an infected reconstruction by a sliding autograft is illustrated by the example in Figure 4.10. The clinical cases show the effectiveness of this technique for the filling of cavities as demonstrated by the rapid incorporation and remodeling.

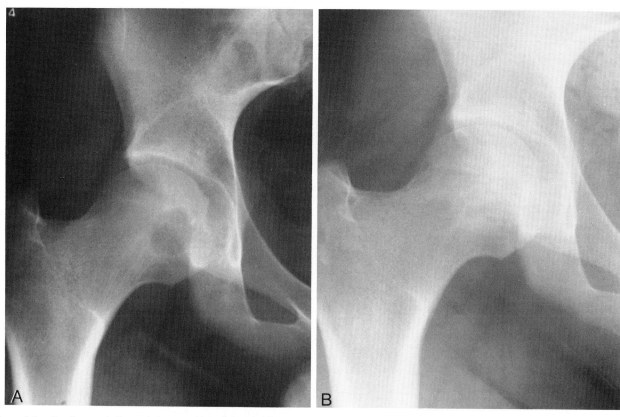

Figure 4.6. Curettage and allogeneic bone grafting of chondroblastoma. *A.* Preoperative radiograph showing a chondroblastoma of the femoral head in an 18-year-old male. *B.* Postoperative radiograph at 4 months demonstrating excellent healing and remodeling.

Use as a Buttress

In this situation, morsellized or small-segment bone allografts are used to support or buttress skeletal structures (Figs. 4.11–4.14) that are either in danger of collapsing after surgical treatment or must be distracted and held in that position as part of the corrective surgery. The first situation arises in fractures involving the articular surface, such as tibial plateau or os calcis fractures. The second indication presents in cases of opening wedge osteotomies (e.g., Macquet osteotomy of the tibial tuberosity) or in anterior spinal fusion procedures (e.g., Cloward cervical fusion). Buttressing of articular surfaces after fractures usually requires morsellized graft while distraction-type buttressing uses cortical-cancellous segments of appropriate shapes and sizes. The use of grafts in the situation of distraction-buttressing is complicated by the additional need to achieve rapid union. As discussed previously, allografts are not indicated to induce union and, therefore, fulfill only partially the required need in these procedures. Moreover, their use in these circumstances is controversial and, therefore, the techniques of distraction-buttressing will not be presented here. On the other hand, the use of morsellized allograft material in articular fractures has a predictably good outcome because, in this situation, it acts as a buttress only and is not expected to induce union. The graft is placed into a vascular bed of metaphyseal-epiphyseal bone and, while it buttresses the articular surface, it acts as an osteoconductive scaffold that permits the ingrowth of host bone. Incorporation is rapid and there is no need for osteoinduction or osteogenesis from the graft because there is an abundance of host osteogenic cells and osteoinductive factors in the surrounding cancellous bone. This is very much like using morsellized allograft bone to fill cavities. The technique of buttressing the articular surface for reconstruction of a tibial plateau fracture with morsellized bone is shown in Figure 4.11 and a clinical example demonstrating the effectiveness of this technique using morsellized allograft material is presented in Figure 4.12. Os calcis fractures are frequent indications for buttressing and the technique of this procedure is shown in Figure 4.13. A clinical example of the use of allograft bone in the os calcis is seen in Figure 4.14. The use of morsellized allograft bone in these circumstances is the best and most common indication for allograft bone in everyday routine orthopaedic practice.

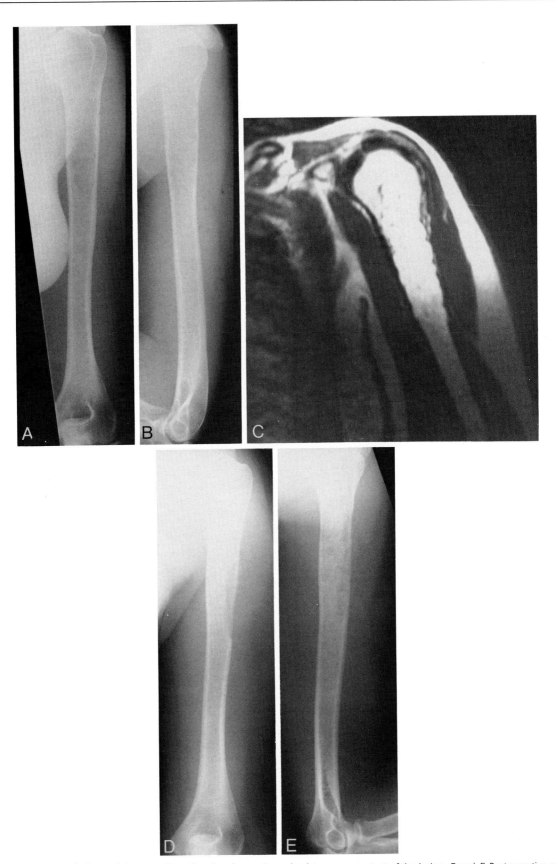

Figure 4.7. Curettage and allogeneic bone grafting of enchondroma. *A* and *B.* Preoperative radiographs of the humerus of a 32-year-old woman showing a large enchondroma. *C.* Magnetic resonance image demonstrat- ing intraosseous extent of the lesion. *D* and *E.* Postoperative radiographs at 2 months after curettage and packing with morsellized allograft sup- plemented with autologous marrow.

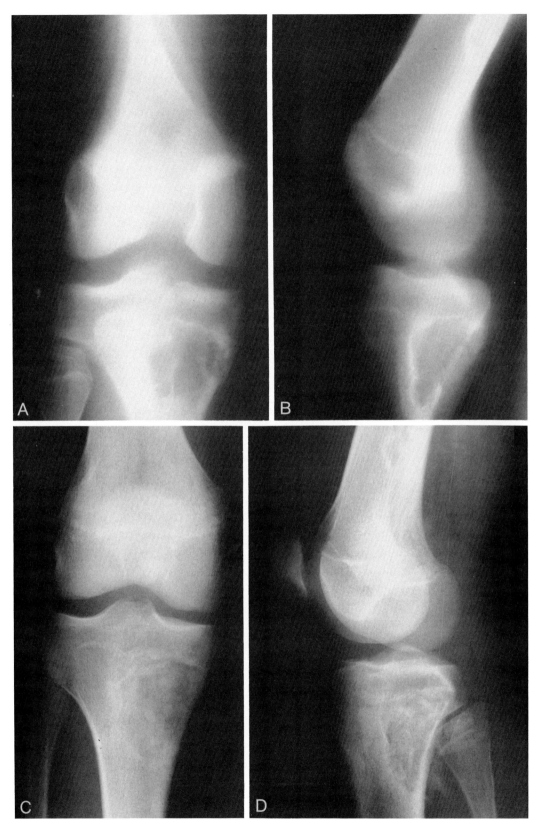

Figure 4.8. Curettage and allogeneic bone grafting of giant cell tumor. A and B. Preoperative anteroposterior and lateral tomograms of the knee of a 20-year-old male showing a giant cell tumor of the proximal tibia with transcortical extension (note the incidental healed fibrous cortical defect of the posteromedial femoral metaphysis). C and D. Anteroposterior and lateral radiographs at 1 month after curettage and reconstruction with morsellized allograft (the femoral lesion was not treated).

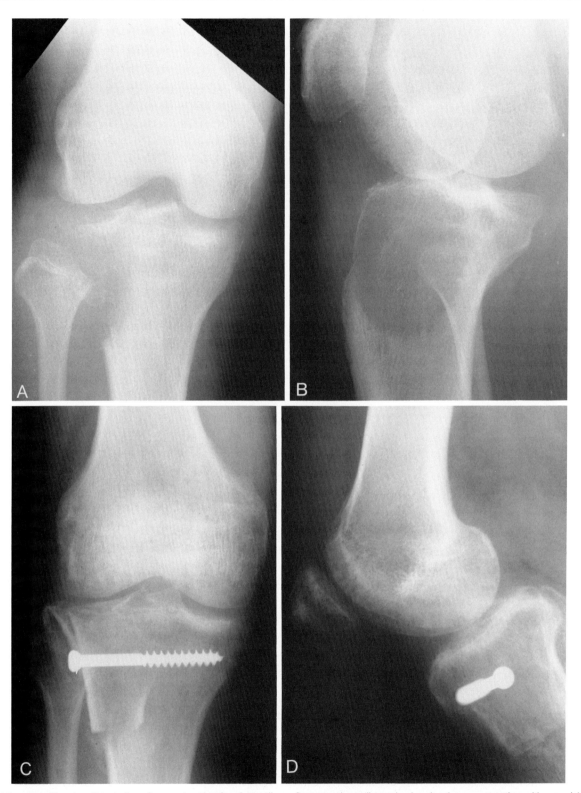

Figure 4.9. Morsellized and strut allograft reconstruction for giant cell tumor. A and B. Anteroposterior and lateral radiographs showing a grade 3 giant cell tumor of the proximal tibia in a 54-year-old man. C and D. Postoperative radiographs showing the reconstruction with a combination of morsellized allograft and cortical strut allograft supporting the articular surface and fixed with a lag screw.

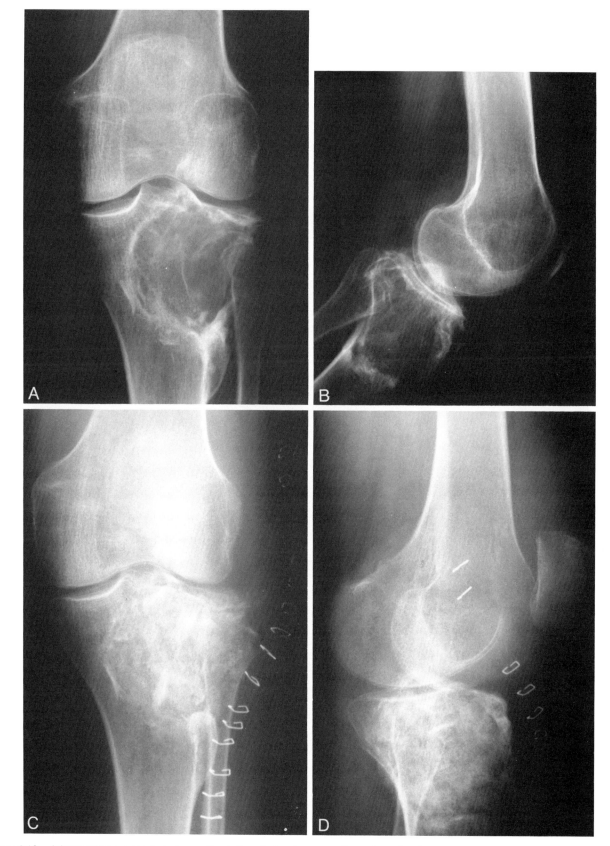

Figure 4.10. Salvage technique of infected morsellized allograft. *A* and *B.* Anteroposterior and lateral radiographs of the knee of a 24-year-old woman showing a recurrent giant cell tumor with a history of two previous curettage procedures with autogenous bone grafting and previous postoperative wound infection. *C* and *D.* Anteroposterior and lateral radiographs at 4 months after curettage and allogeneic bone grafting with persistent infection despite repeat surgical debridements. *E* and *F.* Anteroposterior and lateral radiographs at 2 months after salvage by removal of allograft and sliding cortical autograft reconstruction.

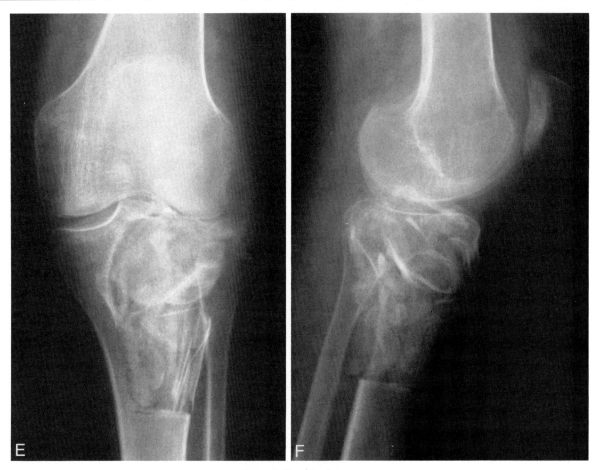

Figure 4.10.   *E* and *F.*

CLINICAL RESULTS AND DISCUSSION

The indications and techniques described are based on clinical experience with morsellized and small-segment allograft reconstructions in general orthopaedic procedures that has been reviewed and presented previously (2). The study included procedures in 183 patients treated by this method for the various indications that were discussed. The results were rated as either a success or a failure defined simply as the bone fulfilling or not fulfilling the function for which it was intended. The outcome with regard to the success rate was as follows: (*a*) filling a cavity: 30 of 32 successful; (*b*) use as a buttress: 95 of 101 successful; (*c*) augmentation of the quantity of autograft bone in spinal fusions: 31 of 33 successful; (*d*) bone graft for nonunions: 4 of 7 successful; and (*e*) to enhance primary union or arthrodesis: 6 of 10 successful. It is clear from these results that allograft bone is not indicated for the treatment of nonunions or for enhancing primary union or arthrodesis. This is in line with what is known about the biology of deep-frozen and freeze-dried allografts, which do not contain osteogenic cells or osteoinductive factors

and, therefore, should not be used as inducers of bone formation.

The filling of cavities is an indication that is backed by sound biological principles. These cavities are generally in metaphyseal cancellous bone, which is extremely vascular and offers an ideal bed for nonosteogenic, nonosteoinductive but osteoconductive materials, such as deep-frozen or freeze-dried allograft bone. This is a unique circumstance in which one would not need to use autograft bone as pointed out by Chalmers (5) more than two decades ago. Many cavities left after the curettage of bone tumors, particularly in the pediatric age group, are very large and the limited availability of autograft bone makes even a better case for the use of morsellized allografts for this indication on a routine basis. The supplementation of bank bone with autograft or autologous marrow most likely speeds up, to some extent, the incorporation and remodeling process by bringing in osteogenic cells and osteoinductive factors. There is no proof for this in clinical practice but the thinking is based on experimental evidence indicating the presence of osteogenic precursor cells in bone marrow (3, 4).

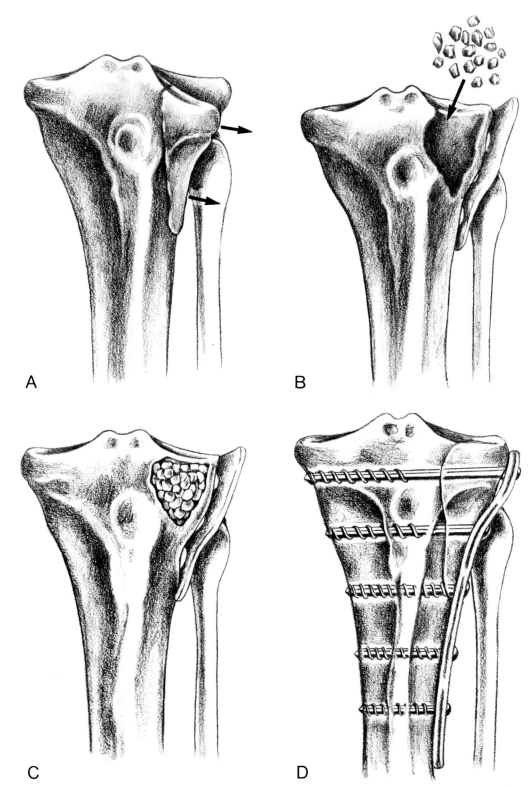

A

B

C

D

Figure 4.11. Technique of buttressing in tibial plateau fractures. *A*. Illustration of depressed fracture of the lateral tibial plateau with vertical fracture component. *B*. Visualization of the depressed articular surface by hinging the vertical fracture fragment ("opening the book"), reduction of the articular surface, and the resulting cavity. *C*. Tight packing of the cavity with morsellized bone graft, which buttresses the articular surface. *D*. Reduction of the vertical component ("closing the book") and internal fixation with a buttress plate.

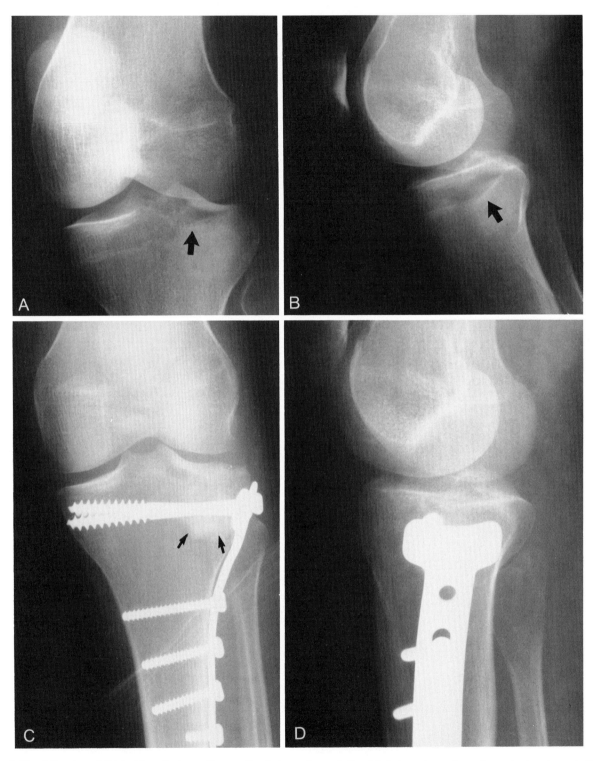

Figure 4.12. Buttressing of tibial plateau fracture with morsellized allograft. *A* and *B.* Anteroposterior and lateral radiographs of the knee of a 25-year-old woman showing depressed fracture of the lateral tibial plateau (*arrows*). *C* and *D.* Early postoperative radiographs showing reduction of the depressed fragment, buttressing of the articular surface with morsellized allograft (*arrows*), and osteosynthesis with buttress plate.

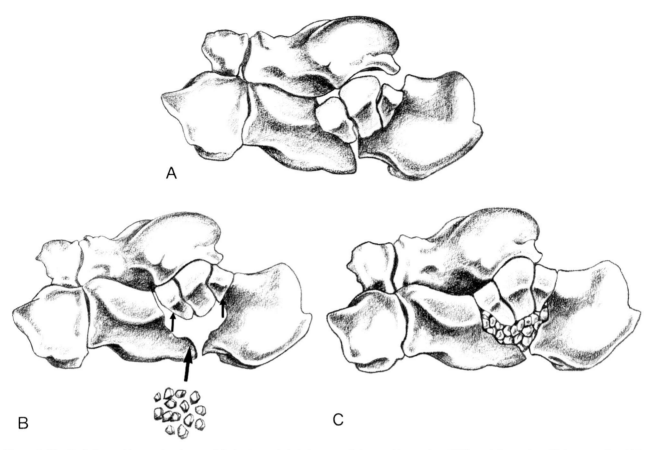

Figure 4.13. Technique of buttressing in os calcis fractures. *A.* Artist's drawing of comminuted joint depression-type fracture of the os calcis. *B.* Elevation of the articular surface by molding fragments against the talus and the resulting cavity. *C.* Filling of the cavity with bone graft, which buttresses the articular surface.

The use of allograft bone as a buttress for supporting articular surfaces in fractures follows the principles described previously for the filling of cavities. The success rate in our series for this indication was 15 of 17 cases. When used in distraction-buttressing, however, the circumstances change because union is also an important consideration. In our experience, the success rates were high with 50 of 51 successful in Macquet osteotomies of the tibial tuberosity and 30 of 33 successful results in Cloward-type cervical spine fusions (2). The use of allografts in spine surgery is a controversial subject and deserves a separate brief discussion.

There is clearly a place for small-segment allograft bone in anterior spine surgery because of its role as a buttress that distracts vertebrae and allows union by functioning as an osteoconductive material. Successful clinical results with high fusion rates have been reported using allograft bone segments for anterior cervical and lumbar fusion (6, 7). However, the use of allograft bone in spine surgery in general is a very complicated matter because of the large variety of fusion techniques and the difficulty

in separating the role of the graft as a buttress and osteoconducting material versus that of an inducer of fusion. Deep-frozen or freeze-dried allografts cannot be inducers of fusion but can augment the quantity of autologous bone used and can act as osteoconductive materials over large surfaces. Thus, their use can lead to fusion in some cases and not in others, depending on the vascularity of the bed into which they are placed. This explains why these allografts can be effective in children when used for posterior spine fusion (8). In addition, the studies of the use of allografts in spine surgery report on a variety of allografts obtained from different sources and processed in different ways. These considerations make it difficult to evaluate studies reporting the use of allograft bone in spine surgery and explain, in part, the variable success rates reported in the literature (9–12). Considering that this particular indication for morsellized allografts is controversial and not well defined at the present time, it is best to classify the use of allografts in spine fusion surgery as needing further study.

In conclusion, the best indications for morsellized

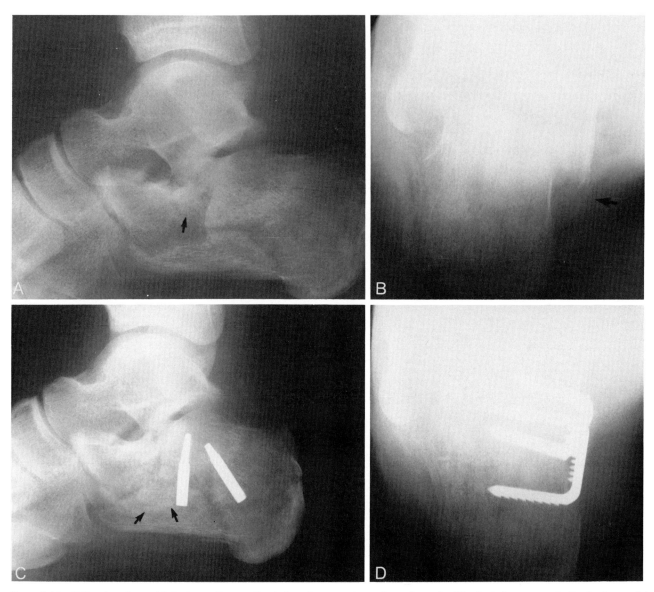

Figure 4.14. Buttressing of os calcis fracture with morsellized allograft. *A.* Lateral radiograph of the foot of a 26-year-old man showing comminuted, joint depression-type fracture of the os calcis (*arrow*) with loss of Bohler's angle. *B.* Axial radiograph of the os calcis demonstrating the widening of the heel and displacement on the medial side (*arrow*). *C.* Lateral postoperative radiograph of the foot after open reduction by the medial approach, elevation of articular surface, buttressing with morsellized allograft (*arrows*), and internal fixation with two staples. *D.* Postoperative axial view of the os calcis demonstrating the anatomic reduction of the medial wall and restoration of the normal width of the heel.

and small-segment allografts in general orthopaedic practice are the filling of cavities and the buttressing of articular surfaces in fractures. Both deep-frozen and freeze-dried bank bone are effective and safe for this purpose, acting as osteoconductive materials that allow ingrowth of host bone and heal and incorporate rapidly if used appropriately.

REFERENCES

1. Frymoyer JW, Howe J, Kuhlmann D. The long-term effects of spinal fusion on the sacroiliac joints and the ilium. Clin Orthop 1978; 134:196.

2. Czitrom AA, Gross AE, Langer F, Sim FH. Bone banks and allografts in community practice. In: Bassett FH III (ed). Instructional Course Lectures. The American Academy of Orthopaedic Surgeons, Park Ridge, IL, 1988; p. 13.
   tional Course Lectures. The American Academy of Orthopaedic Surgeons, Park Ridge, IL, 1988; p. 13.

3. Friedenstein AJ. Determined and inducible osteogenic precursor cells. In: Sognnaes R, Vaughan J (eds). Hard Tissue Growth, Repair and Remineralization. CIBA Foundation Symposium II. Elsevier, New York, 1973; p. 169.

4. Owen M. Lineage of osteogenic cells and their relationship to the stromal system. In: Peck WA (ed). Bone and Mineral Research / 3. Elsevier Science Publishers, Amsterdam, 1985; p. 1.

5. Chalmers J. Bone transplantation. Symp. Tissue Org Transplant, Suppl J Clin Pathol 1967; 20:540.

6. Prolo DJ, Pedrotti PW, White DH. Ethylene oxide sterilization of bone, dura mater, and fascia lata for human transplantation. Neurosurgery 1980; 6:529.

7. Loguidice VA, Johnson RG, Guyer RD, Stith WJ, Ohnmeiss DD, Hochschuler SH, Rashbaum RF. Anterior lumbar interbody fusion. Spine 1987; 13:366.

8. Montgomery DM, et al. Posterior spinal fusion: allograft versus autograft bone. J Spinal Dis 1990; 3:370.

9. Cloward RB. Posterior lumbar fusion updated. Clin Orthop 1985; 193:16.

10. Malinin TI, Brown MD. Bone allografts in spinal surgery. Clin Orthop 1981; 154:68.

11. Nasca RJ, Whelchel JD. Use of cryopreserved bone in spinal surgery. Spine 1987; 12:222.

12. Herron LD, Newman MH. The failure of ethylene oxide gas-sterilized freeze-dried bone graft for thoracic and lumbar spinal fusion. Spine 1989; 14:496.

5

USE OF FRESH OSTEOCHONDRAL ALLOGRAFTS TO REPLACE TRAUMATIC JOINT DEFECTS

Allan E. Gross

The scientific rationale for utilizing fresh rather than preserved osteochondral allografts is as follows. Cartilage harvested without a blood supply within 24 hours of the death of the donor is 100% viable and can be preserved for up to 4 days at 4°C. This has been shown both experimentally and clinically (1–17). The bone, whether fresh or preserved, is not viable because of its inability to survive without immediate vascularization, but it remains structurally intact and mechanically strong until it is replaced by host bone by creeping substitution (14, 15, 18, 19) or until it is weakened and absorbed by invasion of granulation tissue. Freezing, on the other hand, kills the cartilage (20). Even with cryopreservation, the best viability rates that could be achieved varied from 15–50% using glycerol or DMSO (dimethyl sulfoxide) and controlled rates of freezing and thawing (21–26). It has also been shown that freezing decreases the immunogenicity of the bone, but does not ablate it completely (27). Fresh bone is more immunogenic than frozen bone, but there is not enough of a difference to affect the clinical outcome (27). It has been shown that chondrocytes are immunogenic (28) but, when surrounded by matrix, are isolated from the immunocompetent cells and do not sensitize the host.

The indications for fresh osteochondral allografts do not justify the use of immunosuppressive drugs and we, therefore, believed that surgical vascularization of these grafts should not be carried out. Thus, we hoped that fresh osteochondral allografts would provide viable cartilage with the potential to survive transplantation and bone, which although dead, would remain structurally intact until host bone replaced it. Immediate surgical vascularization was not carried out and immunosuppression not used.

The clinical rationale for this program, which was started after the immunology was worked out (27, 28), was that fresh osteochondral allografts could be performed in younger, higher demand patients where implants were not desirable and arthrodesis was not acceptable.

The clinical program started in 1972 at Mount Sinai Hospital, University of Toronto and, as of September 1, 1990, 179 fresh grafts have been performed. Initially, these grafts were performed for unicompartmental osteoarthritis, spontaneous osteonecrosis of the knee, steroid-induced osteonecrosis of the knee, osteochondritis dissecans, and, most commonly, traumatic defects. A review of our first 100 cases revealed that the best indication was for traumatic defects in young patients (29). From January 1972 through September 1, 1990, 119 fresh osteochondral allografts have been performed for traumatic defects of the knee. The surgery should be performed before secondary degenerative changes occur on the opposing pole because the results of bipolar grafts were not nearly as good as unipolar grafts (29).

Based on this review (29), we now perform primarily unicompartmental, unipolar, fresh osteochondral allografts for traumatic joint defects in the knees of people less than 50 years old. We also performed grafts for elbow joint defects (four cases) and a small number of post-traumatic defects of the femoral head (three cases) and talus (four cases). The rest of the chapter, therefore, will deal mainly with our experience in using these grafts for traumatic defects of the knee.

GRAFT PROCUREMENT, HANDLING, AND OPERATIVE TECHNIQUE

Donors are located by the Multiple Organ Retrieval and Exchange program of Toronto and, to be suitable, must meet the criteria outlined by the American Association of Tissue Banks (30). The donors must also be less than 30 years old (and preferably younger) to provide healthy, viable cartilage. Graft procurement is carried out within 24 hours of death, under strict aseptic conditions, with the specimen consisting of the entire joint with the capsule intact. After taking appropriate cultures, the graft is stored in 1 L of sterile Ringer's lactate at 4°C with added cefazolin (1 g), and bacitracin (50,000 U). Tissue typing is no longer performed and no attempt is made to match donor and recipient other than on the basis of size. No immunosuppression is used.

The recipient patient is notified as soon as a donor has been located and immediately is admitted to the hospital as prearranged. Implantation usually is achieved by 12 hours and always within 24 hours of the harvest (graft procurement). This schedule can be adhered to despite the fact that many of the patients come from diverse parts of the United States and Canada.

The transplantation procedure is usually performed in a clean-air room with the operating team wearing body exhaust suits. The patients routinely receive pre- and postoperative prophylactic antibiotics (cefazolin, if no allergy exists). The favored surgical approach is direct midline, which allows easy access for both the transplant and either proximal tibial or distal femoral osteotomy if indicated. Should later salvage procedures be necessary, the same approach is used with little risk of skin complications. Following arthrotomy, the involved damaged articular surface is resected to a good bleeding cancellous bone surface. The donor tissue is then cut to appropriate size and implanted aiming for a tight fit with accurate repro-

duction of normal anatomy. Fixation is augmented by cancellous screws. If the meniscus is irreparably damaged or has previously been excised, it is replaced by an allograft meniscus that is sutured to the capsule of the recipient.

Some changes in technique have evolved since this procedure was last reported. The graft itself is no longer used to correct aligment. This is achieved by osteotomy either prior to or at the time of allograft implantation. This decision depends on whether or not the graft involves the same side of the joint as the osteotomy. For example, a lateral tibial plateau graft can be done simultaneously with a distal femoral varus osteotomy (Figs. 5.1 and 5.2) and a medial femoral condyle graft can be accompanied by a high tibial valgus osteotomy (Figs. 5.3 and 5.4).

The preference is to perform either distal femoral varus or proximal tibial valgus osteotomies. If the realignment procedure involves the same side of the joint as the graft, it should be carried out several months after or prior to transplantation to allow sufficient time for revascularization of host bone (Fig. 5.5). As well, this obviates the technical difficulties of performing these two procedures simultaneously at the same site. The two most common surgical procedures are illustrated in Figures 5.1–5.4.

Postoperatively, the limbs are no longer immobilized but started immediately in the recovery room on continuous passive motion (CPM) to maximize cartilage nutrition and to prevent stiffness. The machines used for CPM have been specially modified to allow positioning in either varus or valgus alignment. Patients are protected from full weight bearing for approximately 1 year by a long leg brace with an ischial ring.

Clinical Material

Between January 1, 1972 and September 1, 1990, 119 fresh osteocartilaginous allografts have been performed for post-traumatic knee joint defects. A recent follow-up study of 55 grafts included 51 patients who had follow-up for more than 2 years. All of the patients were followed prospectively, clinically, and radiographically. A rating score was calculated using a point protocol. These include both subjective and objective data and were previously reported by McDermott and associates (29). In addition, we have performed fresh allografts for four elbows (one distal humerous, two capitellums, one olecranon) four for the ankle, all involving part of the talus, and one distal radius. The data included in this chapter however, will refer primarily to the knee.

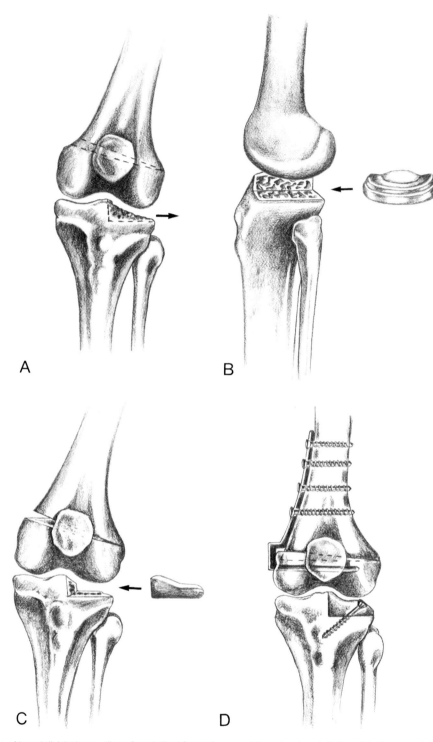

A

B

C

D

Figure 5.1. Illustration of lateral tibial plateau allograft and distal femoral varus osteotomy. *A.* Old lateral plateau fracture with depression of plateau and an associated valgus deformity. *Dotted line* in femur outlines osteotomy. *Dotted line* in lateral tibial plateau outlines planned resection. *B.* Lateral plateau has been resected to a horizontal bed of healthy cancellous bone and the osteochondral allograft is shown ready for insertion. *C.* The allograft is inserted and the distal femoral varus osteotomy performed to correct the deformity. *D.* The allograft is fixed with small cancellous screws and the osteotomy with an offset 90° condylar hip plate.

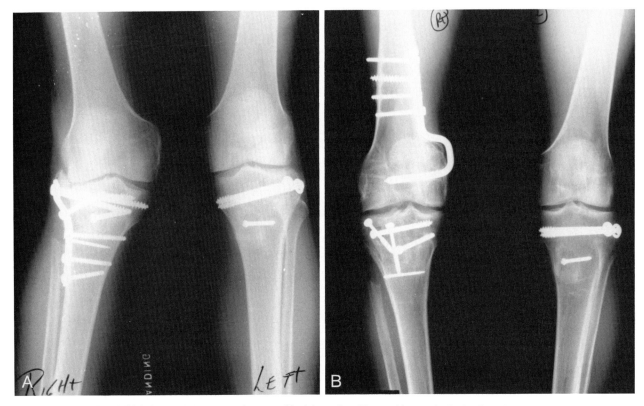

Figure 5.2. Fracture lateral tibial plateau. A. Anteroposterior x-ray of both knees in a 35-year-old man who had suffered bilateral plateau fractures 2 years earlier. B. Anteroposterior x-ray 6 years after reconstruction of a right knee with a fresh lateral tibial plateau allograft and a distal femoral varus osteotomy.

Radiographs were carefully scrutinized. Factors that were examined included joint alignment, fit and fixation of graft, bony union, graft collapse and fragmentation, preservation of cartilage space, and development of osteoarthritis. Pre- and postoperative anteroposterior, lateral, oblique, and skyline views as well as weight-bearing films were utilized for this analysis.

The average age was 37.8 years (range 10–70) with average follow-up of 5.3 years (range 2–16.5 years). There were 33 male patients and 18 female patients. The average interval from injury to graft was 3.9 years (range 2 months–27 years).

Of the 55 allografts, the majority (33) were of the tibial plateau, with 5 medial and 28 lateral (Fig. 5.6). The femoral condyle was involved in 17 cases, eight of them were medial and nine were lateral. Both the femoral condyle and tibial plateau of the same compartment were involved in four cases; these were termed unicompartmental bipolar grafts. One of these was medial and the other three were lateral. One graft was used to resurface the patella.

Twenty realignment osteotomies were carried out in 19 patients who received transplants (Fig. 5.7). Distal femoral osteotomies were performed in 10 patients to achieve

varus and, in two patients, to achieve valgus alignment. High tibial valgus osteotomies were performed in seven patients and varus tibial osteotomy was performed in one patient. Of the 20 osteotomies, nine were carried out prior to or simultaneous with allograft implantation. This practice increased in frequency toward the end of the series.

Menisci were included with 28 of the grafts. Of these, 21 were left attached to their corresponding lateral tibial plateau allograft at time of implantation and five were attached to the medial plateau. Two were actual "free" meniscal allografts at the time of replacement of the lateral femoral condyle.

RESULTS

Clinical Analysis

Patients were rated either as successes or as failures. A successful result required improvement of the rating score by at least 10 points or maintenance of a score of 75 points or higher. Patients were rated as failures if there was any decrease in the rating score or if subsequent salvage surgery was necessary.

Overall, 42 of the 55 grafts or 76% were successful. These had an average preoperative score of 66.5 (range

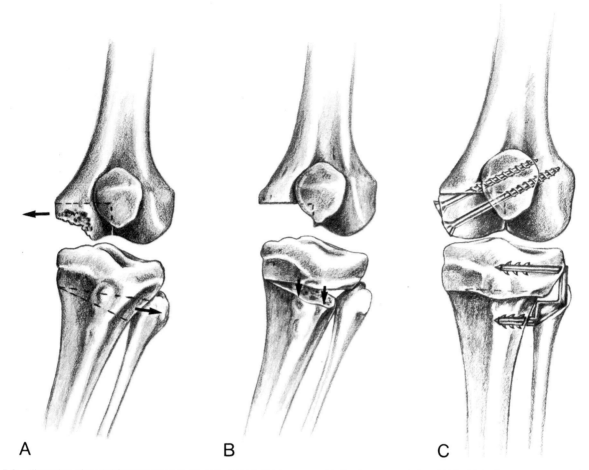

A   B   C

Figure 5.3. Illustration of medial femoral condyle allograft and high tibial osteotomy. *A.* Traumatic loss of medial femoral condyle with secondary varus deformity. *Dotted line* in femur indicates line of resection in preparation for allograft. *Dotted line* in tibia indicates valgus osteotomy. *B.* Diseased condyle has been resected and high tibial valgus osteotomy performed. *C.* Osteochondral allograft has been inserted and held with two cancellous screws. Osteotomy is held with two staples.

31–93) and an average postoperative score of 91 (range 68–100).

Of the 13 failures, four were unicompartmental bipolar grafts, eight were lateral plateau replacements, and one was a medial plateau graft (Fig. 5.8). Four patients have undergone salvage procedures—one arthrodesis at 8 years and three total knee replacements at 2, 4, and 6 years after the original procedure. The other nine grafts were still functioning but were considered failures because of varying degrees of pain or stiffness.

The 17 femoral condylar replacements and the single patellar graft were successful as were four of the five medial plateau grafts and 20 of the 28 lateral plateau replacements. All four bipolar grafts failed. Of the 19 patients who had osteotomies, only four had an unsuccessful result. Of the 28 patients who received meniscal allografts, 21 were successful. However, seven of the 13 failures had an associated meniscal allograft.

Radiographic Review

Every attempt was made to standardize technique but it was obvious during the course of this analysis that perfectly comparable views (Figs. 5.9–5.12) were the exception rather than the rule. This affects serial measurements of parameters, such as height of the bone or cartilage. Radiographic union was derived as establishment of structural continuity between host bone and allograft. Union occurred in all of the 55 grafts. This was usually present by 9–12 months. Restoration of normal bone density (of the allograft) was usually evident within 2–4 years.

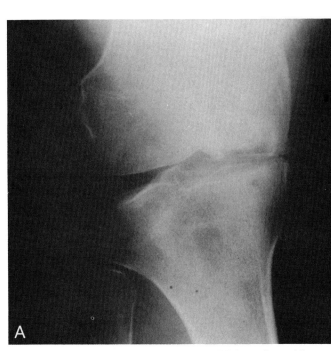

Figure 5.4. Post-traumatic osteonecrosis medial femoral condyle. *A.* Anteroposterior x-ray of the right knee. Post-traumatic osteonecrosis of medial femoral condyle in a 32-year-old woman. *B.* Anteroposterior x-ray of the right knee 9.5 years following fresh osteochondral allograft and high tibial osteotomy. Early degenerative changes are seen but the graft has remodeled without significant collapse and the joint space is well maintained with good alignment.

Adequate x-rays for assessment of bony collapse and cartilage space were available for 54 of the grafts. The joint space was seen to be well preserved in 30 patients, decreased in 10 patients, and absent or arthritic in 14 patients (Fig. 5.13). Virtually all of the grafts were seen to settle at least 1–3 mm; the majority did not collapse further. Fifteen grafts had evidence of collapse greater than 4–5 mm. One graft collapsed completely (Fig. 5.9–5.12 and 5.14).

No actual fractures of grafts were seen. However, six grafts were fragmented adjacent to their articular surface. Whether this represents microfractures or mechanically induced degeneration remains unresolved.

Alignment of the knees was assessed on weight-bearing radiographs of the entire lower extremity. Forty-four patients had adequate x-rays for this. For a lateral compartment graft, ideal alignment is considered to be a femoral-tibial axis of 0 to a few degrees of varus. Conversely, for a medial compartment replacement, ideal alignment is 10° or more of femoral-tibial valgus. Sixteen patients were seen to be ideally aligned, eight of these

by osteotomy (Fig. 5.15). In 28 patients, alignment was judged to be suboptimal. Nine had undergone osteotomy with inadequate correction.

Of the 16 well-aligned patients, there were three failures. Only one of these had had an osteotomy. Eliminating the other two early in the series, where alignment correction was achieved by graft height alone, only one of 14 patients with ideal alignment failed (Fig. 5.15).

Of the 28 poorly aligned patients, there were six failures. Only two of these had had an osteotomy. One osteotomy was performed 3 years after allograft implantation and the other was performed 1 year after the graft with failure to correct alignment adequately (Fig. 5.15). No composite graft failed because of problems with the meniscal allograft. No meniscal allografts have been excised in isolation (Fig. 5.16).

The four osteochondral grafts for the talus were done for post-traumatic osteonecrosis, with three involving the medial corner and one involving the lateral corner. All grafts were press-fit and were done using a transmalleolar

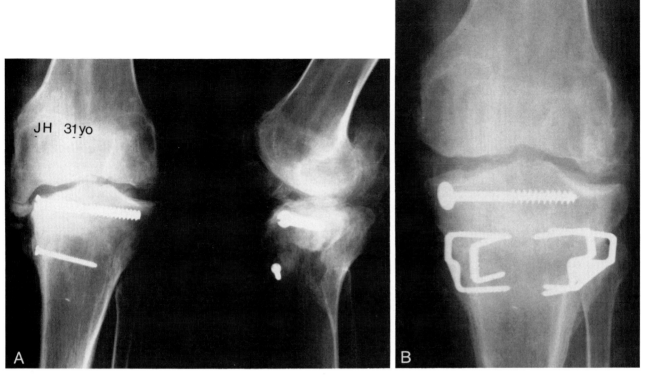

Figure 5.5. Fracture medial tibial plateau. *A.* Anteroposterior and lateral views of left knee in a 31-year-old man who had suffered a fracture of the medial plateau 3 years earlier. *B.* Anteroposterior x-ray of the left knee 5 years following reconstruction with a fresh osteochondral allograft and a valgus high tibial osteotomy. The procedures were staged 1 year apart with the osteotomy being one 1 year after the allograft when the patient was ready to come out of his brace.

approach. At an average follow-up of 60 months, the clinical and radiological reports have been very encouraging. All of the grafts have united with no significant fragmentation or collapse. Three of the four patients are symptom free with good motion and have returned to full activities. The four partial elbow grafts (one distal humerus, two capitellums, and one olecranon), the distal radius, and the three partial femoral head grafts have too short a follow-up for comment at this time.

Histology of Failed Allografts

Despite the fact that all specimens analyzed were retrieved from failed cases, 12 of 18 grafts were observed to contain areas of viable hyaline cartilage (15). Three of these were judged to have substantial amounts (50%) of viable chondrocytes. This evidence was based on morphology, staining techniques, or proteoglycan content, and occasionally, on electron microscopy. Evidence of cartilage viability was present at up to 92 months in these failed specimens. Regarding the bony components, the normal course of events was seen to be replacement of donor by host bone and, in all specimens, complete re-

placement was present by 44 months following implantation.

No evidence of immune rejection was noted in any of the failed cases, even though this was specifically searched for. Chronic synovitis was characteristic with occasional fibrosis of the subsynovial tissue and a mild chronic inflammatory infiltrate. There was no evidence of vasculitis or endothelial cell edema in the marrow vessels. The necrotic bone marrow of the failed grafts elicited little inflammatory reaction and was usually acellular, except in one case. In this patient, with a long history of seronegative arthritis, a marked inflammatory infiltrate was observed within the allograft marrow (15).

Autoradiography of Successful Grafts

Our histological and ultrastructural data on the aforementioned failed fresh osteochondral allografts are consistent with long-term survival of graft cartilage. We, therefore, decided to do a prospective study on four still-functioning, clinically successful grafts (31).

The articular cartilage of four fresh osteochondral allografts was biopsied after transplantation and investigated for viability by autoradiography. The biopsies were

Distribution of Grafts

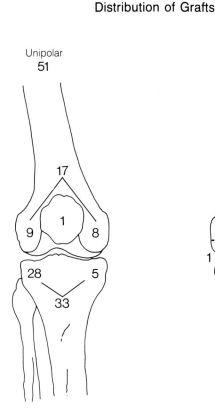

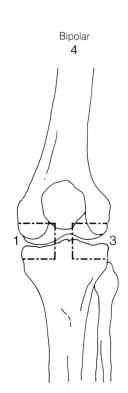

Figure 5.6. Distribution of allografts.

Osteotomies

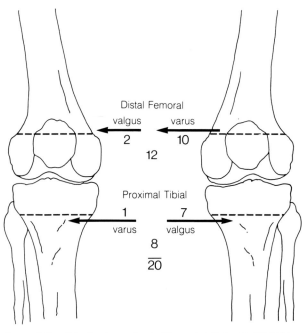

Figure 5.7. Osteotomies performed in conjunction with allografts.

Failures

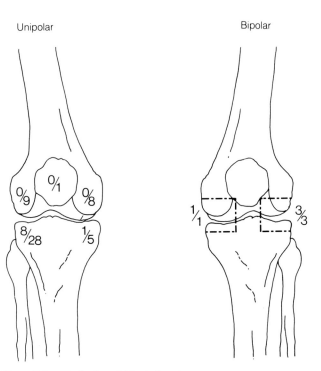

Figure 5.8. Distribution of failed allografts.

tagged with both ^{3}H-cytidine, to label newly synthesized ribonucleic acid, and ^{35}S-sulfate, to label newly synthesized proteoglycan. The cartilage of a lateral humeral condyle graft at 12 months had 96–99% labeled chondrocytes. The articular cartilage of a medial femoral condyle graft at 24 months after transplantation showed 69–78% labeled chondrocytes. The cartilage of a medial tibial plateau graft at 41 months' follow-up had 90% labeled cells; that of a lateral tibial plateau graft at 6 years had 37% labeled chondrocytes. These results demonstrate the ability of articular cartilage on fresh osteochondral allografts to survive after transplantation in humans and provide a rationale for their clinical use.

COMPLICATIONS

Nine complications occurred in eight patients. Three knees required manipulations for stiffness early in the series when postoperative immobilization for 14–21 days was still being used. This complication was not seen following the introduction of CPM. One of these three patients was later diagnosed as having reflex sympathetic dystrophy. Other complications included one wound hematoma, which required evacuation, and one intraoperative rupture of an already frayed patellar tendon, which was successfully repaired immediately. Three patients had

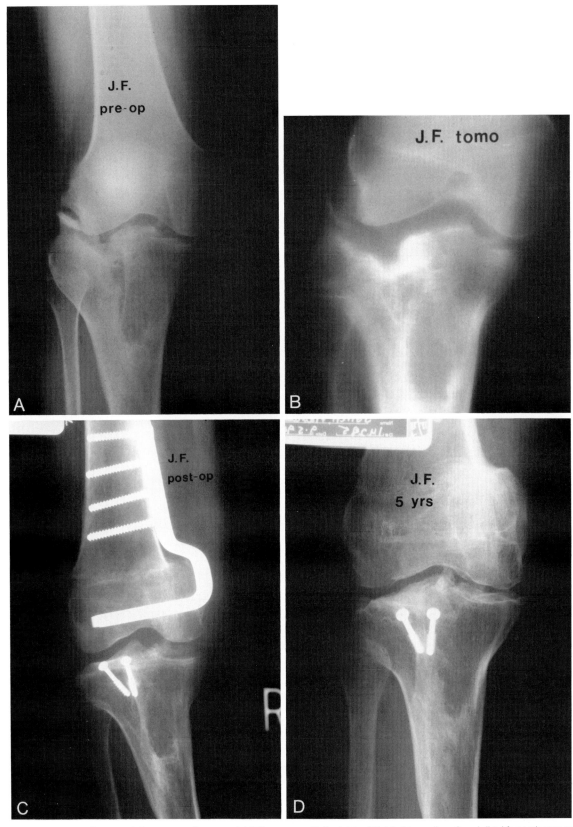

Figure 5.9. Lateral plateau fracture. *A.* Anteroposterior x-ray of right knee showing lateral tibial plateau fracture in a 26-year-old woman. *B.* Anteroposterior tomogram illustrating degree of joint depression and comminution. *C.* Anteroposterior x-ray 6 months following reconstruction with fresh lateral tibial plateau allograft and distal femoral varus osteotomy. *D.* Anteroposterior x-ray at 5 years following reconstruction. The graft is healed with no significant collapse. The hardware has been removed from the femur. There are minimal degenerative changes.

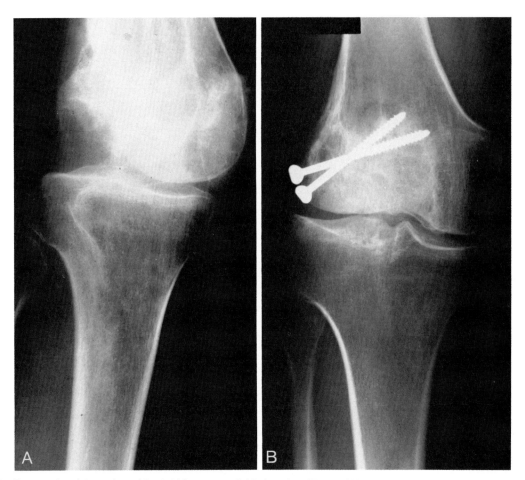

Figure 5.10. Trauma—lateral femoral condyle. *A.* Oblique x-ray of right knee in a 17-year-old boy with traumatic loss of lateral femoral condyle. *B.* Anteroposterior x-ray of right knee 9 years following reconstruction with a fresh lateral femoral condylar allograft.

complications related to the respiratory system. No documented deep vein thrombosis or pulmonary emboli occurred. There were no infections. There were two late deaths unrelated to surgery.

DISCUSSION

Long-term results of fresh, small-fragment osteochondral allografts are encouraging. The best indication is late reconstruction following traumatic loss of joint segments (29, 32, 33). However, patient selection remains a vital consideration. Best results have been seen in highly motivated patients who have no evidence of degenerative arthritis prior to allografting. Some of the unsuccessful results could be directly attributed to poor patient selection.

In our original group of 100 patients, 24 grafts were performed for osteoarthritis with a clinical success rate of only 42% (29). This was thought to be due to the necessity for bipolar grafts (unicompartmental), obesity,

and deformity. Also, these patients were slightly older and did not tolerate the postoperative bracing. The same factors applied to the 11 patients with spontaneous osteonecrosis of the knee; only three obtained successful results. Grafts were also performed for three patients with steroid-induced osteonecrosis, with all three failing, probably due to poor host bone related to blood supply and steroids. Based on our early experience, therefore, we believed that the best patient for this procedure was young and had traumatic loss of one pole (a condyle or a plateau).

The rationale for using fresh rather than stored allografts is based on clinical and experimental evidence supporting the maintenance of viability and function of chondrocytes after fresh transplantation. Currently, experimental work on cryopreservation techniques indicates that relatively high percentages of chondrocytes (50%) survive after freezing and thawing of cartilage in animal models (23–26). However, as yet, there is little objective

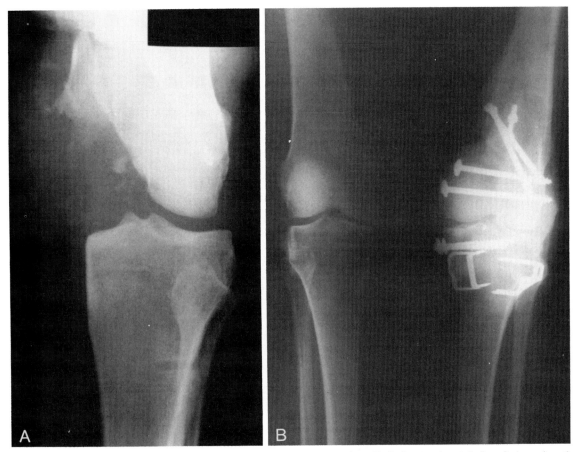

Figure 5.11. Traumatic loss of medial femoral condyle and part of medial plateau. A. Anteroposterior x-ray of left knee in a 33-year-old man who lost all of his medial femoral condyle, his medial ligament, and part of his medial plateau as a result of trauma. B. Anteroposterior x-ray 5 years after reconstruction with fresh osteochondral allografts to replace the medial femoral condyle, the medial tibial plateau, the medial ligament, and the medial meniscus.

objective evidence of prolonged survival of preserved cartilage following implantation in humans. Few reports with histological evidence appear in the literature and, while these are often biopsies of failed cases, the cartilage is usually described as severely degenerated and distinctly abnormal (34–36).

However, even in 12 of 18 failed cases reported by Oakeshott et al. (15), hyaline cartilage survival and matrix production, as late as 9.5 years following transplantation of fresh grafts, was seen. This was demonstrated by staining techniques and electron microscopy. It is likely that, in successful cases, cartilage survival is even better. While intact cartilage is considered immunoprivileged (6), the bony component of the graft is accepted to be immunogenic (18, 27, 37). Antigenicity has been shown to be decreased significantly, although not eliminated completely, by freezing and freeze-drying (both of which adversely affect the cartilage) (27). A definite immune response following transplantation of fresh, frozen, or freeze-dried bone has been well documented (5, 27, 37). However, neither the presence nor the magnitude of this response correlates with clinical success or failure of the graft (37–39). Previous reviews of fresh bone and cartilage transplants have failed to reveal evidence of clinically significant or histologically detectable rejection (14, 40–45). In the literature, only the series of Volkov (46) reported the phenomenon of rejection and this was with frozen grafts. However, clinical rejection has not been identified in 14 years of experience with over 130 fresh grafts at this institution.

Many authors have stated that the fate of the allograft depends heavily on mechanical factors (24, 36, 46–49). Analysis of failed grafts from this center revealed a high association of failure with poorly sized grafts, grafts less than 1 cm in thickness (resulting in

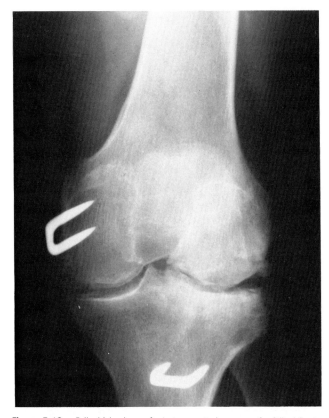

Figure 5.12. Failed bipolar graft. Anteroposterior x-ray of a failed fresh lateral compartment bipolar graft at 8.5 years. This graft was performed for traumatic loss of lateral femoral condyle and secondary degenerative changes on the lateral plateau. At 8.5 years, the joint space is absent in the lateral compartment but the bone stock restored by the allograft is well maintained, facilitating further surgical reconstruction.

fragmentation and fracture), and grafts where internal fixation was not used (15). The present series illustrates the success of unipolar grafts in the knee. Although only a small number of bipolar grafts (four cases) are presented, they were all failures.

The role of osteotomy to realign the joint, especially in weight-bearing extremities, cannot be overemphasized. Of the 19 patients who underwent osteotomy, even when performed late, only four were in the failed group. The preferred realignment procedure to correct valgus deformity is distal femoral varus osteotomy (50). Proximal tibial valgus osteotomy is used to correct varus deformity. Joint surface obliquity and site of the allograft must be taken into consideration. In the present series, only one of 14 grafts in well-aligned extremities failed. Best results can be achieved by adhering to the principles described, including correct sizing, realignment, and fixation to achieve ideal mechanical conditions along with prompt implantation of fresh, healthy cartilage to maximize cell viability.

Substantial evidence in favor of meniscal allotransplantation has come from work with animal models (51). Of the patients in this study, 28 had meniscal allografts and 21 of these continue to do well. The failures were mainly on the basis of malalignment or graft type and none was directly attributable to the meniscus itself. None of the 28 patients has required reoperation because of meniscal tear or detachment.

The use of CPM postoperatively is beneficial. Cartilage nutrition is theoretically improved, helping maintain cell viability. Perhaps better preservation of the matrix is also achieved and, since cartilage is immunologically privileged on the basis of an intact matrix, this would be advantageous. As well, CPM has eliminated stiffness as a complication in this series since its introduction as part of the postoperative protocol. The prompt return of range of motion is related to decreased intra-articular adhesions as seen in animal models (52).

The radiographic results are more difficult to interpret than the clinical results. Previous reviews of allograft series have illustrated that radiographic appearance and clinical result do not necessarily correlate; more specifically, that good function is possible even with an obviously degenerated radiographic appearance (49, 53). Radiographic appearance was worse in patients early in the series when the grafts were used to correct alignment and when internal fixation was often not used or was inadequate. With technical improvements, such as realignment osteotomy to decompress the graft, rigid interfragmentary fixation, and better sizing, radiographic results have improved, at least in the short term. A pattern of typical radiographic progression was identified. The first significant event is host-donor bony union, which is usually complete by 9–12 months and is accompanied by minimal settling of the bony portion (1–3 mm). Virtually all technically adequate grafts were seen to unite.

Grafts should be "decompressed" by realignment osteotomy either at the time of or prior to transplantations. Perhaps consideration should be given to extending the period of protected weight bearing beyond 1 year (the interval currently used), to 2 or 3 years, or until the bony portions return to isodensity. Many of the early cases were performed prior to the recognition of the importance of these factors. Thus, long-term objective assessment of patients treated by adherence to the previously described principles is of considerable interest and part of an ongoing study.

Complications in this series were relatively minor. Because this is a relatively conservative procedure involving minimal bone resection, no "bridges are burned." Subse-

Radiographic Data

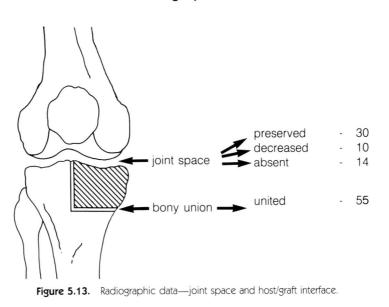

Figure 5.13. Radiographic data—joint space and host/graft interface.

Radiographic Data

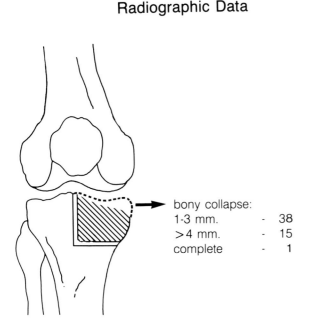

Figure 5.14. Radiographic data—bony collapse.

quent salvage surgery (i.e., arthroplasty or arthrodesis) certainly is not compromised and, conversely, may even be facilitated because deficient bone stock has been replaced.

We are presently doing 10–20 fresh osteochondral allografts per year for traumatic defects of the knee. This group of patients is young with unipolar osteochondral deficits rather than just pure chondral lesions. Thus far, we have been able to meet the needs of patients referred to us from all over North America. A program of fresh

grafts for dealing with chondral lesions of the knee is under way in Atlanta (16). The fresh osteochondral allograft program in San Diego has dealt with defects around the knee and hip (17).

SUMMARY

Long-term follow-up of fresh, small-fragment osteochondral allograft reconstruction of traumatic joint surface defects of the knee revealed 76% to be clinically successful. Best results can be achieved by adhering to the principles described including correct sizing, realignment, and internal fixation to achieve ideal mechanical conditions along with prompt implantation of fresh, healthy cartilage to maximize cell viability. Mechanical factors seem to be more important than immunological factors in determining the fate of the grafts. Correct alignment should be achieved by osteotomy rather than by the graft. Bipolar grafts should be avoided if possible. We have achieved encouraging results with these grafts for unipolar traumatic defects of the knee. We have also been pleased with a very small series of grafts for traumatic defects of the talus.

CONCLUSIONS AND RECOMMENDATIONS

1. Traumatic loss of a joint segment is the best indication for fresh osteochondral allografts.
2. Patient selection is a vital consideration.
3. Mechanical conditions seem more important to successful results than immunological factors.
4. Ideal alignment of the extremity to "unload" the graft is an absolute requirement and, if necessary, should be achieved by osteotomy prior to or simultaneous with allograft implantation.

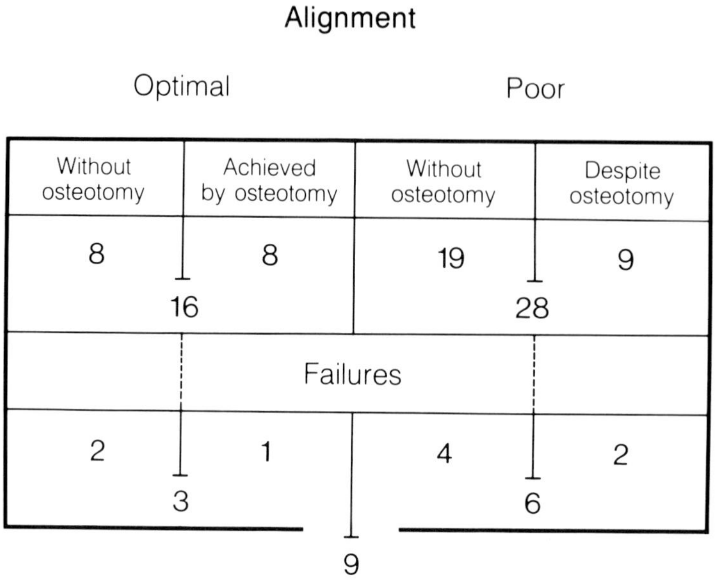

Alignment

Optimal		Poor	
Without osteotomy	Achieved by osteotomy	Without osteotomy	Despite osteotomy
8	8	19	9
	16		28
Failures			
2	1	4	2
	3		6
		9	

Figure 5.15. Relationship of alignment to success.

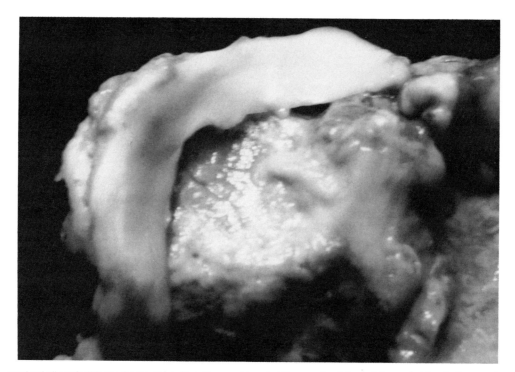

Figure 5.16. Meniscal allograft. This medial meniscal allograft was retrieved at 5 years after failure of the underlying fresh osteochondral allograft. Note the meniscus is structurally intact with a good peripheral repair. The underlying articular cartilage has undergone degenerative changes.

5. Internal fixation of the allograft should be used.
6. Bipolar allografts should be avoided, if at all possible.
7. Menisci can be implanted if the recipient's meniscus is absent or irreparably damaged.
8. CPM is a useful postoperative adjunct.
9. Fresh, small-fragment osteochondral allografts can be successfully used to reconstruct joint surfaces following traumatic, segmental loss.

REFERENCES

1. Campbell CJ, Ishida H, Takahashi H, Kelly F. The transplantation of articular cartilage. An experimental study in dogs. J Bone Joint Surg 1963; 45A:1579–1592.
2. DePalma AF, Tsaltas TT, Mauler GG. Viability of osteochondral grafts as determined by uptake of S^{35}. J Bone Joint Surg 1963; 45A:1565–1578.

3. Lance EM, Fisher RL. Transplantation of the rabbit's patella. J Bone Joint Surg 1970; 52A:145–156.

4. McKibbin B. Immature joint cartilage and the homograft reaction. J Bone Joint Surg 1971; 53B(1):123–135.

5. Paccola CAJ, Xavier CAM, Goncalves RP. Fresh immature articular cartilage allografts. A study on the integration of chondral and osteochondral grafts both in normal and in papain-treated knee joints of rabbit. Arch Orthop Traumat Surg 1979; 93:253–259.

6. Pap K, Krompecher S. Arthroplasty of the knee. Experimental and clinical experiences. J Bone Joint Surg 1961; 43A:523–537.

7. Porter BB, Lance EM. Limb and joint transplantation. A review of research and clinical experience. Clin Orthop 1974; 104:249–274.

8. Rodrigo JJ, Sakovich L, Travis C, Smith G. Osteocartilaginous allograft as compared with autografts in the treatment of knee joint osteocartilaginous defects in dogs. Clin Orthop 1978; 134:342.

9. Thomas V, Jimenez S, Brighton C, Brown N. Sequential changes in the mechanical properties of viable articular cartilage stored in vitro. J Orthop Res 1984; 2:55–60.

10. Craigmyle MBL. An autoradiographic and histochemical study of long-term cartilage grafts in the rabbit. J Anat 1958; 92:467–472.

11. Pritzker KPH, Gross AE, Langer F, Luk SC, Houpt JB. Articular cartilage transplantation. Hum Pathol 1977; 8:635–651.

12. Rodrigo J, Thompson E, Travis C. 4°C preservation of avascular osteocartilaginous shell allografts in rats. Transact Orthop Res Soc 1980; 5:72.

13. Wiley AM, Kosinka E. Experimental and clinical aspects of transplantation of entire hyaline cartilage surfaces. J Am Geriatr Soc 1974; 25:547.

14. Kandel RA, Gross AE, Gavel A, McDermott AGP, Langer F, Pritzker KPH. Histopathology of failed osteoarticular shell allografts. Clin Orthop 1985; 197:103–110.

15. Oakeshott RD, Farine I, Pritzker KPH, Langer F, Gross AE. A clinical and histologic analysis of failed fresh osteochondral allografts. Clin Orthop 1988; 233:283–294.

16. Garret J. Osteochondral allografts for treatment of chondral defects of the femoral condyles: Early results. Proceedings of the Knee Society. Am J Sports Med 1987; 14:387.

17. Meyers M, Akeson W, Convery R. Resurfacing of the knee with fresh osteochondral allografts. J Bone Joint Surg 1989; 71A:704–713.

18. Burchardt H. The biology of bone graft repair. Clin Orthop 1983; 174:28–42.

19. Pelker RR, Friedlaender GE, Markham TC. Biomechanical properties of bone allografts. Clin Orthop 1983; 174:54–57.

20. Simon W, Richardson S, Herman W, Parsons R, Lane J. Long-term effects of chondrocyte death on rabbit articular cartilage in vivo. J Bone Joint Surg 1976; 58A:517–526.

21. Smith AU. Survival of frozen chondrocytes isolated from cartilage of adult mammals. Nature 1965; 205:782.

22. Chesterman PJ, Smith AU. Homotransplantation of articular cartilage and isolated chondrocytes: an experimental study in rabbits. J Bone Joint Surg 1968; 50B:184.

23. Tomford WW, Dugg GP, Mankin HJ. Experimental freeze-preservation of chondrocytes. Clin Orthop 1985; 197:11–14.

24. Tomford WW, Mankin HJ. Investigational approaches to articular cartilage preservation. Clin Orthop 1983; 174:22–27.

25. Schachar NS, McGann LE. Investigations of low-temperature storage of articular cartilage for transplantation. Clin Orthop 1986; 208:146–150.

26. Malinin TI, Wagner JL, Pita JC, Lo H. Hypothermic storage and cryopreservation of cartilage. Clin Orthop 1985; 197:15–26.

27. Langer F, Czitrom AA, Pritzker KP, Gross AE. The immunogenicity of fresh and frozen allogenic bone. J Bone Joint Surg 1975; 57A:216.

28. Langer F, Gross AE. Immunogenicity of allograft articular cartilage. J Bone Joint Surg 1974; 56A:297.

29. McDermott AGP, Langer F, Pritzker KPH, Gross AE. Fresh small fragment osteochondral allografts. Clin Orthop 1985; 197:96–102.

30. Fawcett KJ, Barr HR (eds). Tissue Banking. American Association of Blood Banks, Arlington, VA 1987; pp. 97–107.

31. Czitrom A, Keating S, Gross A. The viability of articular cartilage in fresh osteochondral allografts after clinical transplantation. J Bone Joint Surg 1990; 72A:574.

32. Locht RC, Gross AE, Langer F. Late osteochondral allograft resurfacing for tibial plateau fractures. J Bone Joint Surg 1984; 66A:328.

33. Zukor D, Oakeshott R, Gross A. Osteochondral allograft reconstruction of the knee. Part 2. Experience with successful and failed fresh osteochondral allografts. Am J Knee Surg 1989; 2:182–191.

34. Mankin HJ, Doppelt S, Tomford WW. Clinical experience with allograft implantation. Clin Orthop 1983; 174:69–86.

35. Mnaymneh W, Malinin TI, Makley JT, Dick HM. Massive osteoarticular allografts in the reconstruction of extremities following resection of tumours not requiring chemotherapy and radiation. Clin Orthop 1985; 197:76–87.

36. Mankin HJ, Doppelt SH, Sullivan TR, Tomford WW. Osteoarticular and intercalary allograft transplantation in the management of malignant tumours of bone. Cancer 1982; 50:613.

37. Langer F, Gross AE, West M, Urovitz EP. The immunogenicity of allograft knee joint transplants. Clin Orthop 1978; 132:155.

38. Prolo DI, Rodrigo JJ. Contemporary bone graft physiology and surgery. Clin Orthop 1985; 200:322.

39. Sedgewick AD, Moore AR, All-Duaij AY, Edwards JCW, Willoughby DA. Studies into the influence of carrageenan induced inflammation on articular cartilage degradation using implantation into air pouches. Br J Exp Pathol 1985; 66:445.

40. Aston J, Bentley G. Repair of articular surfaces by allografts of articular and growth-plate cartilage. J Bone Joint Surg 1986; 68B:29–35.

41. Campbell C, Ishida H, Takahashi H, Kelly F. The transplantation of articular cartilage. J Bone Joint Surg 1963; 45A:1579–1592.

42. Goldberg VM, Porter BB, Lance EM. Transplantation of the ca-

nine knee joint on a vascular pedicle. J Bone Joint Surg 1980; 62A:414.

43. Lexer E. Substitution of joints from amputated extremities. Surg Gynecol Obstet 1908; 6:601.

44. Lexer E. Joint transplantation and arthroplasty. Surg Gynecol Obstet 1925; 40:782.

45. Meyers MH. Resurfacing of the femoral head with fresh osteochondral allografts. Clin Orthop 1985; 197:111–114.

46. Volkov M. Allotransplantation of joints. J Bone Joint Surg 1970; 52B:49.

47. Depalma AF, Tsultas TT, Mauler GG. Viability of osteochondral grafts as determined by uptake of 535. J Bone Joint Surg 1963; 45A:1565.

48. Rodrigo JJ, Block N, Thompson EC. Joint transplantation. Vet Clin North Am 1978; 8:523.

49. Urbaniak JR, Black KE. Cadaveric elbow allografts. Clin Orthop 1985; 197:131–140.

50. McDermott AGP, Finkelstein JA, Farine I, Boynton EL, MacIntosh DL, Gross AE. Distal femoral varus osteotomy for valgus deformity of the knee. J Bone Joint Surg 1988; 70A:110.

51. Arnoczky SP, McDevitt CA, Cuzzell JZ, Warren RF, Kristinicz T. Meniscal replacement using a cryopreserved allograft. An experimental study in the dog. Trans Orthop Res Soc 1984; 9:220.

52. Salter RB, Simmonds DF, Malcolm BW, Rumble EJ, MacMichael D, Clements ND. The biological effect of continuous passive motion on the healing of full thickness defects in articular cartilage. J Bone Joint Surg 1980; 62A:1232.

53. Parrish FF. Allograft replacement of all or part of the end of a long bone following excision of a tumour. J Bone Joint Surg 1973; 55A:1.

6

ALLOGRAFT RECONSTRUCTION AFTER TUMOR SURGERY IN THE APPENDICULAR SKELETON

Andrei A. Czitrom

The author gratefully acknowledges the assistance of Drs. F. Langer, A.E. Gross, R.S. Bell, and F.H. Sim for providing some of the clinical examples presented in this chapter.

The wide local resection of bone tumors in the appendicular skeleton for the purpose of limb salvage is currently a well-accepted orthopaedic oncological procedure. Bone and joint defects left after this type of surgery pose a formidable challenge as to how to restore skeletal continuity for the best possible function of the saved extremity. Reconstruction of such skeletal deficits can be performed with autogenous bone grafts (nonvascularized or vascularized), prosthetic implants, or with bone allografts. Nonvascularized and vascularized autogenous bone grafts have been used extensively and successfully for this purpose (1–3). Although they have the best healing potential, autogenous grafts have the disadvantage of limited quantity, possible donor site morbidity, and they cannot be used to restore joint surfaces. Prosthetic implants used in skeletal tumor surgery are usually of the custom type and are preferred over bone grafts by several groups (4, 5). Their limitations, in addition to the waiting time required for the manufacture of a custom prosthesis, are the long-term problems of massive prosthetic replacement including bone loss, loosening, and the potential need for revision. Allografts represent another alternative for the reconstruction of these large bone or joint defects. This chapter discusses the techniques of their use and the clinical results and complications associated with allografts. The author does not intend to suggest that this reconstruction modality is better than others. It is merely one of several methods that can be used to restore bone defects in orthopaedic tumor surgery and is the modality with which the author has had the most experience.

PRINCIPLES OF TUMOR SURGERY IN THE APPENDICULAR SKELETON

Staging

Patients presenting with a bone tumor in the appendicular skeleton require a clinical diagnosis, staging, and biopsy prior to the definitive surgical procedure. The clinical diagnosis most often is based on the detection of a mass but also can be suspected from a history of deep pain. Radiographs, in general, are the most accurate investigatory technique to establish a primary clinical diagnosis. The first steps of staging include imaging studies, such as radiographs, computerized tomography (CT), magnetic resonance imaging (MRI), technetium bone scanning, and angiography, that establish the local and distal extent of the tumor. Ultimately, the staging is completed with the histological diagnosis and grading of the tumor obtained from a biopsy sample. The biopsy can be a needle biopsy or an open biopsy. In either case, the biopsy must be performed along the lines of the eventual extensile exposure used for the resection, away from neurovascular structures, and with minimal contamination of surrounding tissues. Once local and systemic imaging studies are evaluated together with the histological grade of the tumor biopsy sample, the clinical staging is completed according to Enneking's system endorsed by the Muskuloskeletal Tumor Society (6). This allows the classification of the bone tumor into low-grade tumors (I), high-grade tumors (II), or those with evidence of metastatic disease (III). In addition, it reflects the local extent of the tumor with relation to the compartment of origin as either intracompartmental (A) or extracompartmental (B). These considerations are critical for selecting the appropriate margin of surgical treatment.

Surgical Margins

The margins of resection in the surgery of bone tumors can be: (*a*) intralesional, also referred to as "curettage"; (*b*) marginal; or (*c*) wide. Benign tumors (which are less than grade I, i.e., grade 0) are routinely treated by curettage or intralesional excision. Metastatic bone disease,

which represents a special category of tumors in bone to which the staging system previously described does not apply, is generally also treated by intralesional surgery. Benign tumors that are locally aggressive (e.g., giant cell tumors) and low-grade lesions (i.e., parosteal sarcoma) are commonly treated by marginal excision. High-grade tumors require a wide margin of resection to achieve adequate local control. The bone defects created after the different types of resections ultimately depend on the amount of bone removed and are generally larger after wide resections, but can be substantial even after intralesional or marginal surgery. Allograft bone can be used as morsellized graft to fill cavities left after curettage when the structural integrity of the segment is not compromised. When there is compromise of structure, as is commonly the case after marginal and wide resections, large allograft bone segments are required to restore continuity of the skeleton. The use of morsellized allograft material is covered in Chapter 4, which discusses the use of allografts in general orthopaedics. Therefore, this chapter only deals with those reconstructions in tumor surgery that require large allografts. The conditions in which these reconstructions are carried out cover the range from benign lesions (certain giant cell tumors) to high-grade sarcomas and metastatic bone disease.

CLASSIFICATION OF RECONSTRUCTIONS

Allograft reconstructions fall into one of four major categories:

1. *Osteoarticular Allograft*—reconstruction of a joint defect using an allograft that includes an articulating surface (one side of a joint or part thereof);
2. *Allograft-Arthrodesis*—reconstruction of a joint defect by an allograft bone segment to achieve an arthrodesis;
3. *Intercalary Allograft*—reconstruction of a diaphyseal or metaphyseal defect with an allograft bone segment;
4. *Allograft-Prosthesis*—reconstruction of a joint defect by a composite of allograft bone segment and prosthetic implant.

TECHNICAL PRINCIPLES OF RECONSTRUCTION

Reconstruction is planned in conjunction with planning the radical excision and the allograft to be used is selected to match the size of the recipient by the best possible method available, usually by comparing radiographs. The surgical approach and the technique of tumor resection vary according to local anatomy and the characteristics of the tumor. These issues are not discussed here because they are complex and are not within the scope of a text on reconstruction. After completion of the oncological procedure, reconstruction is carried out by the same surgical team (the author's preference) or, in some centers, by a different team. In case of a need for muscle or skin flap coverage, a plastic-microvascular surgical team participates. The allograft is thawed, cultured, and kept in warm physiological saline with antibiotics until use. The resected specimen can be used as a template to shape and sculpt the allograft to fit exactly into the bone defect. The surgical procedure varies according to the type of allograft reconstruction being performed and examples of the different techniques are given later in this chapter. However, there are several common general principles worth summarizing before discussing the individual techniques.

Summary of General Principles

1. Fixation of allograft to host bone must be a rigid osteosynthesis performed according to principles and techniques of the Association for the Study of Internal Fixation (ASIF). In the epiphyseal and metaphyseal regions, this is best accomplished by screws and plates. In the diaphyseal region of long bones, intramedullary fixation is the method of choice with control of rotation provided by step-cuts at the osteosynthesis sites.
2. One must avoid placing screws and screw-holes into the allograft whenever possible because these act as stress risers and are associated with the danger of fracture.
3. Methylmethacrylate is used in the allograft when it is combined with an implant. This rigidly fixes the implant to the allograft (which is a nonliving rigid biological sleeve) and the result is a super-stable composite material. Methylmethacrylate is not used in host bone.
4. The osteosynthesis sites are grafted with morsellized autogenous iliac bone, in all instances, to enhance union of the allograft to host bone.
5. Soft tissues (tendons, ligaments) must be attached to allografts by tight fixation at the proper tension for successful healing and joint stability.
6. Wound closures over allografts must be meticulous to avoid skin sloughs and, therefore, require the frequent use of local or free tissue transfers.

OSTEOARTICULAR ALLOGRAFT RECONSTRUCTION

Osteoarticular reconstruction employs allografts that are fresh or frozen with the help of cryoprotectant agents in an attempt to preserve cartilage viability. Their most common indication is in low-grade, locally aggressive tumors in young adults when curettage is not feasible. It is important to match the size of the allograft to the host because this will minimize joint incongruity, recognizing, at the same time, that a perfect match is not possible. Joint instability is the major functional problem in artic-

ulating grafts and, therefore, particular attention must be devoted to the reattachment of ligaments, tendons, and capsular structures of the host to the allograft bone segment. When these are missing, soft tissue reconstruction can be performed either with allograft soft tissues (ligaments that are left attached to the allograft bone at the time of harvest) or by advancing local host soft tissue structures. Prolonged postoperative bracing is usually required to protect these soft tissue repairs. The advantage of articular allografts is the preservation of joint mobility without prosthetic replacement, which is preferred in young patients with normal life expectancy. The most common site for this type of reconstruction is the knee, followed by the proximal humerus. The following examples illustrate this technique.

Unicondylar Distal Femoral Reconstruction

Partial joint reconstruction is sometimes indicated when a giant cell tumor destroys the articular surface or a low-grade surface lesion is resected with an adequate margin that allows the preservation of the rest of the joint (Fig. 6.1). Osteosynthesis is performed with cancellous lag screws only or in combination with a neutralization plate that functions also as a buttress to prevent vertical displacement.

Total Distal Femoral Replacement

Allograft replacement of the distal femur is indicated after transarticular resections of the distal femur for both low- and high-grade tumors (Fig. 6.2). It is more commonly done in low-grade lesions, such as advanced or recurrent giant cell tumors with intra-articular extension because of reluctance to perform prosthetic replacement or arthrodesis in these patients. Osteosynthesis can be done with a compression plate as shown or with intramedullary fixation and step-cut osteotomies.

Proximal Tibial Reconstruction

The indications for this procedure are the same as for distal femoral replacement. The fibula is either resected at the level of the neck (as shown in Fig. 6.3) or disarticulated after dissection and protection of the peroneal nerve. The collateral ligaments and the patellar tendon are reattached to the allograft with staples. Osteosynthesis is performed with a compression plate.

Proximal Humeral Reconstruction

This procedure has similar indications as the previous articular reconstructions but, because the shoulder is a nonweight-bearing joint, congruity is not as important as

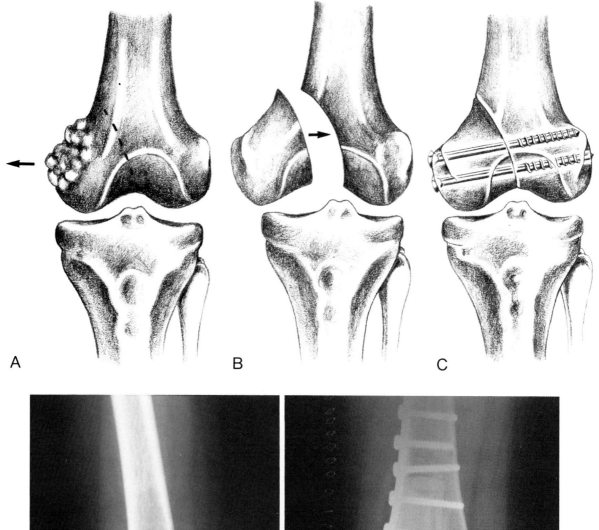

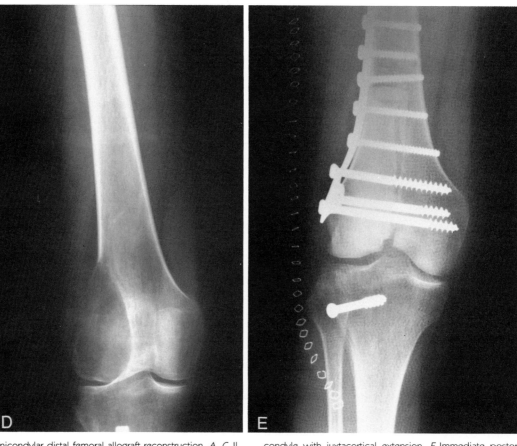

A

B

C

D

E

Figure 6.1. Unicondylar distal femoral allograft reconstruction. *A–C.* Illustrations depicting the resection of the medial femoral condyle and replacement by an articulating allograft fixed with two cancellous screws. *D.* Preoperative radiograph showing a giant cell tumor of the lateral femoral condyle with juxtacortical extension. *E.* Immediate postoperative radiograph showing the reconstruction with a condylar cryopreserved allograft fixed with interfragmental compression screws and a neutralization plate.

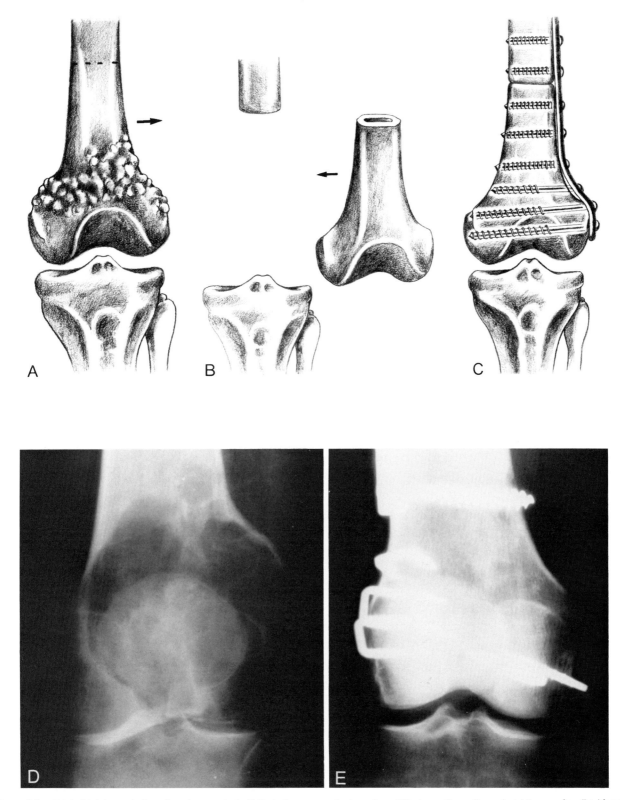

Figure 6.2. Total distal femoral allograft replacement. *A–C.* Illustrations showing resection of distal femur and replacement with articulating allograft fixed with compression plate. *D.* Preoperative radiograph of recurrent giant cell tumor in young female patient with destruction of the articular surface. *E.* Postoperative radiograph at 4.5 years after distal femoral replacement with fresh allograft (note the staples indicating reattachment of ligaments and capsular structures, the maintenance of the integrity of the allograft, and the excellent preservation of the joint space).

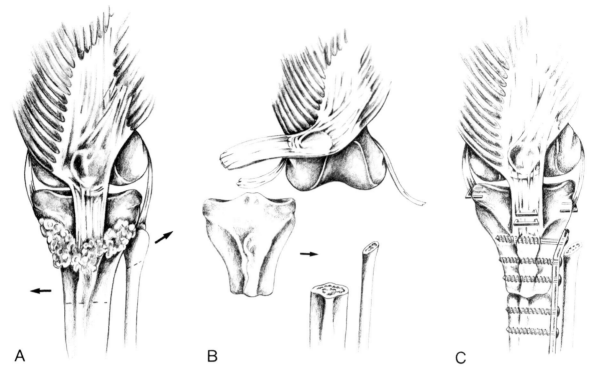

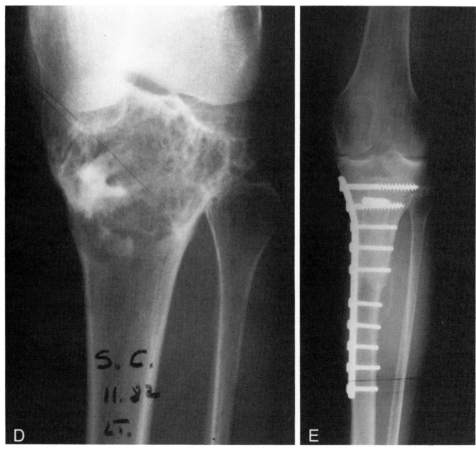

Figure 6.3. Proximal tibial allograft reconstruction. *A–C.* Drawings showing the technique of resection and reconstruction of the proximal tibia. *D.* Radiograph showing recurrent giant cell tumor in the proximal tibia of a 42-year-old woman. *E.* Radiograph at 4 years after en bloc resection and reconstruction with a fresh osteoarticular allograft showing maintenance of the joint space and solid union of the osteosynthesis site (note staple used for reattaching the patellar tendon).

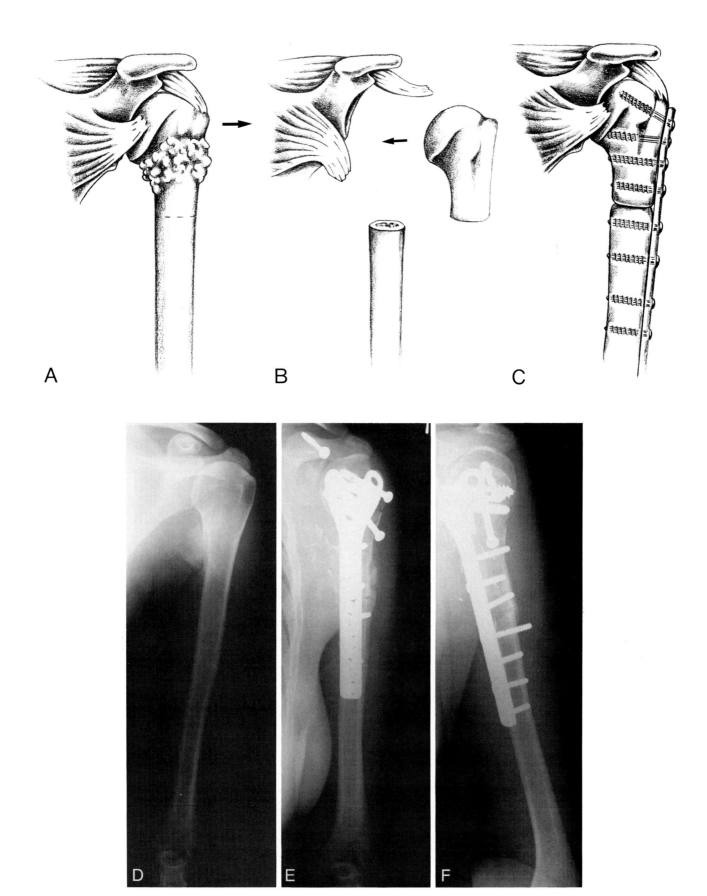

Figure 6.4. Proximal humeral allograft reconstruction. *A–C.* Drawings showing the technique of resection with preservation of musculotendinous units (rotator cuff and subscapularis tendons) that are reattached to the allograft, which, in turn, is fixed with a compression plate. *D.* Preoperative radiograph showing a parosteal sarcoma of the proximal humerus in a 22-year-old woman. *E* and *F.* Postoperative views demonstrating the reconstruction at 4 months (note formation of callus at osteosynthesis site and cancellous screws used for the reattachment of tendons).

in the knee (Fig. 6.4). Proximal humeral allografts function more as spacers to which musculotendinous structures can be reattached and given a chance to unite and to power the joint. Therefore, in this circumstance, the viability of the cartilage is not always essential and frozen osteoarticular grafts can be used.

ALLOGRAFT-ARTHRODESIS RECONSTRUCTION

Allograft-arthrodesis has evolved from the procedure of autograft-arthrodesis and has the advantage of not causing the significant morbidity associated with harvesting large segments of autograft bone. The most common indications are sarcomas that necessitate transarticular or extra-articular resections with extensive excision of soft tissues precluding functional arthroplasty in young, active individuals who have reasonably long life expectancy. The major disadvantage of this procedure is the elimination of mobility that is not readily accepted by some patients, particularly with regard to the knee. Union is not easy to achieve because of the high mechanical stress related to the long lever arms that result after this reconstruction. The use of this procedure in orthopaedic oncology has decreased in recent years concomitant with the increase of reconstructions employing prosthetic implants or allograft-prosthesis composites. However, it remains a viable alternative technique for certain patients and is used most commonly for reconstructions involving the knee and shoulder and, occasionally, the ankle joint. These techniques are illustrated in the following examples.

Allograft-Arthrodesis of the Knee

The best technique for arthrodesing the knee is an osteosynthesis employing intramedullary fixation as shown in the drawings in Figure 6.5. Specially designed long nails are used for this purpose (e.g., Neff nails) and the allograft can be cemented to the nail if the fixation is not rigid without cement. Methylmethacrylate must not be used in the host bone and the ostheosynthesis sites are stabilized by step-cut osteotomies and cerclage wires. Plates and interfragmentary compression screws can also be used as shown in the clinical example but are less optimal than intramedullary fixation.

Allograft-Arthrodesis of the Shoulder

The shoulder is difficult to arthrodese under any circumstances and this is even more true after tumor resection and allograft replacement (Fig. 6.6). Therefore, this technique has limited indications for low-grade tumors in active, young individuals and for some high-grade tumors that necessitate removal of the deltoid and rotator cuff.

The technique employs one or more compression plates that are contoured to fit over the humerus allograft and onto the acromion, spine of the scapula, and/or clavicle with the shoulder in a position that is appropriate for fusion. If soft tissue coverage is not adequate, a local latissimus dorsi rotation flap can be used. The results can be gratifying as shown by the clinical example.

Allograft-Arthrodesis of the Ankle

Although distal tibial sarcomas are often best treated by below-knee amputation, there is a place for limb salvage and arthrodesis in selected patients who do not accept an amputation. Allograft-arthrodesis of the ankle (Fig. 6.7) is difficult primarily because of the lack of adequate soft tissue cover. This necessitates microvascular soft tissue transfer as shown in Figure 6.7. Osteosynthesis is accomplished with compression plates proximally and compression lag screws distally into the talus and os calcis.

INTERCALARY ALLOGRAFT RECONSTRUCTION

This type of reconstruction procedure employs deep-frozen or freeze-dried cylindrical, hemicylindrical, or geometrical allograft segments to reconstruct defects in the diaphyseal or metaphyseal region of long bones. In the author's experience, this is the most successful of all allograft reconstructions in orthopaedic oncology. This is because there is no need to reconstruct joints and there is usually no problem with nonunion or fracture, provided that one follows the general principles outlined earlier in this chapter with regard to rigid osteosynthesis and autogenous bone grafting at the ostheosynthesis sites. The indications for this reconstruction are low- and high-grade sarcomas that involve the metaphyseal or diaphyseal regions of long bones where it is feasible to preserve the joint and lesions of metastatic bone disease in similar areas. The methods used for osteosynthesis are screws, compression plates, or intramedullary nails, depending on the circumstances required by the particular reconstruction procedure. In general, intramedullary fixation is preferred, whenever possible, and attention must be paid to violate the allograft to the least possible extent by unnecessary screw-holes that can act as stress risers to cause fractures. This technique is used in any of the long bones of the appendicular skeleton but only the most common types of intercalary reconstructions will be shown in the following examples.

Geometric Intercalary Reconstruction

Geometric resection and reconstruction (Figs. 6.8 and 6.9) is indicated in low-grade surface lesions, most com-

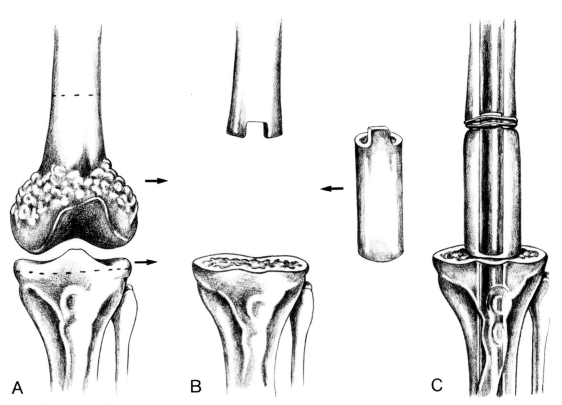

Figure 6.5. Allograft-arthrodesis of the knee. *A–C.* Illustrations depicting preferred technique using intramedullary nail fixation with step-cut osteosynthesis and cerclage wiring to control rotation. *D* and *E.* Antero-posterior and lateral preoperative radiographs showing an osteosarcoma of the distal femur in a 19-year-old male patient. *F.* Initial reconstruction with two plates at 1 month. *G.* Revision of reconstruction because of failure at the proximal osteosynthesis site showing intramedullary fixation with Huckstep-type nail at 1 year (note that union is progressing at both proximal and distal osteosynthesis sites but is not yet complete).

monly, parosteal sarcoma or chondrosarcoma occuring at the diaphyseal-metaphyseal junction of long bones. The resection of these tumors is tricky as it is often difficult to judge the adequacy of the surgical margin. CT and MRI are helpful in planning the geometric resection that achieves a good oncological margin with minimal violation of the integrity of the bone involved. The geometric defect is reconstructed with a fitting, custom-tailored allograft that is fitted like in a jigsaw puzzle and fixed with either lag screws alone (Fig. 6.8) or lag screws in combination with a neutralization plate (Fig. 6.9). These grafts are generally incorporated rapidly as shown by the two clinical examples presented (Figs. 6.8 and 6.9).

Intercalary Reconstruction of the Femur and Tibia

After excision of a diaphyseal segment involved with a primary or metastatic malignant tumor, osteosynthesis of the intercalary allograft used in the reconstruction can be performed by either compression plating or by intramedullary nailing. The plating technique in the femur is illustrated in Figure 6.10, with a clinical example showing its application in a metastatic lesion. Plating of an intercalary allograft in the tibia is shown in Figure 6.11, an example where two plates were required for rigid osteosynthesis because of the proximity of the resection to the ankle joint. Osteosynthesis by intramedullary fixation is preferred over plating because of its superior stability. In addition, it allows the maintenance of the allograft segment's integrity because there are no screws inserted through the allograft. The technique employs step-cut osteotomies and cerclage wiring at the osteosynthesis sites and fixation with a locked intramedullary nail as shown in Figure 6.12. The application of this method for metastatic bone disease is demonstrated by the clinical example in Figure 6.13.

Intercalary Reconstruction of the Humerus

The humerus can also be reconstructed by osteosynthesis using either a compression plate or an intramedullary device. The approach for tumor excision is usually anterior. The plating technique and a relevant clinical example are illustrated in Figure 6.14. Intramedullary fixation is advantageous because it does not

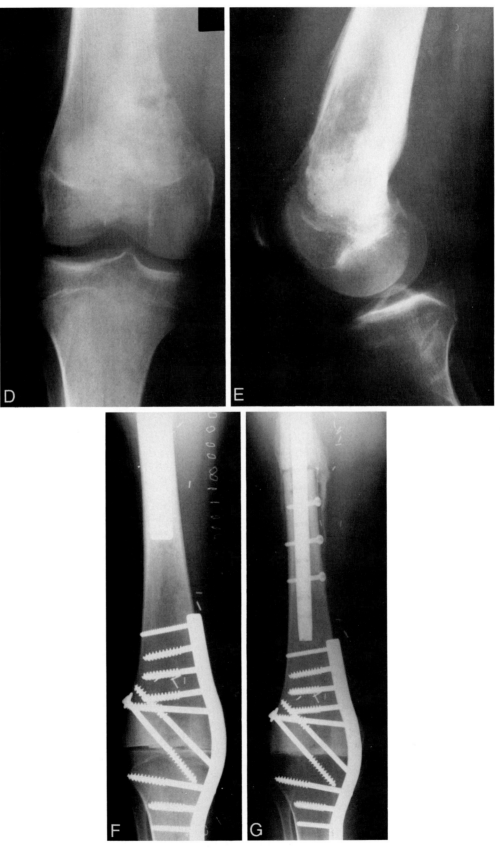

Figure 6.5   *D, E, F,* and *G.*

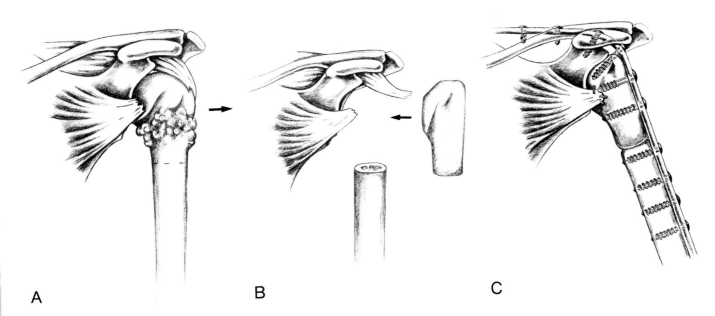

A   B   C

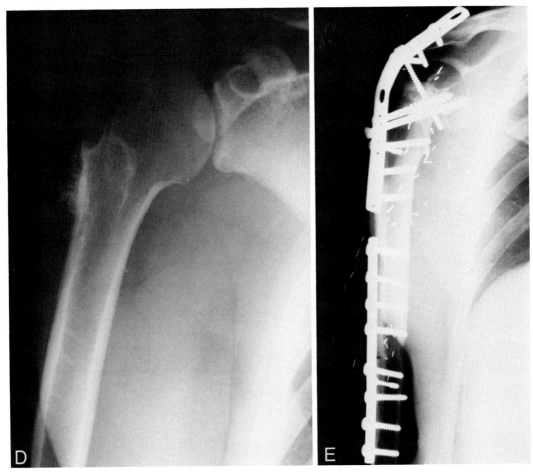

D   E

Figure 6.6. Allograft-arthodesis of the shoulder. *A–C.* Artistic drawing showing the steps involved in allograft-arthrodesis of the shoulder: excision of the proximal humerus, insertion of an appropriately shaped and tailored proximal humeral allograft, and osteosynthesis using a contoured compression plate with proximal fixation into acromion and clavicle. *D.* Preoperative radiograph showing a chondrosarcoma of the proximal humerus in a 31-year-old man. *E.* Radiograph taken 15 months after surgery showing successful arthrodesis with solid union of both proximal and distal osteosynthesis sites.

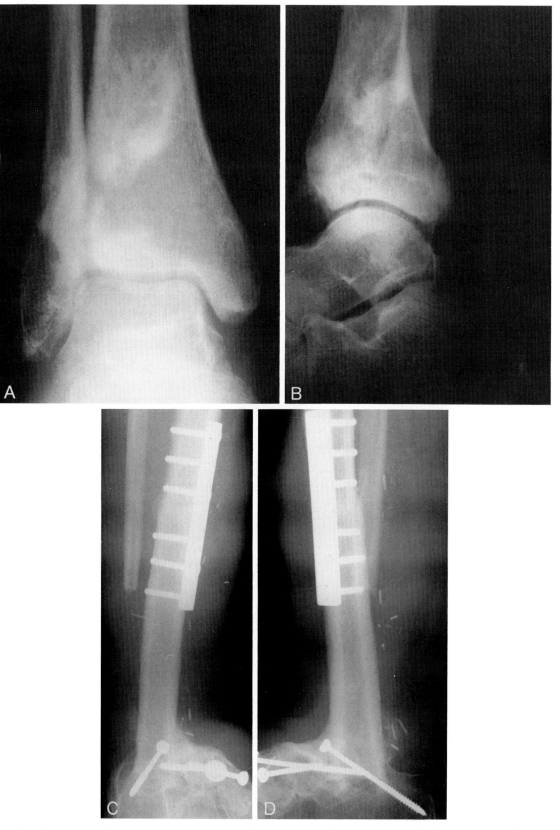

Figure 6.7. Allograft-arthrodesis of the ankle. *A* and *B*. Anteroposterior and lateral radiographs showing an osteosarcoma of the distal tibia in a 49-year-old man. *C* and *D*. Anteroposterior and lateral radiographs demonstrating tibio-talocalcaneal arthrodesis at a 2-year follow-up (note the solid union at both proximal and distal osteosynthesis sites).

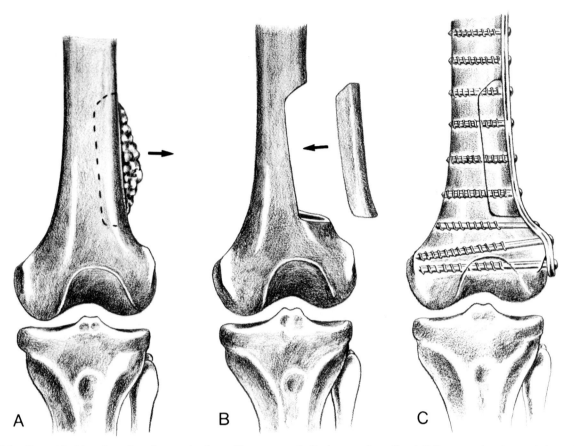

A   B   C

Figure 6.8. Geometric intercalary allograft reconstruction with screw fixation. *A–C.* Drawings depicting the geometric resection of a surface lesion in the distal femur and the reconstruction of the defect with a fitting allograft segment fixed by interfragmental compression screws and a neutralization plate. *D* and *E.* Anteroposterior and lateral radiographs showing a typical parosteal sarcoma of the distal femur in a 21-year-old man. *F.* Computerized tomogram demonstrating the localization of the lesion to the bone surface. *G* and *H.* Bone scan in anteroposterior and lateral projections showing the activity of the lesion. *I* and *J.* Anteroposterior and lateral radiographs at 2 months after geometric excision and reconstruction with allograft segment fixed with lag screws. *K* and *L.* Anteroposterior and lateral radiographs at 10 months showing complete union and extensive incorporation of the allograft.

require the violation of the allograft with screw-holes. However, intramedullary fixation in the humerus is difficult and the available fixation devices do not always give a rigid osteosynthesis. Therefore, methylmethacrylate may need to be used in both allograft and host bone to add stability to the construct and is recommended routinely in cases of metastatic disease. The use of Rush pins is not a new technique and is applicable to intercalary allograft reconstruction as shown in Figure 6.15. A more recent method uses the Seidel locking nail as demonstrated in the clinical example shown in Figure 6.16. Meticulous attention must be paid to the step-cut osteotomies and the wiring technique, no matter what intramedullary device is used.

ALLOGRAFT-PROSTHESIS RECONSTRUCTION

The combination of an allograft and a prosthesis, the "allograft-prosthesis composite implant," is the most ver-

satile and most widely used reconstruction method in orthopaedic oncology. It offers the ability to use standard, off-the-shelf prosthetic components to perform a "custom" joint reconstruction by tailoring the allograft to the size of the defect. This technique, which evolved in the field of tumor surgery, now has widespread use in total joint revision surgery, as discussed in other chapters of this book. The indications for this procedure in orthopaedic oncology are primary and metastatic tumors where the excision includes the joint. Osteoarticular allografts are an alternative in certain low-grade tumors and allograft-arthrodesis is an alternative procedure with the sacrifice of mobility, as discussed earlier. Allograft-prosthesis reconstruction follows the same principles as intercalary reconstruction related to rigid fixation (in this case, by the stem of the prosthetic implant), use of methylmethacrylate in the allograft but not in the host, step-cut osteotomies, cerclage wiring, and autogenous bone graft-

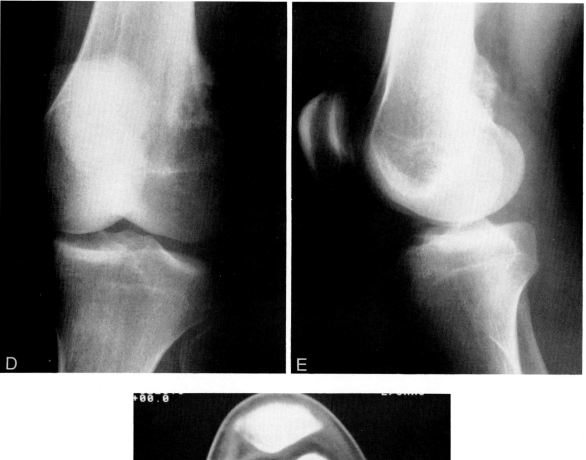

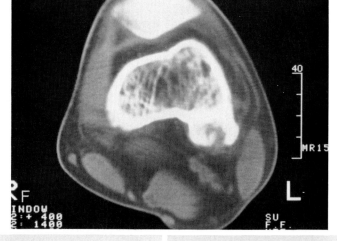

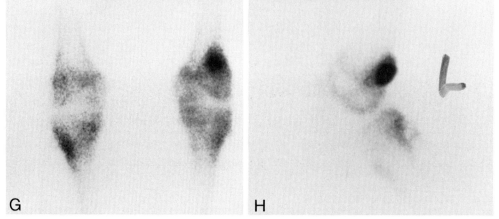

Figure 6.8 *D, E, F, G,* and *H.*

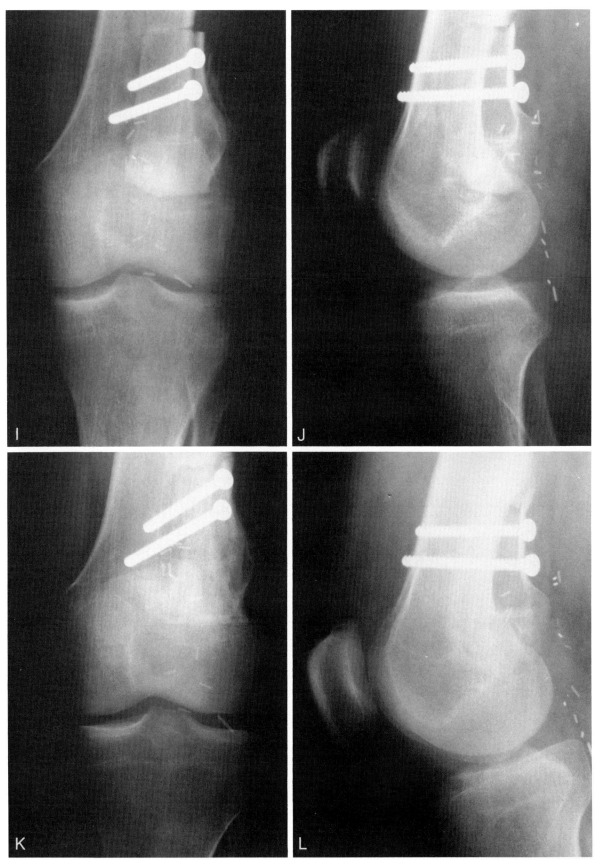

Figure 6.8 *I, J, K,* and *L.*

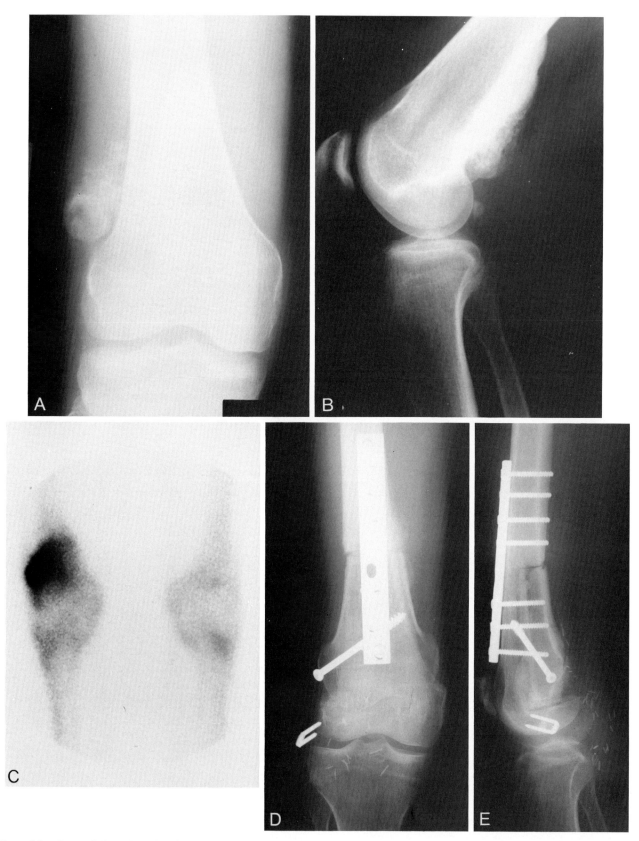

Figure 6.9. Geometric intercalary allograft reconstruction with plate fixation. *A* and *B*. Anteroposterior and lateral radiographs showing another example of a parosteal sarcoma in a 29-year-old man. *C.* Technetium scan showing increased activity in the lesion. *D* and *E.* Anteroposterior and lateral radiographs showing reconstruction at 5 months using a combination of lag screw and plate fixation (note bone formation at osteosynthesis sites).

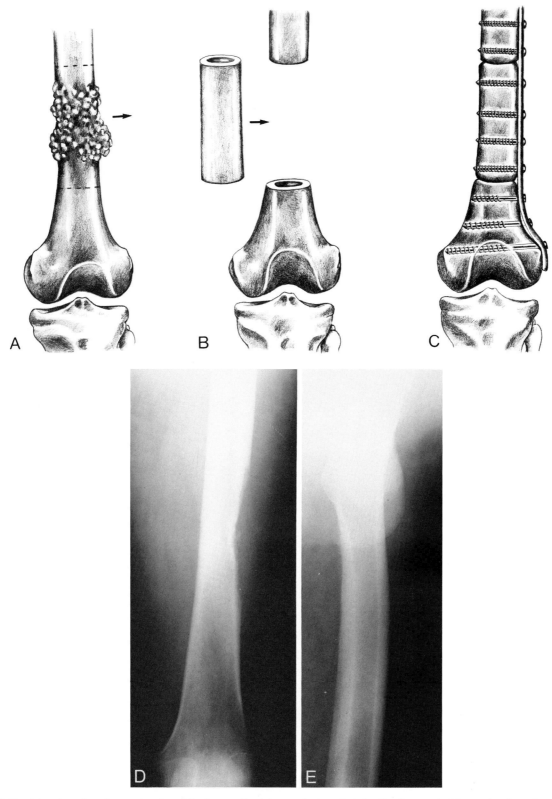

Figure 6.10. Intercalary allograft reconstruction of the femur with plate fixation. *A–C.* Illustrations showing the technique of osteosynthesis with a lateral compression plate. *D* and *E.* Preoperative anteroposterior and lateral radiographs of the femur in a 50-year-old man showing extensive diaphyseal destruction from metastatic renal cell carcinoma. *F* and *G.* Postoperative radiographs at 2 weeks showing the plate osteosynthesis of the allograft segment. *H* and *I.* Postoperative radiographs at 4 months showing formation of callus.

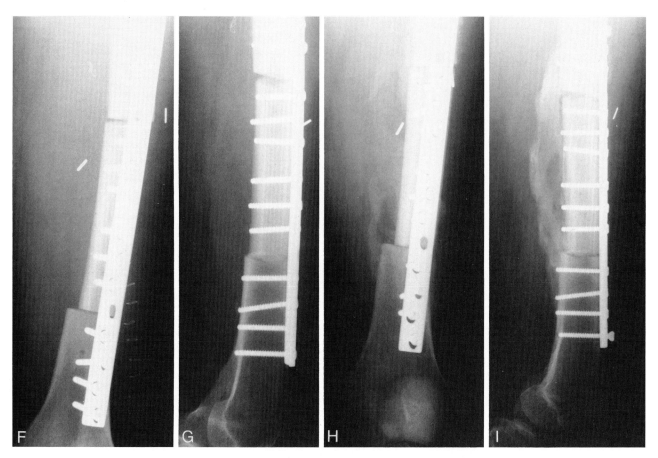

Figure 6.10. *F, G, H,* and *I.*

ing at the osteosynthesis sites. The technique is used in the appendicular skeleton most commonly in the proximal femur, distal femur, proximal tibia, and proximal humerus; reconstructions at these sites are shown in the following examples.

Allograft-Prosthesis Reconstruction of the Proximal Femur

The technique (Fig. 6.17) is similar to that used in the revision of total hip arthroplasties with proximal femoral deficiency (Chapter 8). It is interesting that, although the method was developed by tumor surgeons, it is being perfected today by total joint surgeons who perform the volume of operations and have the follow-up required for obtaining the information related to the efficacy of these techniques. The greater trochanter, which is preserved and reattached in revision surgery, can also be detached in a significant number of tumor excisions. Otherwise, the leftover abductors are reattached to the allograft. A long-stem femoral component is cemented to the allograft segment and fixed by press-fit into host bone. The use of step-cuts and cerclage wiring gives rigid os-

teosynthesis. The acetabular component is fixed directly by screws or cemented into a reinforcement ring, which is held by long cancellous screws as in the clinical example shown in Figure 6.17. This technique is useful not only in primary tumors but it also has a frequent application in metastatic disease involving the proximal femur.

Allograft-Prosthesis Reconstruction of the Distal Femur

The distal femur is the most frequent site of involvement by primary malignant tumors of the appendicular skeleton. Although the use of allograft-prosthesis composites is useful for distal femoral reconstruction (Fig. 6.18), this is the location where one can equally effectively use an articulating allograft or a custom/modular prosthetic implant. Allograft-prosthesis reconstruction in the distal femur is technically problematic because of the difficulty of combining the prosthetic component with rigid osteosynthesis. In addition, when an unconstrained prosthesis is used, as shown in the example in Figure 6.18, the capsular and ligament reconstruction required can be difficult technically and may not give the stability that is

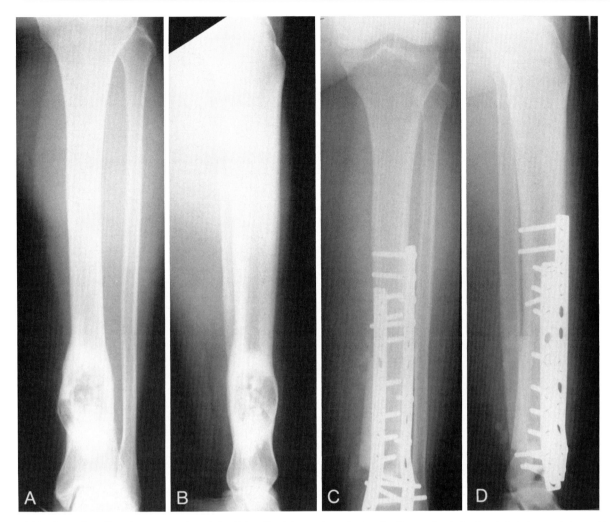

Figure 6.11. Intercalary allograft reconstruction of the tibia with plate fixation. *A* and *B*. Anteroposterior and lateral radiographs of the tibia of a 46-year-old woman showing fusiform swelling due to what ultimately turned out to be fibrous dysplasia. *C* and *D*. Anteroposterior and lateral views after resection and allograft reconstruction with double plate osteosynthesis.

wanted. For all of these reasons, one must use critical judgment when choosing this reconstruction procedure over a custom or modular, partially constrained prosthesis. The technique shown in the drawing represents a special femoral prosthesis (J & J) that has a stem shaped like an intramedullary nail, which is inserted in a retrograde fashion through the allograft and the host femur and allows the attachment of the surface component by a screw. Alternatively, a regular intramedullary nail is used and the total knee femoral component is cemented to the allograft as shown in the clinical example presented (Fig. 6.18).

Allograft-Prosthesis Reconstruction of the Proximal Tibia

The use of an allograft-prosthesis composite has an advantage in the proximal tibia (Fig. 6.19) over prosthetic replacement because it gives a central attachment site for the reinsertion of the patellar tendon. Thus, it is advantageous to have the allograft in place even when using a partially constrained prosthesis. The stem of the tibial component of the prosthesis is cemented to the allograft and fixed to host bone by press-fit and step-cut osteosynthesis with cerclage wiring. The patellar tendon can be reattached by staples to the allograft bone, by suturing it to allograft tendon, or by performing a wire-osteosynthesis between host and allograft patella (a technique described by Dr. G. Delepine, Paris, France).

Allograft-Prosthesis Reconstruction in the Proximal Humerus

This is a versatile and readily applicable reconstruction in both primary and metastatic tumors, which frequently occur in the proximal humerus. In the shoulder, resto-

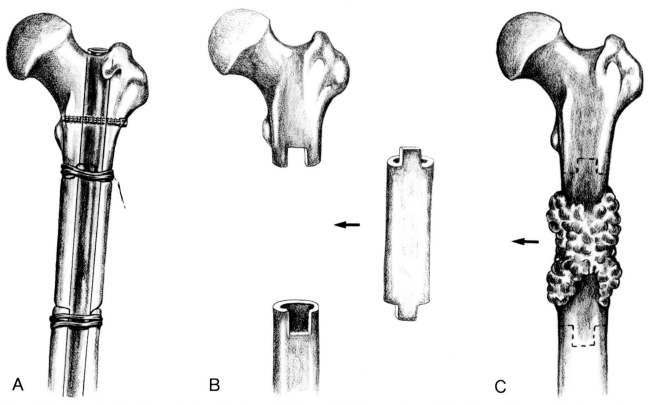

A   B   C

Figure 6.12. Intercalary allograft reconstruction of the femur with intramedullary nail fixation. *A–C.* Illustrations showing resection and reconstruction with step-cut osteotomies, cerclage wiring, and osteosynthesis with locked intramedullary nail. *D* and *E.* Clinical example of failed fixation after closed intramedullary nailing for lymphoma in 53-year-old woman.

F–H. Anteroposterior and lateral views of femur and lateral view of knee showing the intercalary reconstruction at 3 months (note the rigid osteosynthesis with nail locked proximally and distally, step-cuts, and cerclage wires).

ration of motion is the primary goal and it depends on functioning of the rotator cuff and subscapularis musculotendinous units, which can be reattached to and can unite to allograft bone. The technique of osteosynthesis follows the rules described for other allograft-prosthesis reconstructions, i.e., long-stem prosthetic component cemented in the allograft and press-fitted in host bone with step-cut osteotomies and cerclage wiring to control rotation. Alternatively, the stem can be cemented on its entire length as shown in the examples of two cases of metastatic disease in Figure 6.20. When the defect is large and a long-stem component is not available, control of rotation can be secured by adding a plate, as in the clinical example of reconstruction for an osteosarcoma shown in Figure 6.21.

CLINICAL RESULTS AND COMPLICATIONS

There are numerous clinical reviews, most of them published over the last decade, describing the results and complications of allograft reconstruction after the excision of bone tumors (7–21). Generally, these studies are retrospective evaluations of series of patients treated in

a particular center by this surgical modality over a period of time. While earlier reports were merely descriptions of cases treated by this surgical procedure, as experience grew, the clinical reviews have proceeded to analyze the effectiveness of allograft reconstruction. The parameters used for judging the relative efficacy of the procedure are a combination of assessments of functional end results, analyses of common complications (infection, fracture, nonunion), and late problems (joint instability, degenerative arthritis) that can lead to failure. The functional assessment methods follow either the system devised by Enneking (22) or a slightly different protocol used by Mankin et al. (10). According to these evaluations, the rate of acceptable (excellent or good) functional results is generally at the 70–80% level. The incidence of complications is generally high with infection, fracture, and nonunion occurring in 5–15% of cases. The late problems of joint instability and degenerative arthritis in osteoarticular replacements run at about 5%.

The difficulty with interpreting the results of allograft reconstruction is the fact that most clinical series include several methods of reconstruction used at a variety of

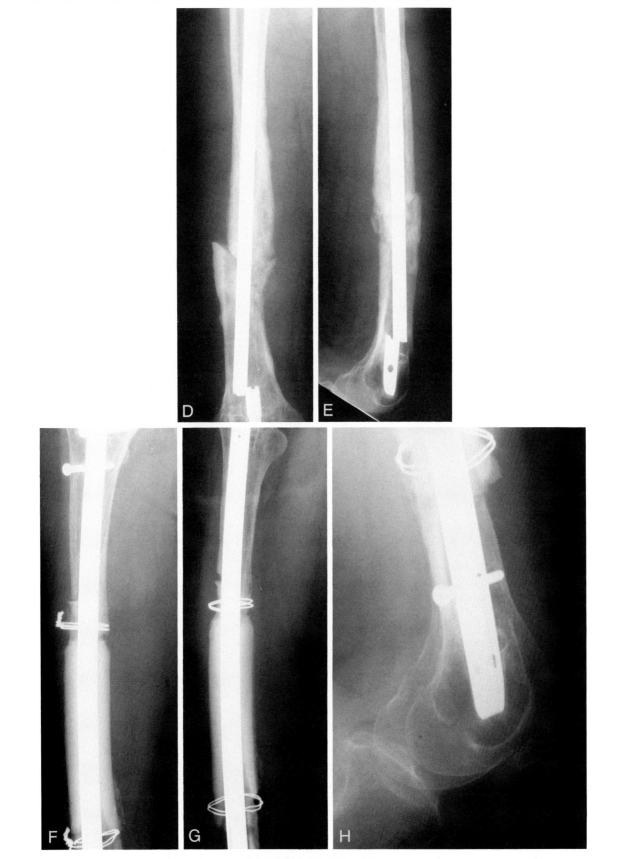

Figure 6.12 *D, E, F, G,* and *H.*

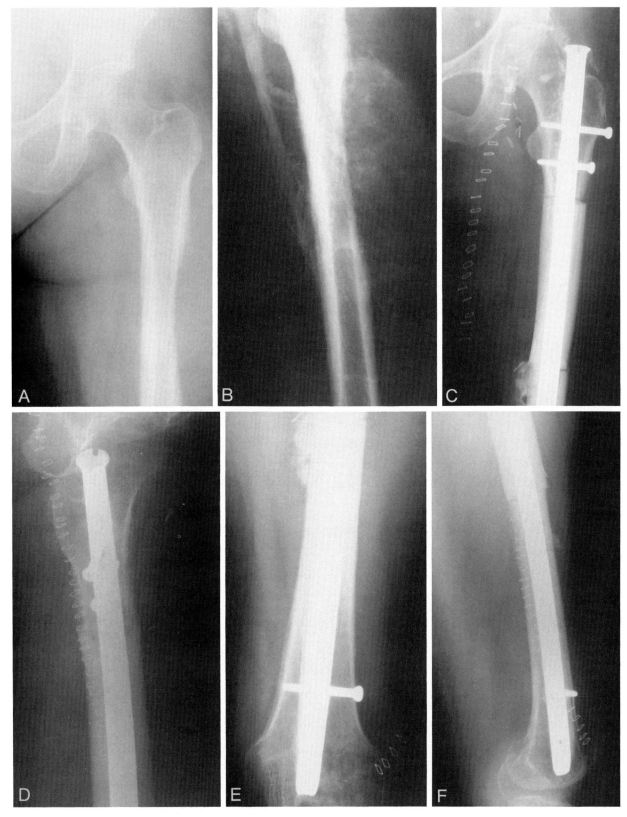

Figure 6.13. Intercalary reconstruction of the femur in metastatic disease. A. Anteroposterior radiograph of the femur showing large area of diaphyseal destruction by small-cell lung carcinoma in a 44-year-old woman. B. Venous phase of preoperative angiogram showing the large soft tissue mass. C–F. Anteroposterior and lateral radiographs taken 1 week after marginal resection and reconstruction with intercalary allograft and locked Universal nail.

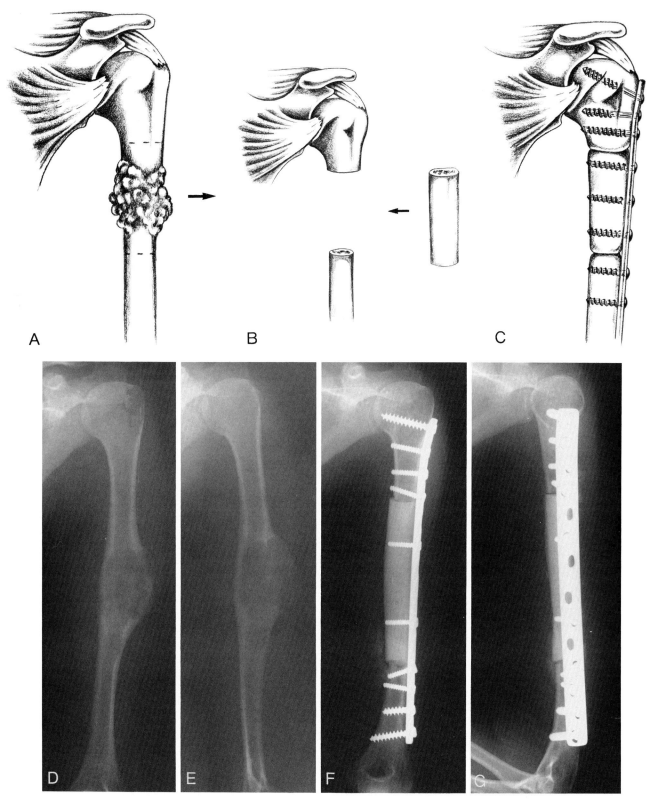

Figure 6.14. Intercalary reconstruction of the humerus with plate fixation. A–C. Drawings showing intercalary resection and reconstruction using plate osteosynthesis. D and E. Preoperative radiographs showing a chondrosarcoma of the humerus in a 63-year-old woman with multiple en-chondromatosis. F and G. Postoperative radiographs showing intercalary reconstruction and plate osteosynthesis at 3 months (note beginning of consolidation at the osteosynthesis sites).

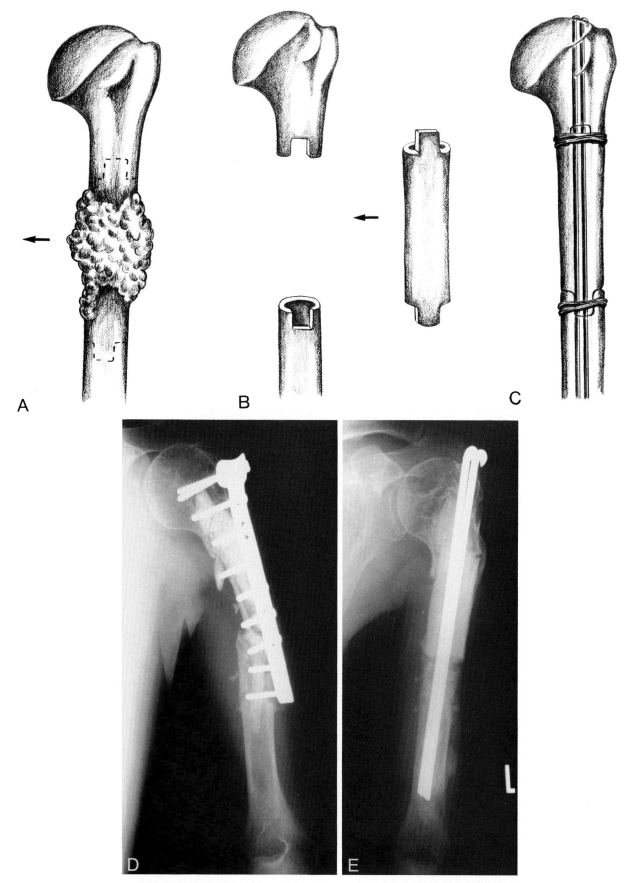

Figure 6.15. Intercalary reconstruction of the humerus with Rush pin fixation. *A–C.* Illustration showing technique of resection and reconstruction with step-cut osteotomies, cerclage wires, and intramedullary Rush pins, which generally must be supplemented by methylmethacrylate in both allograft and host bone. *D.* Radiograph showing failure of fixation of pathological fracture from metastatic renal cell carcinoma repaired with plate and methylmethacrylate in a 57-year-old man. *E.* Radiograph taken 16 months after excision and intercalary reconstruction with allograft, Rush pins, and methylmethacrylate showing solid fixation and no evidence of recurrence.

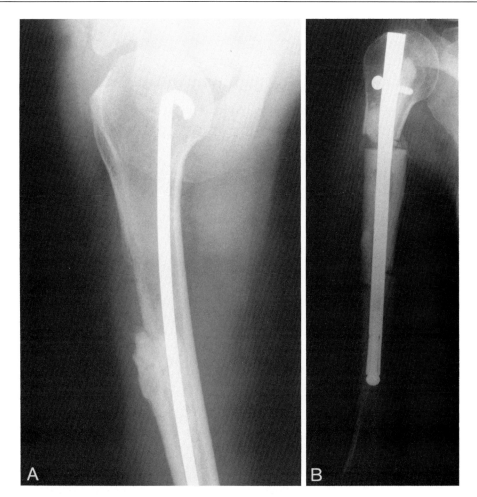

Figure 6.16. Intercalary reconstruction of the humerus with locked nail. *A.* Radiograph of the humerus in a 40-year-old woman with metastatic carcinoma of the lung showing recurrence proximal to the area curetted and plugged with methylmethacrylate at the time of insertion of a Rush rod, which did not give rigid fixation. *B.* Radiograph at 6 months after segmental resection and intercalary allograft reconstruction with Seidel locking nail and methylmethacrylate.

sites within the appendicular skeleton. It is evident that the type of reconstruction, the method of osteosynthesis, the extent of surgery, the condition of the host, the site of allograft replacement, and many other variables can have a significant effect on both function and complication rates. Clinical experience has taught us some general rules with regard to the presence or absence of special problems that can affect the outcome of different types of reconstruction. Thus, osteoarticular reconstruction is uniquely associated with problems of joint instability and late degenerative change. Intercalary replacement has better functional results than other types of reconstruction because it does not violate joints. Allograft-arthrodesis is difficult to judge in terms of functional result because it eliminates the factor of mobility. Allograft-prostheses have the unique problem of prosthetic loosening that is not encountered in other allograft procedures. While this experience is valuable, it does not represent scientific proof

as to the efficacy of these procedures in skeletal reconstruction. Recent approaches in clinical studies that attempt to define more precisely the outcome after allograft reconstruction have centered upon the analysis of defined reconstruction methods at specific skeletal sites or of specific complications of this procedure. These studies are worth reviewing briefly as they provide information that is of value when selecting this modality of surgical treatment.

Knee

We have recently reviewed our experience with allograft reconstructions of the knee in two studies that examined separately the outcome of fresh osteoarticular grafts used for advanced giant cell tumors and that of deep-frozen, irradiated bone used as intercalary, arthrodesis, or prosthetic composite grafts in primary malignant tumors (23, 24). The long-term review of fresh osteoarticular allo-

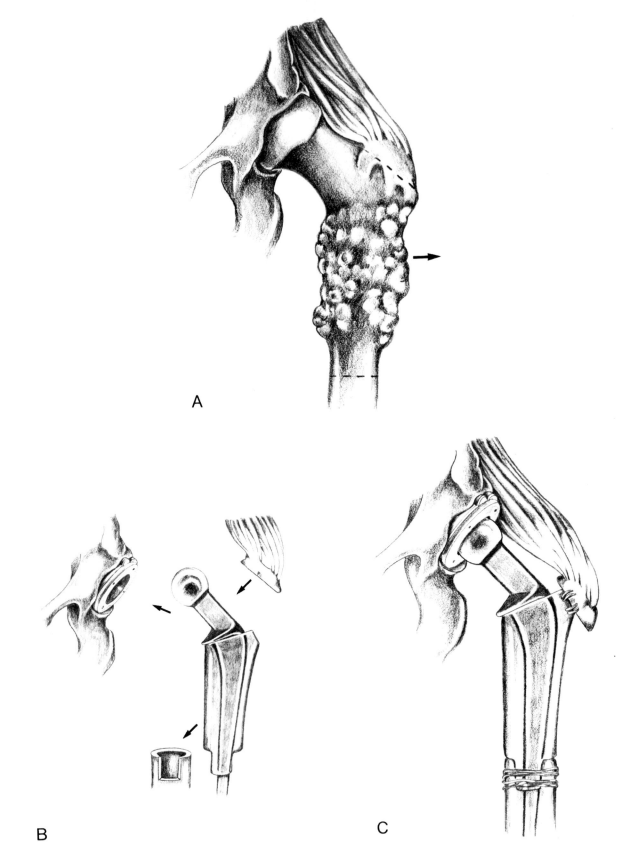

A

B

C

Figure 6.17. Allograft-prosthesis reconstruction in the proximal femur.
A–C. Artist's drawings of the proximal femoral resection and reconstruction
showing the preservation and reattachment of the abductors and the
technique of osteosynthesis with a long-stem femoral component and a
step-cut osteotomy with cerclage wiring at the host-allograft junction. *D*
and *E.* Anteroposterior and lateral radiographs of the hip in a 41-year-old
woman showing an angiosarcoma of the femoral neck. *F.* Early postoperative radiograph after proximal femoral resection and reconstruction with
allograft-prosthesis showing step-cut osteosynthesis fixed with long-stem
femoral component and cerclage wires (note fixation of femoral stem to
allograft by methylmethacrylate and to host bone by press-fit and the use
of a cemented cup and a Mueller ring with cancellous screws for fixation
in the acetabulum).

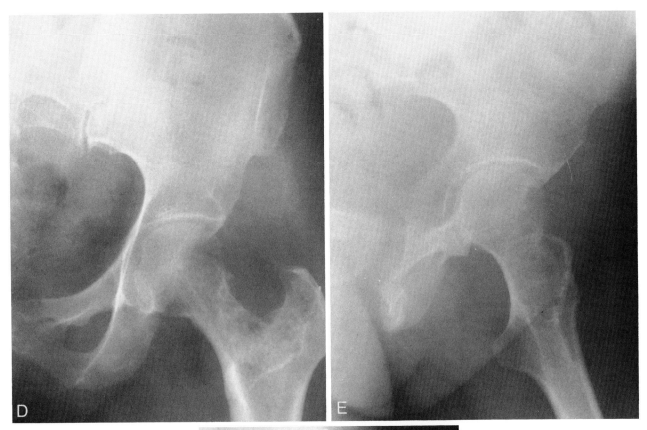

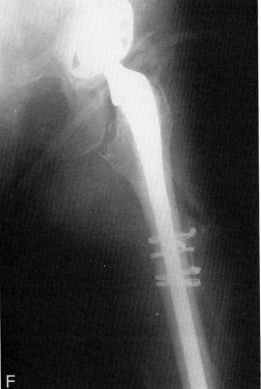

Figure 6.17   *D, E,* and *F.*

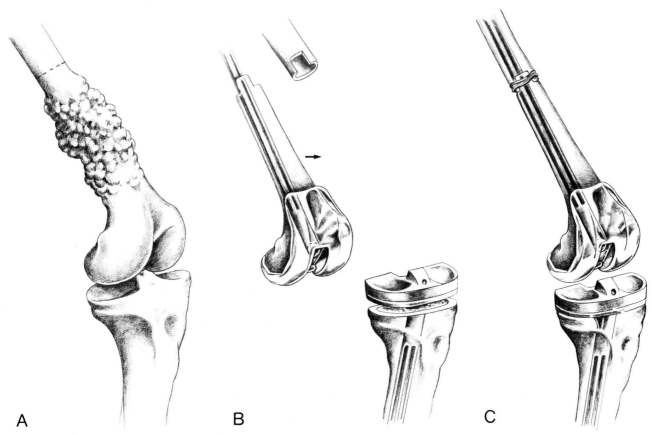

A   B   C

Figure 6.18. Allograft-prosthesis reconstruction in the distal femur. A–C. Illustrations showing technique of distal femoral resection and reconstruction with special Johnson and Johnson femoral allograft-prosthesis. The stem is inserted retrograde after reaming the medullary canal, methylmethacrylate is used in the allograft, and osteosynthesis is done by step-cut osteotomies and cerclage wiring. The surface component is attached with a screw to the stem and articulates with a regular tibial component. D and E. Anteroposterior and lateral radiographs of the knee showing a

chondrosarcoma of the distal femur in an 18-year-old female patient. F. Computerized tomogram showing the lesion with cortical breakthrough and a soft tissue mass. G and H. Anteroposterior and lateral views of the distal femur at 9 months showing reconstruction with unconstrained prosthesis combined with allograft and retrograde intramedullary nail (note the step-cut osteosynthesis with cerclage wires, the use of methylmethacrylate in the allograft, and the wires used for the reconstruction of the posterior capsule and ligaments).

grafts (mean follow-up of 8 years) showed satisfactory function (good or excellent) in 60% of cases. Joint instability was a significant problem in 30% of these reconstructions. The complications in this small group of 16 patients who all had benign giant cell tumors were: one infection (6%), one nonunion (6%), and five fractures (31%). The high fracture rate is related to the long follow-up time and shows that these massive allografts remain susceptible to fractures indefinitely. The failure rate in this series, judged by the need to remove the allograft was 19% (three of 16 cases). It is interesting that the joint spaces remained well preserved radiologically in all but one patient, suggesting that fresh articular cartilage remains viable and functional after allotransplantation as shown formally for small osteochondral grafts (25). Our review of reconstructions at the knee in primary malignant tumors showed the usual rates of satisfactory func-

tion and major complications as in previous series but we observed interesting differences in outcome when comparing failure rates of different types of reconstruction. Thus, intercalary reconstructions fared significantly better than allograft-arthrodeses or allograft-prostheses, which had a 50% failure rate mainly as a result of infections, skin slough, and fractures. These findings have made us more cautious and selective in employing allograft-prosthesis composites for distal femoral reconstruction where we prefer to use a modular knee-replacement system. A recent review describes the various choices available today for mobile knee reconstruction (26).

Proximal Femur

Allograft reconstruction methods for the proximal femur have been the subject of a review that compared allograft-prostheses with cryopreserved osteoarticular allografts

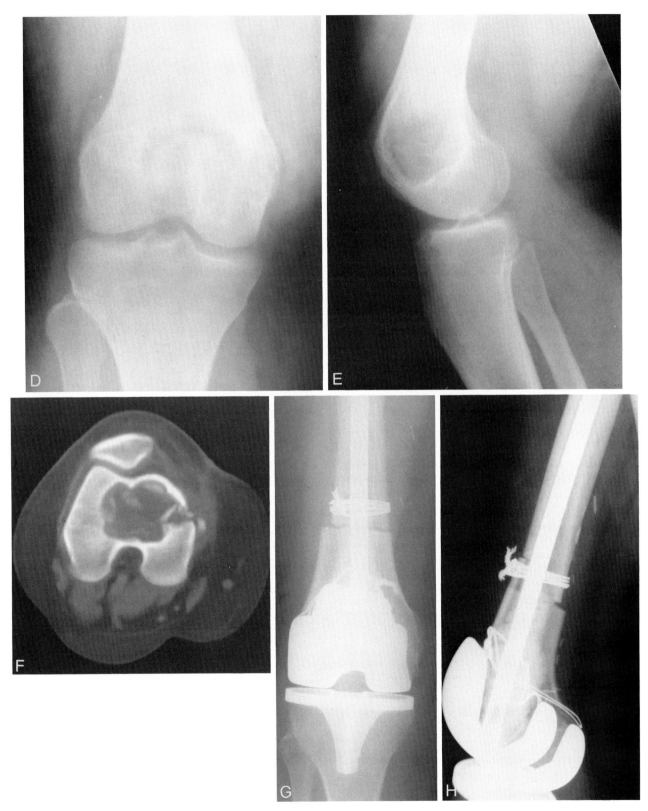

Figure 6.18 *D, E, F, G,* and *H.*

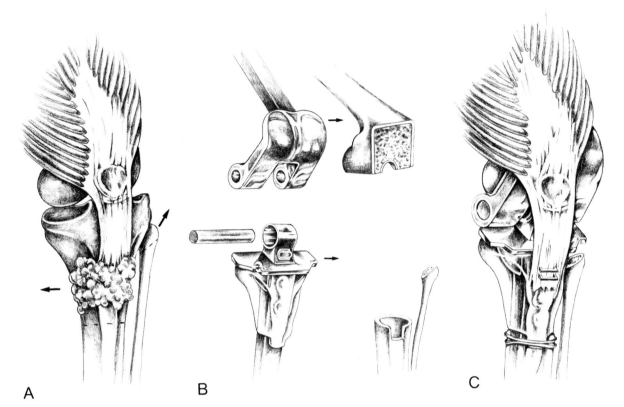

A   B   C

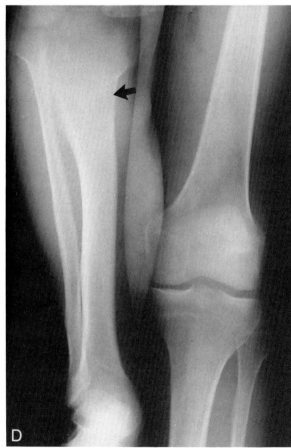

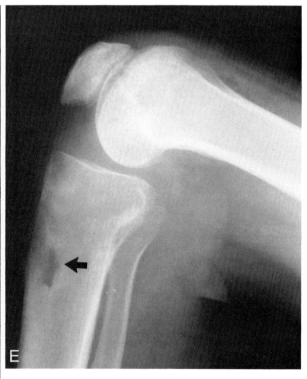

Figure 6.19. Allograft-prosthesis reconstruction of the proximal tibia. *A–C.* Illustrations depicting technique of resection of proximal tibia and replacement by a partially constrained prosthesis combined with an allograft. The tibial stem is cemented to the allograft and osteosynthesis is by press-fit of the long stem, step-cuts to control rotation and cerclage wiring. The patellar tendon is re-attached to the allograft by staples. *D* and *E.* Anteroposterior and lateral radiographs showing a fibrosarcoma of the proximal tibia (*arrow*) in a 47-year-old man (note the extreme flexion deformity of the right knee). *F* and *G.* Magnetic resonance images in coronal and sagittal planes demonstrating intraosseous extent of the tumor. *H* and *I.* Anteroposterior and lateral radiographs of the knee and proximal tibia taken at 6 weeks after reconstruction with allograft-prosthesis (note the osteosynthesis by methylmethacrylate fixation of the stem in the allograft, press-fit in the host bone, step-cuts, and cerclage wires).

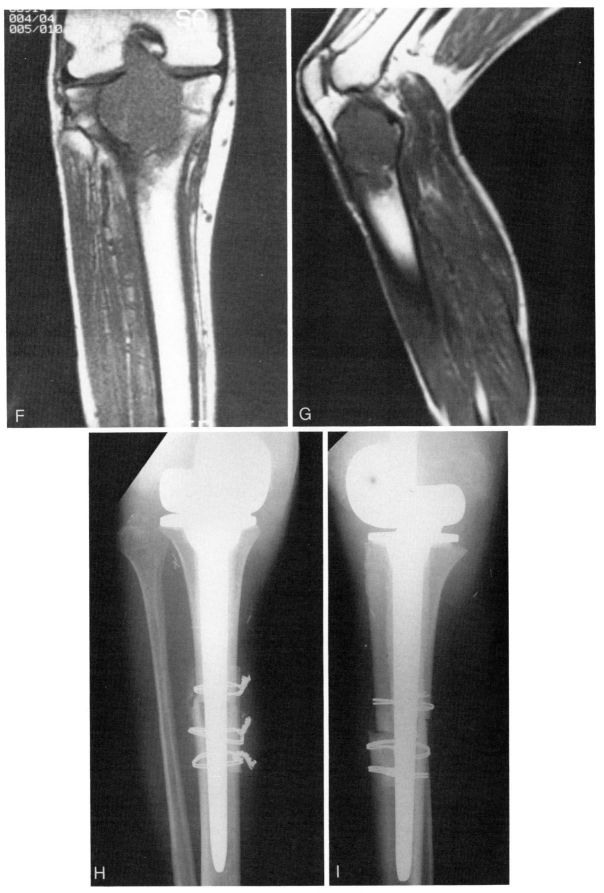

Figure 6.19 *F, G, H,* and *I.*

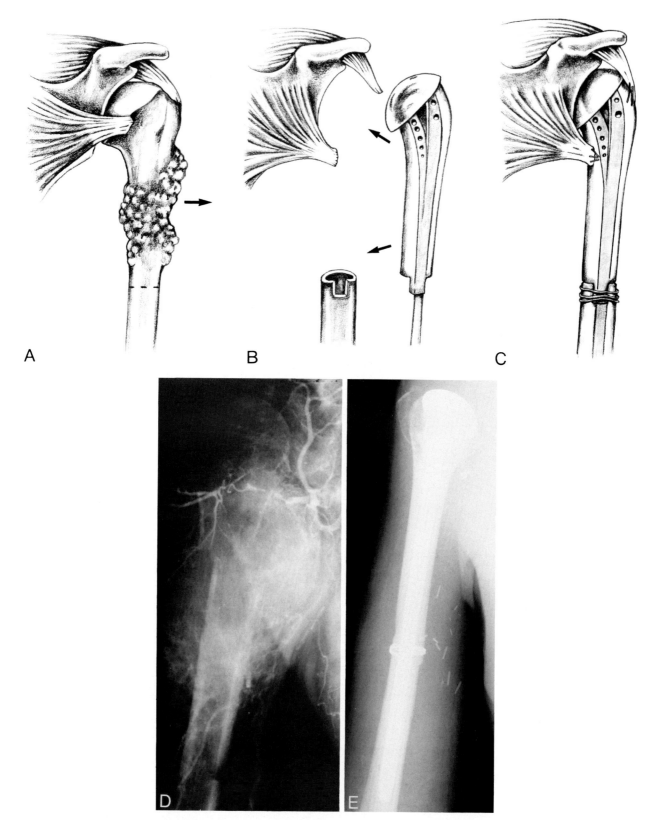

A   B   C

D   E

Figure 6.20. Allograft-prosthesis reconstruction in the proximal humerus with long-stem Neer prosthesis. *A–C.* Illustrations showing the resection of the proximal humerus, reinsertion of rotator cuff and subscapularis tendons into allograft, and reconstruction using long-stem humeral component cemented to allograft, press-fitted into host bone, and stabilized by step-cut and cerclage wiring at osteosynthesis site. *D.* Preoperative angiogram showing pathological fracture of the humerus and large tumor mass (metastatic adenocarcinoma) in 69-year-old man. *E.* Postoperative radiographs at 2 months showing reconstruction with long-stem Neer prosthesis and step-cut osteosynthesis. *F.* Preoperative radiograph showing pathological fracture of proximal humerus and destruction by metastatic carcinoma of the breast in 54-year-old woman. *G.* Postoperative radiographs at 1 month showing reconstruction with long-stem prosthesis cemented into both allograft and host bone.

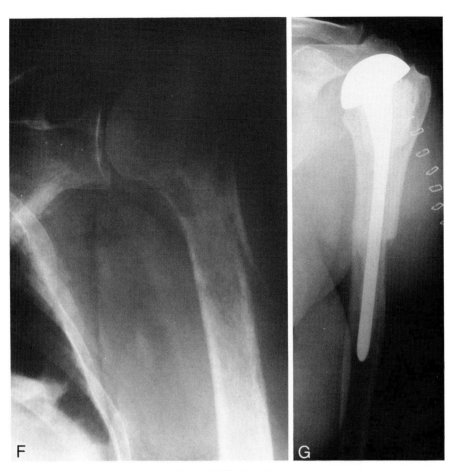

Figure 6.20 *F* and *G*.

(27). The overall satisfactory function in both groups was 80% with an unusually high infection rate of 20% attributed to the magnitude of these operations and to the fact that many of the patients had malignant tumors. Although the two groups studied were not easily comparable, the results of this study showed a lower complication rate and a better success rate (75% compared with 60%) in the allograft-prosthesis group, prompting those investigators to increase the use of composite replacements for proximal femoral reconstruction. Our experience with allograft-prosthetic composite replacements in the proximal femur has been gratifying in both primary tumors and metastatic disease (unpublished results). It is clear, however, that this is just one of many different modalities available for reconstruction at this anatomic site (28).

Proximal Humerus

A recent report has analyzed the experience with cryopreserved osteoarticular allografts for proximal humeral reconstruction in a group of 20 patients, most of whom had benign or low-grade tumors (29). As in other studies, the satisfactory functional results were in the 65–70% range, but it is worthwhile to note that abduction of the shoulder beyond 45° was not restored despite reconstruction procedures of the deltoid and rotator cuff. Most failures were due to infection, the incidence of which was 15%. It is noteworthy that proximal humeral allografts have a high fracture rate (35%) and a low nonunion rate (5%), findings that the authors attribute to the more rapid revascularization and resorption due to reattachment of the rotator cuff and other muscles to the graft. This also results in a relatively high incidence of resorption about the humeral head (25%), suggesting that perhaps an allograft-prosthesis composite would be a better choice of reconstruction at this particular site. This is supported by published experience on the use of this method (30). The various choices of reconstruction methods in the proximal humerus are described in a recently published overview (31).

Infection

This most devastating complication of allograft reconstruction procedures has been investigated in a comprehensive study by the group at the Massachusetts General

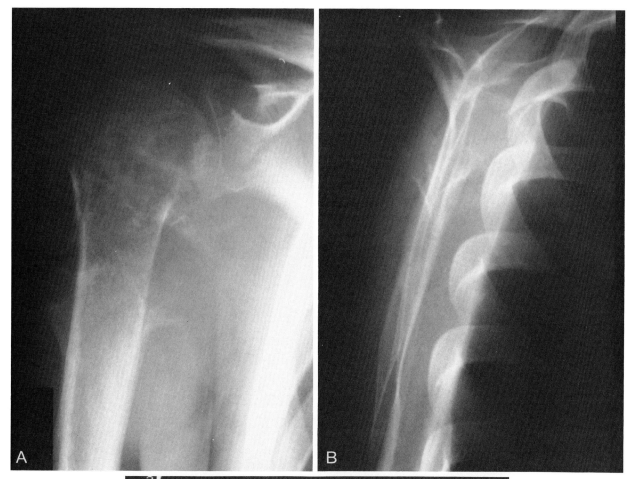

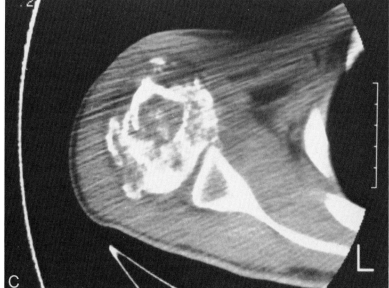

Figure 6.21. Allograft-prosthesis reconstruction in the proximal humerus with regular Neer prosthesis and plate. *A* and *B*. Anteroposterior and lateral radiographs of proximal humerus showing an osteosarcoma in a 19-year-old male patient. *C*. Computerized tomogram showing bone destruction and soft tissue mass in the area of the proximal humerus. *D* and *E*. Anteroposterior and lateral radiographs taken at 2 weeks after reconstruction showing technique with standard Neer prosthesis cemented into the allograft and plate fixation for the control of rotation. *F* and *G*. Anteroposterior and lateral radiographs taken 2 years after the reconstruction showing union at the osteosynthesis site and good maintenance of the integrity of the allograft.

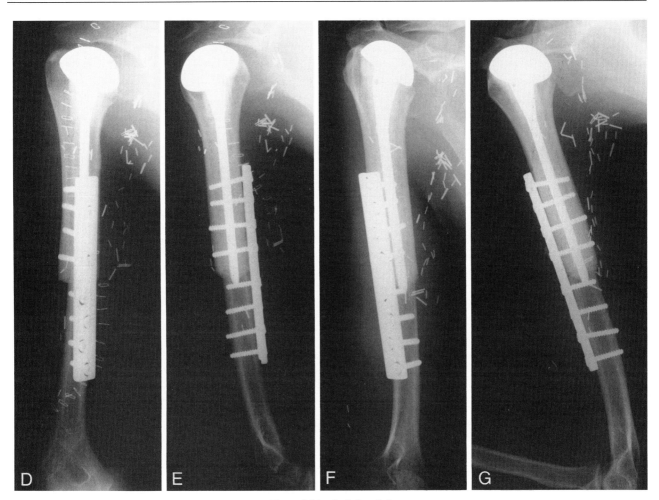

Figure 6.21 *D, E, F,* and *G.*

Hospital (32). Their collection of cases is the largest of all allograft reconstruction series and lends itself to a detailed analysis of factors associated with an overall infection rate of 12% in 283 procedures. Transfer of infection with the graft was found in only one case (0.3%) demonstrating that possible graft contamination is not the cause of high infection rates after this reconstruction procedure. Extensive surgery can be a cause of infection as demonstrated statistically in a subgroup of patients undergoing distal femoral reconstruction. The authors speculate that large allografts are a "locus resistentiae minoris," susceptible to local or systemic infectious agents with the possible contribution of immune mechanisms due to tissue incompatibility. This hypothesis is by no means proven but it is noteworthy that nonunion rates are higher in patients who have an infection suggesting that these two complications can be associated with one another in a possibly immunoreactive host. The possible effect of chemotherapy on infection rates was not demonstrated as only very few patients in this series received it. Overall,

infection is the most devastating complication of allograft reconstruction as shown by the fact that 82% of infected allografts resulted in failures in this study. It is of interest, however, that infected allografts are not a contraindication for a new allograft reconstruction because this can be done successfully using a staged procedure and systemic antibiotics. A recent report on the clinical incidence of infections related to the use of bone allografts from the same group examined a different series of 324 reconstructions using grafts from one bone bank (33). This study confirms that contamination of the allograft is not a factor in causing infection in most cases. The presence of infection after allograft reconstruction in this study was related to the use of large allografts (no infections were recorded after small allografts) and all infections occurred in patients with malignant tumors (10%) or who had a revision joint replacement (5%), suggesting that the extensive surgical dissection increases the risk of clinical infection. When soft tissue complications or factors related to possibly contaminated allografts are excluded, the infection rate in patients with malignant bone tumors drops to 5% and is comparable to infection rates recorded in patients receiving metallic prosthetic implants for reconstruction after the excision of bone tumors (4, 5).

Fracture

Interesting information about fractures of allografts used in the reconstruction after tumor excisions has come recently from a study by the Massachusetts General Hospital group that analyzed in depth this particular complication (34). It is based on an analysis of 43 fractures in 274 patients who received massive allografts after tumor excision. The risk for fracture begins after the first 6 months after surgery, peaks after 2–3 years (mean 28.6 months), and is practically nil after 4 years. This suggests a biological stability of allografts after union and accomodation to normal weight-bearing or functional demands despite the lack of extensive remodeling or revascularization. Fractures do not correlate with any potential risk factors except with the incidence of nonunion of allografts. This unexpected correlation suggests that instability and micromotion in an ununited graft may play a role in causing mechanical fatigue with subsequent fracturing. Chemotherapy has no apparent effect inasmuch as only six of 43 patients with fractures in this study received adjuvant treatment. The classification of fractures into three categories: type I (rapid dissolution of the graft), type II (fracture of the shaft), and type III (fragmentation of the joint) is useful to devise appropriate treatment modalities. Type I fractures (which are rare) require replacement of the graft; type II fractures can be treated by osteosynthesis and autogenous bone grafting; and type III fractures are managed by conventional prosthetic replacement into allograft bone. It is interesting that type II fractures can actually heal by conventional techniques used to treat living bone, albeit they do not do it with a predictable success rate (30% union). Overall, allograft fractures can be salvaged successfully in 80% of cases making this complication one of the least problematic ones in this type of reconstructive surgery.

Nonunion

The issue of delayed union of allografts in patients receiving concomitant neoadjuvant or adjuvant chemotherapy has been investigated recently by Delepine et al. (35). These studies demonstrate that chemotherapy delays bone union of allografts to host bone, particularly when methotrexate is used. The average healing time at the allograft-host osteosynthesis site in this study was 75 days in the absence of chemotherapy. This increased to 175 days on

adriamycin-endoxan and to 246 days on a T10 protocol using methotrexate. These findings confirm experimental and clinical studies looking at the effect of chemotherapeutic agents on bone healing in autogenous systems (36–38). Delayed union can be treated readily by autogenous bone grafting and, therefore, is not as much of a problem as other complications seen in allograft surgery. While chemotherapy delays union, it has no apparent effect on the ultimate rate of other major complications and, therefore, allograft reconstruction with concomitant neoadjuvant or adjuvant chemotherapy is not contraindicated (39).

CONCLUSION

Allograft reconstruction in orthopaedic oncological surgery is clearly a valuable method to restore skeletal defects. Its use demands attention to surgical detail and technical principles that are characteristic to this modality of treatment and the discussion of which, by necessity, can only be limited in a text like this. As experience grows, more and more pitfalls and technical failures can be avoided, thereby increasing the success rate and decreasing the complication rate of this procedure. This requires an open and critical attitude when analyzing the clinical results of this and of alternative modalities of reconstruction. The ultimate aim is an individualized choice of reconstruction for the particular problem and for the specific patient, be it allograft, prosthetic replacement, autograft, or a combination of these techniques.

REFERENCES

1. Enneking WF, Eady JL, Burchardt H. Autogenous cortical bone grafts in the reconstruction of segmental skeletal defects. J Bone Joint Surg 1980; 62A:1039.
2. Weiland AJ, Moore JR, Daniel RK. Vascularized bone autografts. Experience with 41 cases. Clin Orthop 1983; 174:87.
3. Wood MB. Free vascularized bone transfers for nonunions, segmental gaps, and following tumor resection. Orthopedics 1986; 9:810.
4. Bradish CF, Kemp HBS, Scales JT, Wilson JN. Distal femoral replacement by custom-made prostheses. Clinical follow-up and survivorship analysis. J Bone Joint Surg 1987; 69B:276.
5. Sim FH, Beauchamp CP, Chao EYS. Reconstruction of musculoskeletal defects about the knee for tumor. Clin Orthop 1987; 221:188.
6. Enneking WF. A system of staging musculoskeletal neoplasms. Clin Orthop 1986; 204:9.
7. Ottolenghi CE. Massive osteo and osteo-articular bone grafts: technique and results of 62 cases. Clin Orthop 1972; 87:156.
8. Parish FF. Allograft replacement of part of a long bone following

excision of a tumor: report of twenty-one cases. J Bone Joint Surg 1973; 55A:1.

9. Volkov MV, Immaliyev AS. Use of allogenous articular bone implants as substitutes for autotransplants in adult patients. Clin Orthop 1976; 114:192.

10. Mankin HJ, Doppelt S, Tomford W. Clinical experience with allograft implantation. The first ten years. Clin Orthop 1983; 174:69.

11. Gross AE, McKee N, Farine I, Czitrom A, Langer F. Reconstruction of skeletal defects following en-bloc excision of bone tumors. In: Uhtoff HK (ed). Current Concepts of Diagnosis and Treatment of Bone and Soft Tissue Tumors. Springer-Verlag, Berlin, Heidelberg, 1984; p. 163.

12. Makley JT. The use of allografts to reconstruct intercalary defects of long bones. Clin Orthop 1985; 197:58.

13. Mnaymneh W, Malinin TI, Makley JT, Dick HM. Massive osteoarticular allografts in the reconstruction of extremities following resection of tumors not requiring chemotherapy and radiation. Clin Orthop 1985; 197:76.

14. Dick HM, Malinin TI, Mnaymneh W. Massive allograft implantation following radical resection of high grade tumors requiring adjuvant chemotherapy treatment. Clin Orthop 1985; 197:88.

15. Aho A. Half joint transplantation in human bone tumors. Int Orthop 1985; 9:77.

16. Poitout D, Novakovitch G. The use of allografts for replacement of major defects in bone. Int Orthop 1987; 11:169.

17. Delloye C, de Nayer P, Allington N, Munting E, Coutelier L, Vincent A. Massive bone allografts in large skeletal defects after tumor surgery: a clinical and microradiographic evaluation. Arch Orthop Trauma Surg 1988; 107:31.

18. Alho A, Karaharju EO, Korkala O, Laasonen EM, Holstrom T, Muller C. Allogeneic grafts for bone tumor. Acta Orthop Scand 1989; 60:143.

19. Delepine G, Hernigou P, Goutallier D, Delepine N. Orthopaedic results of 87 massive allografts in reconstructive surgery for bone cancers. In: Aebi M, Regazzoni P (eds). Bone Transplantation. Springer-Verlag, Berlin, Heidelberg, 1989; p. 331.

20. Mnaymneh W, Malinin T. Massive allografts in surgery of bone tumors. Orthop Clin North Am 1989; 20:455.

21. Czitrom AA, Langer F, Bell RS, Shahin AM. Allograft reconstruction for bone metastases. In: Langlais F, Tomeno B (eds). Limb Salvage—Major Reconstructions in Oncologic and Nontumoral Conditions. Springer-Verlag, Berlin, Heidelberg, 1991; p. 733.

22. Enneking WF. Modification of the system for functional evaluation of surgical management of musculoskeletal tumors. In: Enneking WF (ed). Limb Salvage in Musculoskeletal Oncology. Churchill Livingstone, New York, 1987; p. 626.

23. Bell RS, Davis A, Allan DG, Langer F, Czitrom AA, Gross AE. Fresh osteochondral allografts for advanced giant cell tumors at the knee. J Bone Joint Surg (Br) (submitted for publication).

24. Bell RS, Davis A, Langer F, Czitrom AA, Gross AE. Reconstruction of primary malignant knee tumors using irradiated allograft bone. J Bone Joint Surg (Br) 1991; (in press).

25. Czitrom AA, Keating S, Gross AE. The viability of cartilage in fresh osteochondral grafts after clinical transplantation. J Bone Joint Surg 1990; 72A:574.

26. Kneisl JS, Finn HA, Simon MA. Mobile knee reconstruction after resection of malignant tumors of the distal femur. Orthop Clin North Am 1991; 22:105.

27. Jofe MH, Gebhardt MC, Tomford WW, Mankin HJ. Reconstruction for defects of the proximal part of the femur using allograft arthroplasty. J Bone Joint Surg 1988; 70A:507.

28. Johnson ME, Mankin HJ. Reconstruction after resections of tumors involving the proximal femur. Orthop Clin North Am 1991; 22:87.

29. Gebhardt MC, Roth YF, Mankin HJ. Osteoarticular allografts for reconstruction in the proximal part of the humerus after excision of a musculoskeletal tumor. J Bone Joint Surg 1990; 72A:334.

30. Rock M. Intercalary allograft and custom Neer prosthesis after en bloc resection of the proximal humerus. In: Enneking WF (ed). Limb Salvage in Musculoskeletal Oncology. Churchill Livingstone, New York, 1987; p. 586.

31. Cheng EY, Gebhardt MC. Allograft reconstruction of the shoulder after bone tumor resections. Orthop Clin North Am 1991; 22:37.

32. Lord CF, Gebhardt MC, Tomford WW, Mankin HJ. Infection in bone allografts. Incidence, nature and treatment. J Bone Joint Surg 1988; 70A:369.

33. Tomford WW, Thongphasuk J, Mankin HJ, Ferraro MJ. Frozen musculoskeletal allografts. A study of the clinical incidence and causes of infection associated with their use. J Bone Joint Surg 1990; 72A:1137.

34. Berrey H, Lord F, Gebhardt MC, Mankin HJ. Fractures of allografts. Frequency, treatment, and end-results. J Bone Joint Surg 1990; 72A:825.

35. Delepine N, Delepine G, Hernigou P, Hassan M, Desbois JC. Bone union of allografts and chemotherapy. Consideration about 55 consecutive cases. In: Aebi M, Regazzoni P (eds). Bone Transplantation. Springer-Verlag, Berlin, Heidelberg, 1989; p. 333.

36. Burchardt H, Glowczewskie FP, Enneking WF. The effect of adriamycin and methotrexate on repair of segmental cortical autografts in dogs. J Bone Joint Surg 1983; 65A:103.

37. Friedlaender GE, Tross RB, Doganis A, Kirkwood JM, Baron R. Effects of chemotherapeutic agents on bone. I. Short-term methotrexate and doxorubicin (adriamycin) treatment in a rat model. J Bone Joint Surg 1984; 66A:602.

38. Winkelmann W, Jurgens H. The influence of pre- and postoperative polydrug chemotherapy on bone healing in tumor surgery. In: Aebi M, Regazzoni P (eds). Bone Transplantation. Springer-Verlag, Berlin, Heidelberg, 1989; p. 335.

39. Czitrom A, Capanna R, Donati D, Bacci G, Campanacci M. Segmental allograft reconstruction concomitant with neoadjuvant chemotherapy. In: Langlais F, Tomeno B (eds). Limb Salvage—Major Reconstructions in Oncologic and Nontumoral Conditions. Springer-Verlag, Berlin, Heidelberg, 1991; p. 95.

7

ALLOGRAFTS IN PELVIC ONCOLOGY SURGERY

Robert S. Bell and Cameron B. Guest

Bone tumors arising in the pelvis present particular difficulties in both diagnosis and treatment (1–22). The large internal capacity of the pelvis often permits tumors to grow to substantial size prior to diagnosis and, all too frequently, the early symptoms of a deep-seated pelvic tumor are misinterpreted as sciatic or degenerative lumbar spine pain (Fig. 7.1). When a primary or secondary tumor is eventually diagnosed in the pelvis, a variety of factors can make appropriate treatment difficult. The fascial compartments of the pelvis are not as well defined as they are in the extremities and extracompartmental tumor origin and spread beyond fascial boundaries is the rule rather than the exception. Biopsy is often difficult since the usual surgical approach to the pelvis may involve exposure of neurovascular structures that would be contaminated by open biopsy techniques. The proximity of neurovascular and visceral structures complicates the resection of pelvic tumors and may result in intraoperative complications. Finally, the importance of the pelvis in transferring load from the lower extremity to the spine makes reconstruction of the bony defect remaining following tumor resection both critically important in determining functional outcome and difficult to achieve.

In this chapter, we will review the role that allograft bone can assume in pelvic reconstruction of primary and secondary neoplasms. To place the issues of reconstruction in an appropriate context, some general aspects of oncological management of pelvic tumors will be discussed further.

STAGING AND BIOPSY OF THE PATIENT WITH A PELVIC TUMOR

Staging

All patients with primary or secondary pelvic tumors should undergo systemic and local staging. Most symptomatic lesions in the pelvis result from metastatic spread of a carcinoma and, in general, these patients will present with a history of known primary cancer elsewhere. Patients presenting with pelvic lesions and no history of primary

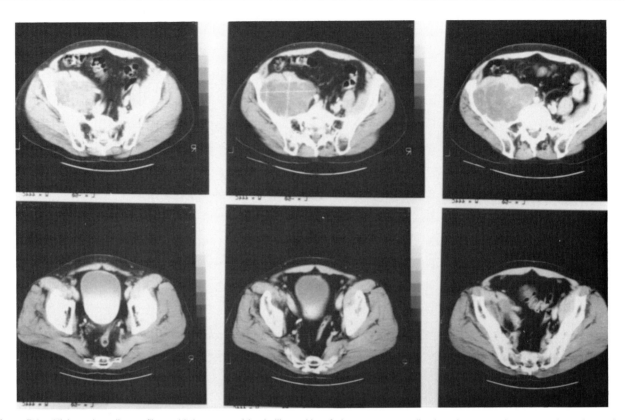

Figure 7.1. High-grade malignant fibrous histiocytoma arising in ilium with soft tissue mass extending into the retroperitoneum and anterior to the sacrum. The patient is free of local and systemic disease 52 months after local resection and adjuvant chemotherapy.

tumors elsewhere should, however, be suspected of having a primary tumor, especially if the bony lesion is solitary. Physical examination (with particular attention to the lymph nodes, thyroid, breast, and prostate) as well as a complete blood count, erythrocyte sedimentation rate, calcium, phosphorus, alkaline and acid phosphatase (or prostate specific antigen), serum immune electrophoresis, urinalysis, chest x-ray, mammogram, and abdominal ultrasound will serve to identify most primary carcinomas in patients presenting with metastatic disease without a history of a known cancer. Further systemic investigations should include a total-body technetium bone scan, which is useful in determining the bone remodeling activity at the lesion in the pelvis and in determining the existence of other bony lesions (metastatic from a primary carcinoma or, much less commonly, metastatic or metachronous disease associated with a pelvic bone sarcoma).

Following the initial history, physical examination, and simple laboratory and radiographic investigations, the clinician should have a reasonably accurate concept as to the etiology of the pelvic lesion. If there is a history of a primary tumor elsewhere, or if a probably primary

site is identified during the initial work-up, there may be no need for a diagnostic biopsy. If, however, no primary carcinoma is identified or if the radiographic changes in the pelvis are typical of a primary (as opposed to metastatic) bone tumor, biopsy is indicated; but first, local and systemic radiographic staging should be completed. Chest CT should be performed prior to biopsy to identify early pulmonary metastatic lesions and CT and/or MRI (23) of the local site should be utilized to determine the extent of the pelvic lesion and the most appropriate approach for biopsy.

The next step in staging a primary tumor of the pelvis requires tissue sampling to determine a pathological diagnosis. The surgical technique used in biopsying a pelvic primary tumor can either facilitate or markedly complicate the eventual definitive resection.

Biopsy

It is a well-accepted principle of primary bone tumor surgery that the surgeon who is likely to perform the eventual tumor resection should also do the biopsy and the pelvis is one of the most important anatomical examples of this truism (24, 25). Pelvic sarcoma resections are difficult procedures at best and, if complicated by an inappropriate biopsy, may be entirely impossible due to tumor contamination. In assessing the location of pelvic lesions prior to biopsy, the surgeon can divide the bony pelvis into safe and unsafe zones for an open biopsy. Lesions arising in the ilium, supra-acetabular region, sacrum, or the medial portions of the superior/inferior rami can be biopsied through straightforward open procedures. Tumors arising in the anterior or posterior columns of the acetabulum present particular problems for biopsy, however.

Many pelvic lesions can be biopsied through a simple subperiosteal iliac wing approach. Tumors of the ilium or the supra-acetabular bone can be biopsied through an iliac incision with muscle stripping of the inner or outer table. Lesions presenting with an outer or inner iliac table soft tissue mass should be approached for biopsy by stripping the gluteus or iliacus muscles, respectively. If the lesion is intraosseous without a soft tissue mass, care should be taken while broaching the cortex to avoid needless tumor contamination of normal soft tissues. The most frequent intraosseous location without cortical breakthrough is in the supra-acetabular bone. These lesions are best approached by a careful elevation of the gluteus minimus from the bone. Using the muscle to contain biopsy hematoma and then resecting this muscle at the definite resection permits the surgeon to conserve the gluteus medius as an abductor.

Sacral lesions should always be biopsied through a posterior (rather than a transrectal) approach. Transrectal biopsy not only contaminates the rectum with tumor (requiring colostomy for adequate tumor resection), but also may result in bacterial contamination of the sacral lesion.

The anterior pelvis (pubic ramus and medial portion of the superior and inferior pubic ramus) can be safely reached through transverse incisions that can later be incorporated in an ilioinguinal excision. The presence of the sciatic nerve and the femoral neurovascular structures make open biopsy of the posterior and anterior acetabular column regions difficult to achieve without hindering the eventual sarcoma resection. For lesions arising in these areas, we prefer needle biopsy under fluoroscopic or CT guidance to minimize the surgical exposure necessary for biopsy. It is a critical mistake, for example, to expose and displace the femoral nerve and vessels during an open biopsy of a tumor arising in the anterior acetabular column. Although exposure of the vessels may be necessary to protect these structures during open biopsy, the contamination of nerve and vessel by tumor

exposed during the biopsy markedly complicates later tumor resection.

Clinical Staging

Following biopsy and evaluation of the local and systemic radiological studies, the lesion should be staged using Enneking's system adopted by the Musculoskeletal Tumor Society (26–29). This would apply to primary (as opposed to metastatic) bone tumors.

Based on the pathological interpretation of the biopsy, the lesion should be graded as 0, I, or II. Grade 0 lesions have no potential for metastasis (e.g., enchondroma, osteocartilaginous exostosis, fibrous dysplasia); grade I lesions have a low risk of metastases; and grade II lesions have a high risk of metastases. Grade III primary bone tumors are those that have metastatic disease evident at presentation. In addition to the pathological grade of the tumor, radiographs should be analyzed to determine whether the lesions are isolated to the compartment of origin (A lesions) or are extracompartmental (B lesions).

The clinical staging is critical in deciding what treatment is necessary. In deciding what type of operation is indicated for primary pelvic tumors, consideration of both the anatomical site of origin and the histology of the tumor is necessary.

OPTIMAL ONCOLOGICAL MANAGEMENT OF PRIMARY PELVIC NEOPLASMS

Three basic options are availabe in planning limb salvage surgical removal of a primary pelvic tumor: intralesional removal, marginal resection, or wide resection. In general, tumors with very low risk of metastasis (grade 0 lesions, such as enchondroma, for example) can be treated with intralesional curettage, often in combination with adjuvant treatment of the tumor bed (phenol or liquid nitrogen). However, low-grade tumors with a high risk of local recurrence (for example, giant cell tumor), are perhaps better managed by wide or marginal excision if the lesion arises in "disposable" portions of the pubis (e.g., ilium, ischium). The difficulty of treating recurrent, locally aggressive lesions in the pelvis often suggests that marginal excision is a better treatment than curettage since local recurrence risk is lower. However, resection of benign lesions should not be undertaken if a substantial functional deficit will result.

The most common low-grade malignant lesion of the pelvis is the grade I chondrosarcoma (Fig. 7.2) These tumors, although unlikely to metastasize early in their

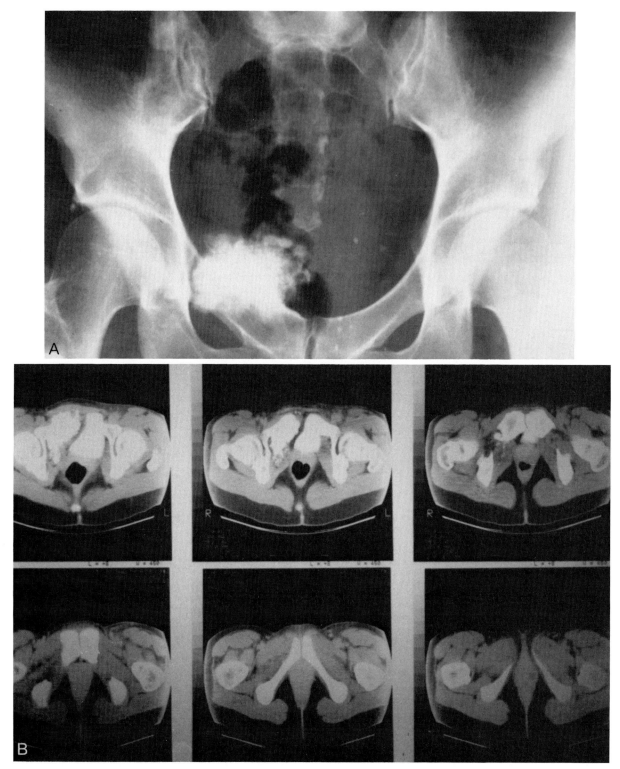

Figure 7.2. A–E. Low-grade chondrosarcoma arising (probably in a solitary osteochondroma) from the superior pubic ramus and extending to the quadrilateral plate. Reconstruction with a hemiacetabular allograft with cryopreserved articular cartilage was complicated by myositis ossificans but, at 42-month follow-up, the patient maintains 50° of hip flexion, walks with one cane, and suffers minimal pain.

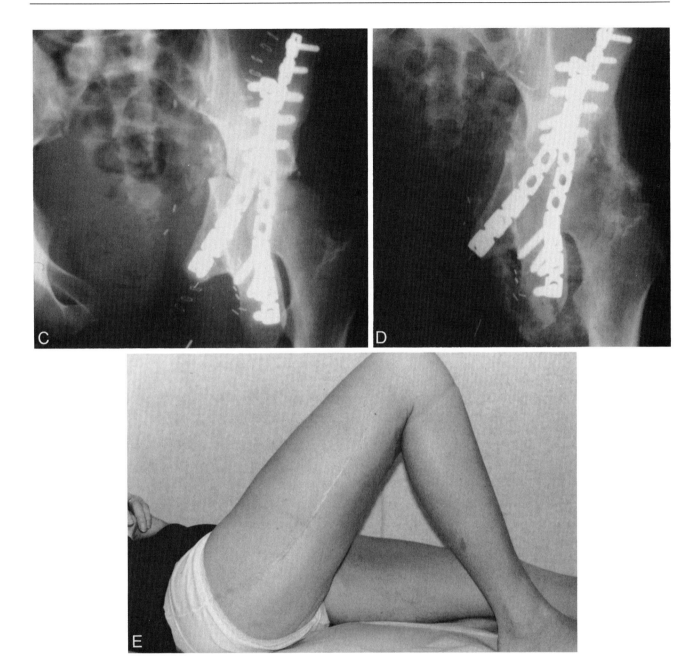

Figure 7.2. *C, D,* and *E.*

course, have a high risk of local relapse if not completely excised and may eventually metastasize if not controlled locally. These lesions are best treated by wide excision. Not infrequently, adequate resection may result in pelvic instability or compromise the acetabular bone stock requiring reconstruction of the defect.

High-grade lesions of the pelvis are particularly difficult tumors to resect. Generally, these lesions present at IIB stage with extension of the tumor into the soft tissues. Since these tumors require wide resection to pre-

vent local recurrence, extracompartmental spread is a negative prognostic feature for adequate excision. Although amputation by hemipelvectomy is preferable to an inadequate wide resection, the soft tissue extension from high-grade sarcomas often results in a medial soft tissue mass abutting the retroperitoneal space. The surgical margin for amputation of this lesion is often no better than the margin achieved by an internal hemipelvectomy (limb salvage surgery).

High-grade bone sarcomas are often responsive to

chemotherapy and administration of chemotherapeutic drugs prior to surgery (neoadjuvant treatment) may cause substantial shrinkage in the extraosseous mass (30–32). Well-established protocols for osteosarcomas and Ewing's sarcomas have demonstrated a definite adjuvant role for cytotoxic drugs in these two diseases. Preoperative or postoperative radiotherapy is frequently employed in Ewing's sarcoma to facilitate local resection and to decrease the risk of local recurrence. High-grade chondrosarcoma, on the other hand, is not known to respond to chemotherapy and preoperative, neoadjuvant treatment is not generally employed in this disease.

OPERATIVE APPROACHES FOR RESECTION OF PELVIC SARCOMAS

The surgical approach to intralesional removal of bone tumors is generally straightforward and will not be discussed further. Selecting the best approach to limb salvage resection of malignant primary bone tumors is, however, frequently a major factor in preoperative decision-making. Two basic approaches to pelvic lesions (the ilioinguinal and iliofemoral approaches) will be described.

The ilioinguinal approach is very useful for the resection of lesions arising anterior to the acetabulum and especially for tumors that require extensive retroperioto-

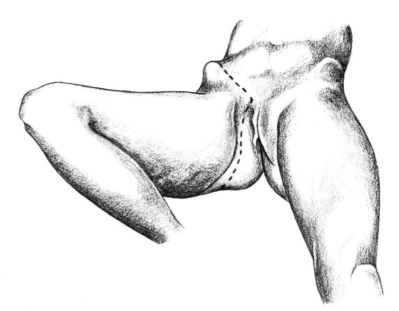

Figure 7.3. Medial view of extended ilioinguinal approach. The incision runs laterally along the iliac crease and then is directed posteriorly from the pubic tubercle to the ischium. The posterior extension of the standard ilioinguinal approach permits exposure of the ischium and inferior pubic ramus.

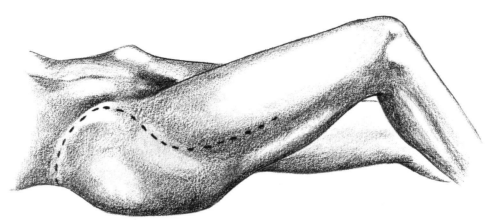

Figure 7.4. Lateral view of the iliofemoral approach. Following stripping of the outer table of the ilium and trochanteric osteotomy, excellent exposure of the sciatic notch and posterior column is afforded but limited access to the medial pelvis is available.

neal dissection of medial soft tissue extension or division of the anterior pelvis at the symphysis or through the contralateral hemipelvis. The iliofemoral approach, on the other hand, provides less exposure to the medial and midline structures but offers better exposure of the posterior column.

Ilioinguinal Approach

The ilioinguinal approach is predominantly used for tumors of the anterior column, anterior pelvis, or lesions that extend to the quadrilateral plate. Exposure of the posterior column is only available after dislocation of the hip and/or resection of the femoral head. If wide exposure to the posterior column is necessary in reconstruction (e.g., for plating the posterior column in an allograft acetabular reconstruction), a second posterior Kocher-Langenbeck incision can be used as long as the superior gluteal artery is carefully protected during dissection. This vessel supports the skin bridge between the two wounds and is critical to uncomplicated wound healing.

In the approach to an anterior pelvic tumor, the retroperitoneal exposure is performed first. The abdominal wall muscles are detached from the ilium and the femoral nerve and vessels are dissected and freed from the anterior column. Prior exposure of the neurovascular structures at the time of biopsy markedly complicates this step. The bladder is packed away from the symphysis and the dissection plane is deepened medial to the obturator internus (which covers the medial quadrilateral plate). The obturator nerve and vessels are identified and either ligated or dissected to the obturator foramen. If the ischium is to be resected, we carry the medial incision posteriorly through the groin and parallel to the inferior pubic ramus to the ischium (Fig. 7.3). Depending on the extent of the adductor soft tissue mass, the adductors can be detached at a variable distance from the outer pelvis. The psoas tendon is identified, divided, and allowed to retract proximally after placement of a "tagging" suture for later repair. If the surgeon plans to dislocate the hip (as opposed to en bloc, extra-articular resection of the joint), the capsule is now divided and the femoral head is displaced anteriorly.

In the ilioinguinal approach, there is easy access to osteotomy of the symphysis pubis or the pubic rami. By subperiosteal stripping of the outer iliac table (if no lateral soft tissue mass is evident), the sciatic notch can be easily exposed and the ilium can be divided using a Gigli saw. By continuing the infero-medial dissection plane medial to the ischium, both the sacrotuberous and the sacrospinous ligaments can be divided. After the ham-

strings have been detached from the ischium (with or without attached bone), the only remaining structures to divide are the pelvic floor muscles. Using this approach, resection of the pelvis from the sacrum to the symphysis pubis can be achieved.

Iliofemoral Approach

This approach is more appropriate for lesions of the ilium that have lateral soft tissue extension or for tumors arising in or around the acetabulum that require extraarticular en bloc excision of the hip. The chief deficiencies of this approach are that (a) division of the pelvis far medial to the acetabulum is difficult; (b) a large posterior flap is turned from the outer iliac table, which is largely dependent on the gluteal vessels for blood supply. If the gluteals are damaged or resected, there is a substantial risk of wound complications.

A curvilinear incision is made parallel to the iliac crest turning distally down the leg a variable distance from the superior iliac spine (Fig. 7.4). Retroperitoneal dissection (or subperiosteal dissection, if there is no medial soft tissue mass) is carried out and the femoral neurovascular structures are pushed in a medial direction. The glutei (if not invaded by tumor) are then dissected from the outer table while protecting (if possible) the gluteal vessels. To relax the gluteal muscles and neurovascular strucures, the trochanter may be osteotomized and displaced posteriorly. Trochanteric osteotomy is particulary useful if extra-articular hip resection is intended.

Reflection of the gluteal flap permits access to the posterior column by dissecting superficial to or deep to the external rotators. The sciatic nerve is often freed from the tumor during this dissection. Posterior osteotomy can be accomplished at the sciatic notch or further back at the sacroiliac joint. Although it is possible to retract the medial flap as far as the symphysis pubis, in most cases, the superior pubic ramus is divided medial to the acetabulum and the inferior pubic ramus is divided anterior to the ischium.

PLANNING RECONSTRUCTION—AN ANATOMICAL APPROACH

In determining whether reconstruction of the bony pelvis is required, Enneking's zonal classification of the pelvic skeleton (33) is worthwhile (Fig. 7.5). Zone I lesions arising proximal to the acetabulum may require resection of all or a portion of the ilium with resultant destabilization of the posterior pelvic ring. If only a small portion of the sacroiliac joint remains intact, fusion of this joint

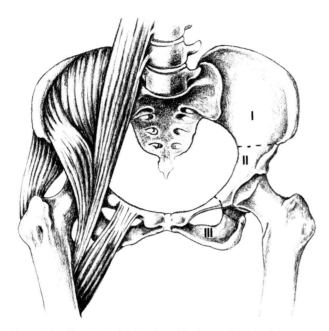

Figure 7.5. Enneking's classification of the bony origin of pelvis tumors. Periacetabular (zone II) lesions represent the most common indication for reconstruction using allograft.

is generally successful. If the weight-bearing zone between acetabulum and sacrum is totally deficient, we prefer to use an autogenous graft harvested from the ilium to bridge this defect (Fig. 7.6). Although allograft could be utilized to bridge the skeletal deficit, our preference is to avoid the use of allograft in the pelvis unless there is no other option.

For patients who have small but complete deficiencies of the posterior pelvis, we have resorted to sacroiliac pseudarthrosis as definitive management. The resected posterior gap is not reconstructed and autogenous bone grafts are placed in the gap between the residual ilium and the sacrum. Patients are permitted progressive weight bearing starting about 1 month postoperatively. With time, a stable pseudarthrosis of the resected region will develop. Four patients whom we have treated in this manner have gone on to a pain-free result (Fig. 7.7).

Zone III lesions arise from the anterior pelvis medial to the acetabulum. We have not generally reconstructed these deficits unless the acetabulum is also deficient. The intact sacroiliac ligaments, as well as the stout sacrotuberous and sacrospinous ligaments serve to stabilize the residual pelvis. Often, patients will complain of posterior pelvic pain when starting to ambulate following surgery. This pain generally resolves over the first year postoperatively. In our initial series of patients undergoing pelvic resection, seven patients with anterior defects were

noted to have no pain or minor pain at one-year follow-up.

Tumors that require acetabular resection (Enneking zone II) present one of the most difficult reconstructive challenges in orthopaedic oncology (34–41). Transmission of force from the lower extremity to the spine through a mobile yet stable articulation is the goal and a variety of techniques can be utilized to reconstruct the defect left by acetabular excision. Basically, four options are available: prosthetic replacement, fusion, pseudarthrosis, or allograft implant composite.

The most commonly used prosthetic component is the iliofemoral prosthesis. If sufficient bone stock remains in the ilium to stabilize the implant, this "saddle" prosthesis can result in excellent stability and mobility (42). The prosthesis is dependent, however, on the availability of sufficient iliac bone oriented in horizontal position to permit stable articulation of the prosthesis.

Arthrodesis of the femur to the residual ilium or ischium offers the advantage of avoiding prosthetic or allogeneic material in reconstructing a stable linkage between spine and pelvis (5, 14). Although fusion, by definition, eliminates motion between the pelvis and the lower extremity, the mobility of the lumbar spine is sufficient to permit flexion and extension, as well as some rotation of the pelvis and leg. If sufficient bone remains after tumor resection to permit fusion of the femoral head to the ilium without marked leg shortening, this procedure is probably optimal for acetabular reconstruction. The patient avoids the long-term risks of allograft or prosthetic implantation and does not require periarticular musculature to maintain hip stability. Indeed, one of the major advantages of arthrodesis compared with either a prosthesis or allograft implant is that, if no abductor or flexor muscles remain after tumor resection, the patient with a fused hip can ambulate with a minimal limp.

The chief drawbacks of arthrodesis relate to limb shortening and difficulty in achieving fusion. Periarticular lesions frequently involve the hip joint, requiring extra-articular resection of the proximal femur as well as the acetabulum. If the superior acetabulum dome and ilium are also resected, iliofemoral fusion will result in dramatic limb shortening. Although ischiofemoral arthrodesis can be utilized in this situation, fusion to the ischium is considerably more difficult to achieve.

Although iliofemoral arthrodesis is technically more straightforward (with available Cobra-plate fixation hardware) than the ischiofemoral operation, even this fusion is difficult to achieve. Indeed, in most series, the fusion

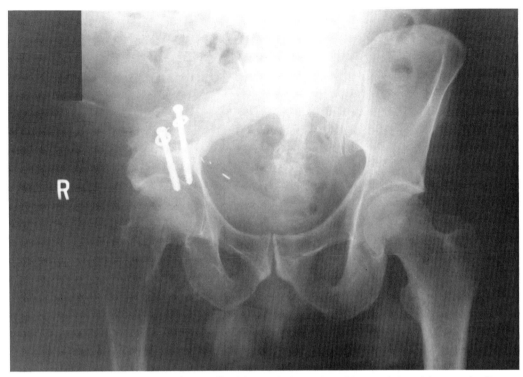

Figure 7.6. A grade II chondrosarcoma arising at the sacroiliac joint required resection of the sacral ala and the posterior ilium as well as the sacroiliac joint. The superior iliac crest was used to stabilize the posterior pelvis.

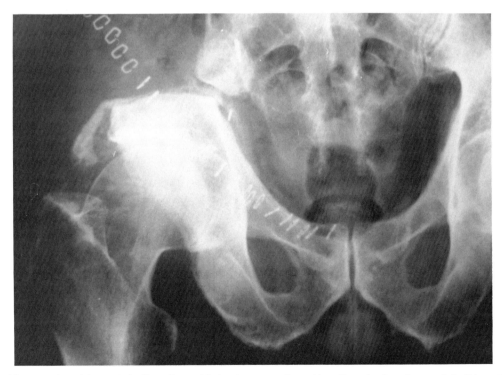

Figure 7.7. After resection of the posterior ilium, the acetabular dome was allowed to collapse back on the sacral ala. This acetabular-sacral pseudarthrosis resulted in minimal pain and about 3 cm of limb length discrepancy.

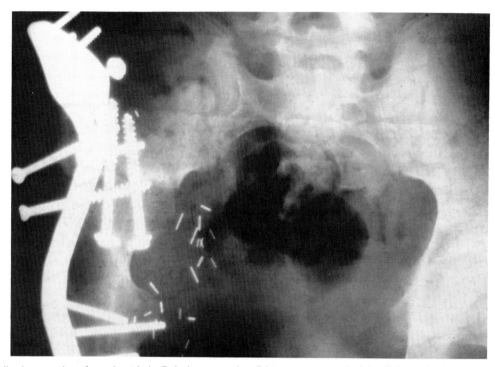

Figure 7.8.   Following resection of a periacetabular Ewing's sarcoma that did not penetrate to the joint, iliofemoral arthrodesis was achieved with intrafragmentary fixation and a neutralizing Cobra plate.

rate is about 50%. Although iliofemoral pseudarthrosis is said to provide a reasonable result, the chance of pain on weight bearing is greater with pseudarthrosis than with a solid fusion.

In general, following a transarticular resection with preservation of the femoral head and neck and a reasonable portion of the ilium, we would recommend an iliofemoral fusion using intrafragmentary fixation neutralized by a Cobra plate (Fig. 7.8). If, however, the femoral neck is excised in the course of tumor resection or if iliofemoral fusion will result in more than 5.0 cm of shortening, we would suggest that the patient undergo allograft implant composite reconstruction. In this situation, if the composite graft fails, the alternative procedures for reconstruction (saddle prosthesis, ischiofemoral arthodesis, flail hip) would still be available after removal of the graft.

As mentioned previously, there are relatively few indications for the use of allograft bone in reconstructing the pelvis following primary tumor excision. We would not recommend using allograft for lesions that do not involve the acetabulum and, even in periacetabular tumors, we prefer an iliofemoral fusion if the femoral head is intact and only a small portion of ilium is resected.

However, a substantial proportion of periacetabular

lesions do involve either total joint resection (including the intra-articular proximal femur), or a substantial proportion of the ilium. In these cases, allograft reconstruction of the resected bony defect offers a remarkably versatile reconstruction. It should be recognized, however, that the use of allografts in pelvic reconstructive surgery is a relatively new technique and that long-term clinical follow-up is not yet available.

The advantage of allograft reconstruction is that the bone can be tailored to fit virtually any internal hemipelvectomy defect and that secure immediate fixation can be achieved using straightforward techniques in most cases. Once the allograft reconstruction has been completed, a standard total hip arthroplasty can be performed in the usual fashion (43–45).

PLANNING OF THE PELVIC ALLOGRAFT RECONSTRUCTION: PREVENTING COMPLICATIONS

In planning allograft reconstruction of the pelvis, the surgeon should remember the three most frequent complications of the procedure: local recurrence, infection, and dislocation (46). In our initial consecutive series of 12 patients undergoing allograft pelvic reconstruction, four patients were noted to have positive microscopic resection margins (i.e., had undergone marginal resections) in the region of the medial, anterior soft tissues close to the bladder and prostrate. Three of these patients recurred at the local site of surgery and, in retrospect, should have undergone bladder resection en bloc with the bony removal. Careful analysis of the CT and MRI scans is essential in planning both the soft tissue and bone resection margins to avoid marginal surgery.

The availability of allograft for reconstruction facilitates planning of the osteotomies used to resect the pelvic tumor, since, with allograft, it is possible to reconstruct a defect extending from the sacroiliac joint to the symphysis. It is not necessary to "skimp" on the bony resection margins to perform the reconstruction. We generally plan our osteotomies several centimeters from the furthest extent of tumor involvement.

If a local recurrence is undoubtedly the most serious local complication of allograft reconstruction of a periacetabular tumor, infection surely ranks as the second most disturbing setback. Infection can be due either to graft or to intraoperative contamination (47–51). In most allograft bone harvest protocols, the pelvis is the last bone to be removed. Surgical fatigue and the potential for perineal or anal contamination of the graft increases the risk of allograft infection during harvest. Because of these risks, we routinely irradiate pelvic allografts (2.5 megarads) prior to utilization to eliminate the chance of donor infection.

The extensive incisions necessary for periacetabular tumor excision increases the risk of wound contamination intraoperatively by the patient's own skin flora or from operating room contamination. To decrease these risks, we instruct our patients (if not allergic) to wash the pelvic area twice daily with pHisoHex soap for at least 4 days prior to surgery. We routinely perform this surgery within a laminar flow clean air environment using body exhaust equipment. Patients receive 1.0 g of cephalosporine intravenously every 8 hours starting prior to endotracheal intubation and continuing 48 hours after surgery. Urinary catheters are always inserted in the operating room under sterile conditions and are removed on the third or fourth postoperative day. Finally, we pay meticulous attention to wound closure and, not infrequently, we utilize vascularized tissue transfer to underlay the skin incision. As a general rule, we strive to avoid leaving any dead space within the wound and try to avoid closing unsupported skin over an allograft.

Dislocation of the hip postoperatively can be avoided by two features related to preoperative planning. Orientation of the acetabulum can be extremely difficult once a portion of the pelvis is removed and orientation is much more simple if the allograft pelvis is about the same size

as the resected bone. We always attempt to match size on standardized preoperative radiographs. The other factor that assists hip stability relates to the treatment of the hip capsule during allograft harvest. If the hip capsule is detached from the trochanter and is left attached to the acetabular rim, this capsule can be utilized in reconstruction to stabilize the femoral prosthetic component or to reconstruct the hip capsule if the allograft is used in osteoarticular fashion.

As mentioned previously, it is probably better to resect many periacetabular tumors through an extended ilioinguinal approach if the tumor extends to the anteromedial pelvis. This generally does not complicate allograft fixation if the entire acetabulum is being replaced. On one occasion, we have found it necessary to make a separate Kocher-Langenbeck approach to the acetabulum. In this case, a cryopreserved allograft was used as an osteoarticular graft (Fig. 7.2). Access to the posterior column was necessary for fixation and was not available through the ilioinguinal approach. In most cases involving resection of the entire acetabulum, fixation will be provided by intrafragmentary screws placed through the superior acetabulum or dome region and this area is readily accessible through the ilioinguinal incision.

ACETABULAR RECONSTRUCTION USING AN ALLOGRAFT IMPLANT COMPOSITE OR OSTEOARTICULAR ALLOGRAFT

Technical Aspects and Postoperative Management

The allograft is generally unwrapped and thawed approximately one-half hour prior to the completion of tumor resection. The surgeon supervises allograft unwrapping by experienced members of the operating room nursing staff. The usual fragments of soft tissue and bone are obtained for culture and the graft placed in warm half-strength Betadine solution.

Optimal preparation of the pelvic allograft requires that the resected specimen be present in the operating room while the allograft is cut to fill the skeletal defect. Particular attention must be paid to the orientation of the proximal iliac cut, since varying this osteotomy in the flexion or abduction planes may result in acetabular malorientation, leading to dislocation. Two reference planes are used in directing the iliac allograft osteotomy: a plan through the acetabular dome (for abduction and adduction) and a plane through the sacroiliac joint (for flexion-extension) (Fig. 7.9). An attempt is then made to duplicate exactly the plane of the osteotomy through the patient's

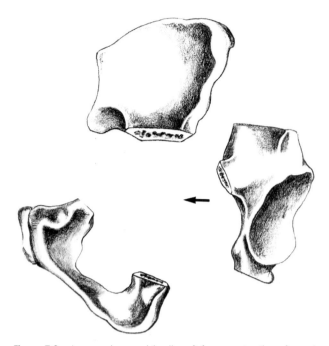

Figure 7.9. In preparing a pelvic allograft for reconstruction of a peri-acetabular defect after tumor resection, the transiliac osteotomy is crucial. The distance from this osteotomy to the joint determines limb length and soft tissue tension across the hip. The plane of the osteotomy provides the flexion and abduction orientation of the socket.

ilium. Three cuts in the allograft pelvis are required in most cases: the iliac, the ischial, and the superior pubic. Since the iliac osteotomy will be rigidly fixed and determine both the acetabular position and the soft tissue tension across the hip, it is crucial that this osteotomy be exact.

While planning and performing the allograft osteotomies, the resected specimen serves as an invaluable template. However, it must be recognized that the pelvic specimen is contaminated by tumor and should not be handled. We place the specimen on a separate Mayo stand where it can be easily visualized but handled as little as possible. As soon as the surgeon is satisfied with the preparation of the allograft, the specimen is passed off for pathological evaluation.

The size of the allograft rarely matches exactly the size of the skeletal deficit left by tumor excision exactly. Maximal attention is always focused on the iliac osteotomy, where excellent fit and rigid internal fixation is a necessity. The distance from the iliac osteotomy to the acetabulum should duplicate the resected specimen to restore optimal soft tissue tension across the hip. If a portion of the autogenous ischium remains after tumor excision, it is reattached to the allograft to provide a new origin for the hamstrings. These muscles may provide the

only source of active hip extension if the gluteus maximus has been defunctioned or resected.

We do not emphasize fixation of the anterior pelvis. The superior pubic ramus frequently presents a problem in that it is difficult to fit around the femoral vessels and nerve during allograft insertion. Since fixation through the anterior column or pubic ramus is rarely rigid, we generally tend to remove the superior pubic ramus of the allograft close to the socket. This facilitates relaxation of the neurovascular structures and eliminates allograft bone under the anterior skin closure.

Once the allograft has been fitted into the skeletal defect, a decision must be made as to whether the graft is used as an allograft implant composite or as an osteoarticular graft. If the graft is frozen without cryopreservation or if it has been irradiated, there is little or no rationale for using an osteoarticular reconstruction since the acetabular cartilage is dead and will go on to degenerate. If, however, the surgeon is using fresh or a cryopreserved acetabulum, it may be reasonable simply to reduce the femoral head (if it remains following tumor excision) into the allograft socket, if and only if, both fit and orientation are perfect. In this case, fixation of the allograft will require intrafragmentary screw insertion peripheral to the articular surface and capsular repair will be utilized to hold the joint reduced (Fig 7.2 and 7.10).

In most situations requiring acetabular resection, the femoral head will have been removed or the allograft-femoral head fit is insufficient for an osteoarticular graft. In these cases, we generally use an allograft implant composite reconstruction. If the femoral head is resected to permit reconstruction (as opposed to resected for tumor excision), it is kept as a bone graft. Indeed, in some cases of partial acetabular excision, the femoral head can be used as an autogenous graft that obviates the necessity for using allograft (Fig. 7.11).

Following appropriate fitting of the allograft, the articular cartilage is removed to permit cement fixation of the acetabular component of a total hip replacement. This step should be accomplished prior to fixation to prevent unnecessary shear stresses on the fixation. We prefer to cement the acetabular component (rather than utilizing a bipolar component), since optimal fixation can be achieved through screws placed in the acetabular dome and also since placement of the acetabular component promotes a more stable total hip orientation.

While reaming the allograft, care should be taken to remove only cartilage and not subchondral bone. Indeed, we generally remove the soft tissue from the

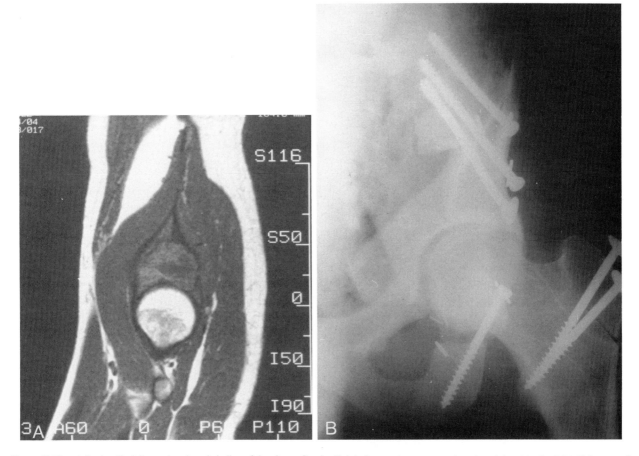

Figure 7.10. A fresh articulating osteochondral allograft has been fixed with intrafragmentary screws placed peripheral to the joint. This type of osteoarticular reconstruction is rarely used since the size match of the allograft is rarely adequate for joint preservation.

acetabulum using periosteal elevators rather than the usual centrifugal reamers. Intrafragmentary screws are then placed across the iliac osteotomy (Figs. 7.12 and 7.13). In most recent cases, we have avoided the use of neutralization plates since three or four screws through the acetabular dome and into the ilium are remarkably stable. It is our impression that buttress plates do little to improve this fixation and may weaken the allograft. Neutralization plates were used in our initial cases, however (Figs. 7.14–7.16). We continue to utilize plates to buttress screws placed in the ilium when large defects require proximal fixation.

If the iliac osteotomy is too far proximal to permit stabilization with screws placed through the acetabular dome, intrafragmentary screws are inserted through acetabular reconstruction plates. This distributes the forces on the allograft more evenly and decreases stress concentration at the screw hole (Figs. 7.17 and 7.18).

In our initial experience, we attempted to maintain the integrity of the pelvic ring by reconstructing the anterior pelvis using screws from the allograft pelvis into the contralateral anterior column. In each case, fracture of the allograft occurred lateral to the point of fixation, without an increase in postoperative symptoms (Figs. 7.14 and 7.15). Because positioning of the medial allograft under the femoral neurovascular structures complicates allograft insertion, we now rely on fixation to the ilium and ischium (if it remains following tumor resection).

Prior to cementing the acetabular component, the trial femoral component should be inserted and the soft tissue tension and acetabular version and hip stability assessed. If the soft tissues are very lax (either because of muscle excision or inadvertent proximal positioning of the acetabulum), consideration should be given to increasing the cement mantle of the acetabular component and placing the component in a more horizontal position.

In younger patients, we generally employ a bone ingrowth femoral component unless the patient has received or will receive chemotherapy or irradiation (Fig. 7.13). If adjuvant cytotoxic treatment is being employed,

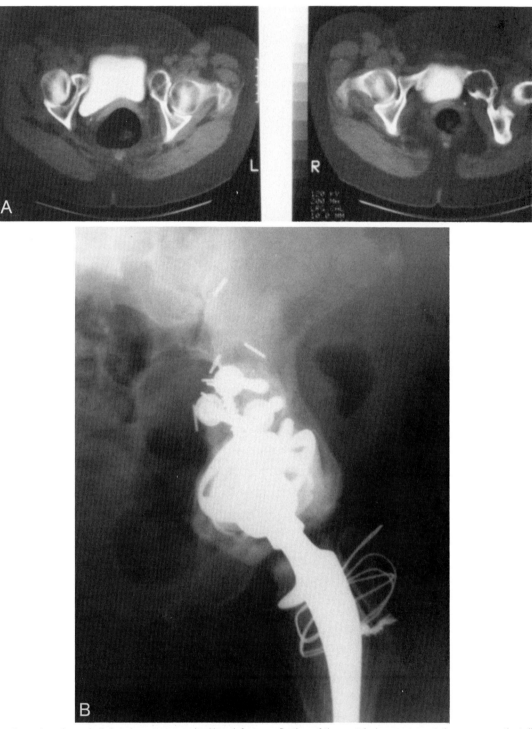

Figure 7.11. Resection of a grade II chondrosarcoma resulted in a defect in the anterior column and quadrilateral plate. Because the joint was not involved, the femoral head was utilized as a bone graft to supplement fixation of the acetabular component. In a young patient, iliofemoral arthrodesis or osteoarticular allograft hemijoint replacement would have been utilized.

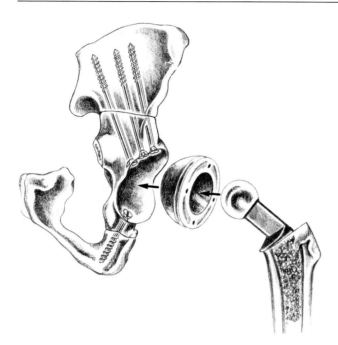

Figure 7.12. Our current technique for fixation of a whole acetabular allograft utilized intrafragmentary transarticular screws to stabilize the iliac and ischial osteotomies. Fixation to the superior pubic ramus is avoided since it is rarely stable and since maintenance of the allograft superior ramus often interferes with the external iliac vessels and femoral nerves.

the femoral component is cemented using standard techniques of cement preparation and pressurization.

Two further techniques are generally employed to increase the stability of the allograft implant composite. It should be recognized that factors which increase the risk of hip dislocation include the circumferential resection of hip capsule in combination with the hip flexor, abductor, adductor, and extensor muscles. In addition to placing the acetabulum into a horizontal position, we frequently advance the trochanter and use a long-necked femoral component to increase residual soft tissue tension. Care should be taken, however, in monitoring tension in the sciatic nerve. In some cases, this is the only soft tissue left that traverses the hip joint and excessively lengthening the hip will simply damage the nerve.

If the hip capsule has been retained on the pelvic allograft, it should not be resected prior to reconstruction. The allograft should be fixed and the socket cemented in place with the capsule intact. The capsular tissue is then sutured tightly around the neck of the femoral component. If the capsule has been resected during allograft harvest, Dacron vascular graft is cemented to the periphery of the acetabular component. It can then be tied tightly around the femoral neck or

attached to the femur through drill holes. Although this capsular prosthesis cannot maintain hip stability indefinitely, it serves to maintain the hip in joint while a fibrous pseudocapsule forms. If the allograft capsule is conserved, care should be taken to determine the level of the bone-labrum junction accurately, prior to cementing. In one of our cases, lateral positioning of the acetabular component resulted because capsule obscured the bony landmarks of the socket (Fig. 7.13).

As a final step in bone reconstruction, bone graft harvested from the femoral head (if not resected with the tumor) or from the ilium, is packed around the iliac osteotomy site. Perforations of the allograft are minimized and the allograft cortex is not violated.

Attention to soft tissue closure is crucial to the success of the operation. Frequently, tumor excision requires that all muscles anterior to the hip capsule and acetabulum (iliopsoas, sartorius, and rectus femoris) have been resected. In this situation, we think that it is inappropriate simply to close the skin over the allograft total hip composite. Instead, vascularized tissue transfer (usually rectus abdominis), is used to provide stable tissue that eliminates dead space and lines the skin closure over the graft. Our routine protocol for pelvic allograft reconstruction emphasizes that intra-operative consultation with the plastic reconstructive service be obtained prior to wound closure.

At the time of wound closure, suction drains are inserted and left for 2–5 days. The patients are generally nursed on air mattresses to eliminate the necessity for frequent turning. Bed rest in an abduction splint with 2 lb of skin traction is maintained for 1–6 weeks depending on the stability of the hip joint and the trochanteric fixation. If prolonged bed rest is planned, prophylactic Coumadin is initiated following drain removal. Although we recognize that this is inadequate prophylaxis for deep vein thrombosis, we are reluctant to initiate anticoagulation prior to surgery for obvious reasons. Impedence plethysmography is used routinely starting on the third postoperative day to monitor the development of thrombi. Surprisingly, to date, we have detected only one patient with thigh thrombosis. There have been no recognized pulmonary emboli.

Tough weight-bearing ambulation is initiated once the hip is judged to be stable. Touch weight bearing with crutches or a walker is maintained until the proximal iliac osteotomy is radiographically united (usually 4–6 months). Postoperative rehabilitation is individualized and dependent upon the musculature remaining following tumor resection. Particular difficulty is encountered in the re-

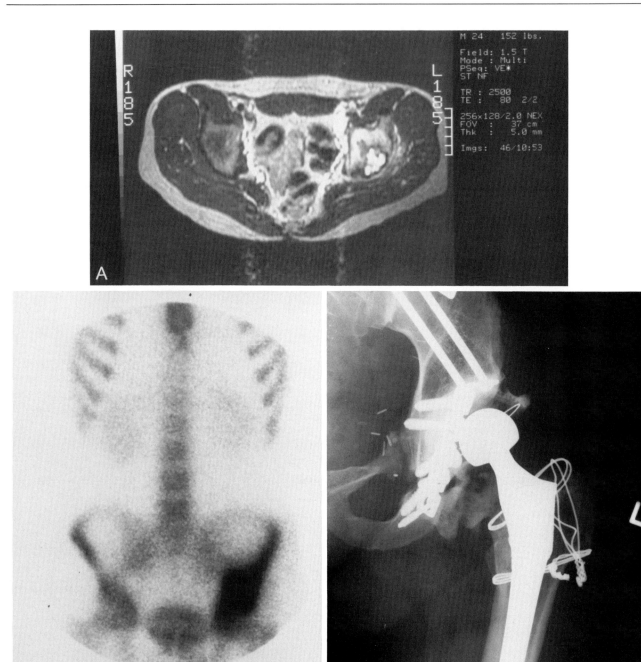

Figure 7.13. A grade II periacetabular chondrosarcoma required extra-articular resection extending to the posterior ilium. At 2 years, the iliac osteotomy is healed and the patient walks with one cane and no pain. Maintenance of the hip capsule interfered with acetabular implant position resulting in lateral placement of the cup.

habilitation of patients who have undergone resection of the hip flexors. These patients must learn to initiate forward limb propulsion with pelvic rotation and have difficulty with floor clearance during swing phase. We generally fit a 1-inch lift to the contralateral shoe to facilitate swing-through of the involved extremity.

If the femoral nerve and hip flexors are involved by tumor (or if the femoral nerve is contaminated by inappropriate biopsy of an anterior column tumor), rehabilitation is extremely difficult and the patient generally will not achieve an acceptable functional result. If possible, we would prefer to perform an iliofemoral arthrodesis in these patients, relying on later limb lengthening procedures to correct major limb length discrepancy.

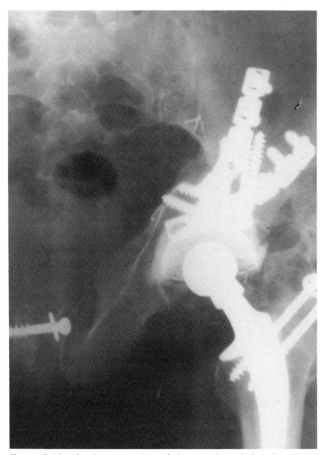

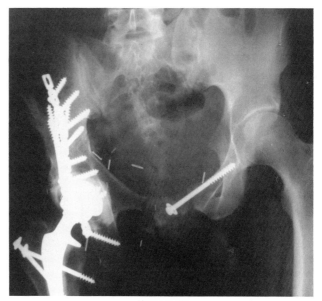

Figure 7.15.

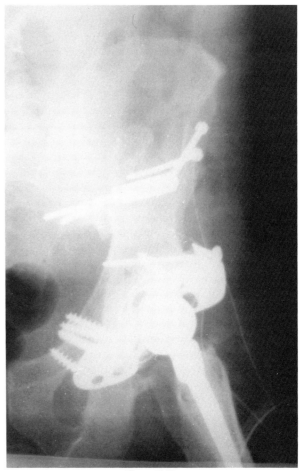

Figure 7.16.

Figure 7.14–16. Reconstruction of three periacetabular chondrosarcomas utilizing buttress plate fixation of the allograft. Although all patients walk well at 38, 52, and 88 months follow-up, respectively, we now avoid buttress plates since all iliac osteotomies fixed with intrafragmentary screws have healed rapidly.

RESULTS OF ALLOGRAFT RECONSTRUCTION FOLLOWING ACETABULAR RESECTION

At the University of Toronto Musculoskeletal Oncology Unit, we have performed 12 allograft reconstructions of pelvic defects following tumor resection with minimum clinical follow-up of 20 months (range 21–91 months). Another five patients who had shorter follow-up periods have not been included in this review. Ten cases have used allograft implant composites and two patients have undergone osteoarticular reconstructions (*see* Tables 7.1 and 7.2). Three further patients have undergone reconstruction of partial acetabular excisions using femoral head autografts. In the past 3 years, another 18 patients have undergone pelvic tumor excision and have been treated without allograft.

Although complications have been frequent in this series, the overall results have been acceptable. Four pa-

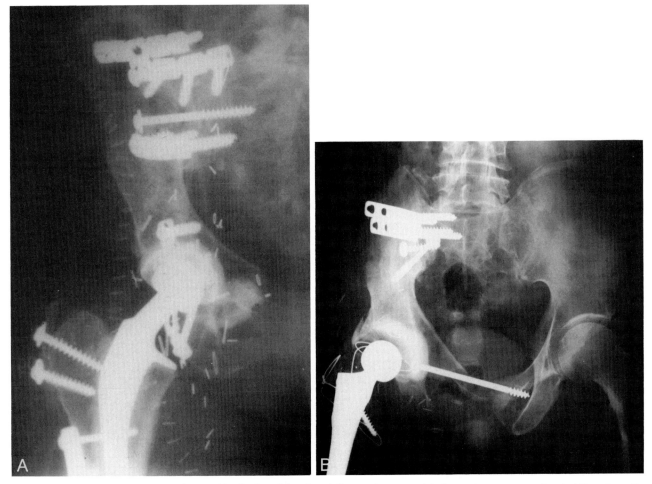

Figure 7.17. A and B. For reconstruction requiring fixation of the allograft ilium to the sacrum, intrafragmentary screws are inserted through small pelvic reconstruction plates to distribute better the load on the allograft.

tients with allograft reconstructions have been resected with positive margins and two of these people (both with high-grade sarcomas) died with both local and systemic disease recurrence. One patient with positive margins remains disease free at 7 years' follow-up and one patient remains disease free 2 years after a second resection of a local wound recurrence.

Three patients (one of whom died with both local and systemic recurrence) developed allograft infection. Removal of the allograft with a resultant flail hip was necessary in one patient. One patient functions with a chronic infection and changes her dressings daily. She will eventually require allograft removal.

Four patients have developed dislocations of the allograft implant composite and one of these patients required trochanteric advancement for eventual stability. All patients have eventually gone on to a stable articulation.

To date, no revisions of the mechanical construction

have been necessary. The first patient in our series (who now has been followed for 8 years), suffered an allograft fracture at 6 years after surgery, but this healed and he is now fully ambulatory.

At present, eight of ten patients surviving following allograft implant composite reconstructions are fully ambulatory using one cane. We insist that all patients utilize canes indefinitely. One patient requires two canes and another patient is limited to ambulation with crutches following allograft removal.

We used the Musculoskeletal Tumor Society Assessment (52–54) score to evaluate outcome in nine surviving patients with intact allografts (two patients have died and one allograft has been removed due to infection). Four patients achieved overall good or excellent results, two were fair, and three were poor. As mentioned, the usual causes of poor results related to muscle weakness, with poor scores in stability and strength. There were no results below good on analysis of pain or emotional ac-

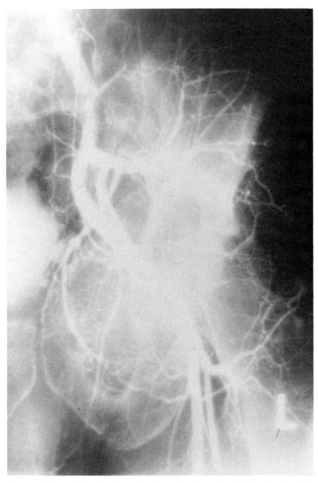

Figure 7.18. Embolization of periacetabular metastatic lesions is often complicated by multiple sources of tumor vessels.

ceptance and all but three patients rated good or excellent on functional ability (Table 7.2).

Serial radiographs have been obtained at 3-month intervals in most patients. All iliac osteotomies have healed within 4–12 months (the patients are kept touch weight bearing on crutches until the osteotomies have healed). With the exception of one patient who developed a stress fracture at 6 years, there have been no mechanical failures of the reconstruction. This patient went on to heal spontaneously and is not fully ambulatory. All allografts appear equal in density to the surrounding host bone with the exception of the patient undergoing allograft removal for sepsis. The graft in this patient became osteopenic as the infection progressed.

In assessing functional results, the key determinate of function would seem to be the muscle remaining after tumor excision. Patients with deficient hip flexors and abductors have significant difficulty in relearning ambulation but generally succeed in achieving a stable

gait using one or two canes and pelvic propulsion of the lower extremity. In general, patients with deficient femoral nerves are particularly compromised since the combination of weak hip flexion and weak quadriceps is particularly difficult to overcome. As mentioned previously, we prefer to use iliofemoral arthrodesis in these patients if possible.

In summary, pelvic allografts should be reserved for those patients requiring resection of the acetabulum who cannot be reasonably managed with iliofemoral fusion. Although this procedure should still be considered as a clinical experiment, early results appear generally promising.

RECONSTRUCTION OF ACETABULAR SECONDARY (METASTATIC) TUMORS

Metastatic tumors involving the acetabulum are diagnosed much more frequently than primary tumors but they rarely require reconstructive surgery. Of the tumors that frequently metastasize to bone, breast cancer and prostatic cancer are generally responsive to radiation or hormonal therapy. Longevity in patients with metastatic lung carcinoma is generally too limited to warrant major reconstructive surgery of the hip. In general, palliative surgery is reserved for patients who are in good general health, with a solitary symptomatic metastasis (or limited metastases elsewhere) that has proven resistant to medical and radiation management.

The type of metastatic tumor that most often presents in this fashion is renal cell carcinoma. Although the pace of disease is highly variable with this malignancy, bone metastases are frequent and often cause marked lytic destruction. Renal cell metastases rarely respond to either irradiation or chemotherapy, leaving surgery as the only palliative option.

It should be recognized that, in the vast majority of cases, acetabular reconstruction for metastatic disease is palliative rather than potentially curative. Therefore, wide resection of the lesion is not required and curettage is generally adequate for disease control. The resultant skeletal defect is, therefore, much smaller than following primary tumor resection and allograft bone is not often needed.

APPROACH TO THE PATIENT WITH METASTATIC DISEASE OF THE PELVIS

In most cases, patients presenting with symptomatic periacetabular or pelvic metastases are known to have primary cancer elsewhere and biopsy is not usually required. If, however, the patient presents with a solitary lesion

Table 7.1.
Results of Prospective/Retrospective Study of Limb Salvage Surgery/Allograft Reconstruction for Periacetabular Neoplasms

Pt.	Age/Sex	Diagnosis	Stage	Resection	Margin	Complications
1	61/M	Chondrosarcoma	IIB	IA/IIA/III	Wide	None to date
2	40/M	Chondrosarcoma	IIB	IA/IIA/III	Marginal	Late fracture (healed)
3	39/F	Chondrosarcoma	IB	II/III	Wide	Acute dislocation (stable, long-term)
4	32/F	Chondrosarcoma	IA	IA/IIA/III	Wide	None to date
5	29/M	Chondrosarcoma	IB	II/IIIA	Wide	Wound necrosis (successfully treated with soft tissue transfer)
6	38/M	Ewing's sarcoma	IIB	IA/IIA/IIIA	Marginal	Dislocation, local recurrence, dead of disease 8 months post-operatively
7	49/M	Chondrosarcoma	IB	I/IIA/IIIA	Marginal	Local recurrence (resected with no further recurrence) cup dislocation at 26 months with revision THR and acetabular autograft
8	50/F	Chondrosarcoma	IIB	IIA/III	Wide	Dislocation; required trochanteric advancement; (stable, long-term) deep vein thrombosis; infection at 25 months
9	16/M	Osteosarcoma	IIB	IIA/IIIA	Marginal	Acute dislocation, acute infection; required amputation, skin slough, local recurrence, systemic recurrence, dead of disease 12 months postoperatively
10	62/F	Chondrosarcoma	IB	IA/IIA	Wide	Chronic infection; will require revision procedure or amputation in future, allograft removed at 39 months
11	25/M	Osteosarcoma	IIB	IA/IIA	Wide	None
12	26/F	Osteosarcoma	IIB	IA/IIB	Wide	None

without a known primary, complete staging and biopsy should be carried out to ensure that the patient does not have a primary bone sarcoma.

If the diagnosis is not at issue, evaluation of the patient's symptoms is the critical feature in determining treatment. It should be recognized that palliative surgery for metastatic disease is reserved for patients who have pain and functional loss that has not been improved with nonsurgical modalities. Accordingly, it is critical that an accurate objective analysis of the patient's symptoms is obtained initially and serially monitored. We have found that recording of the analgesic requirements and use of a visual analogue pain score is useful in monitoring sympton control.

Most patients respond to irradiation, hormonal therapy, or chemotherapy management with marked symp-

tomatic improvement. Indeed, occasionally, symptoms will improve following treatment of a metastatic, lytic malignency despite the fact that the lesion has not changed radiographically. We tend to treat only those metastatic pelvic tumors that are symptomatic no matter what the radiographic appearance.

If a patient is not responsive to pain management with nonoperative treatment and presents with severe symptoms from a metastatic periacetabular tumor, the next issue to be decided is whether the patient can tolerate and benefit from surgery. Pelvic reconstructive procedures entail major surgery with prolonged recovery time and it is crucial that the patient is both well enough to withstand surgery and has a sufficiently good prognosis to benefit from hip reconstruction.

In general, patients with extensive visceral metastases

Table 7.2.
Functional Results of Periacetabular Limb Salvage Surgery (For Nine Surviving Patients)

Pt.	Follow-up[a]	Motion	Pain	Stability	Deformity	Strength	Emotional	Function	Overall	Score
1	22	P	G	P	E	P	G	F	P	12
2	96	G	E	P	E	P	E	E	P	23
3	39	F	E	G	E	G	E	E	G	27
4	24	E	E	E	E	E	E	E	E	35
5	30	G	E	E	P	E	E	E	G	28
6	8[b]	F	E	P	E	P	E	P	P	16
7	36[c]	F	E	G	G	G	E	F	F	21
8	24	G	G	G	G	F	G	F	F	17
10[d]	39	P	G	P	F	P	G	F	P	8
11	21	E	E	G	E	G	E	G	G	29
12	28	F	E	P	P	P	G	F	P	10

[a]Follow-up times noted are in months.
[b]Patient evaluated prior to death at 8 months.
[c]4 months postrevision.
[d]Allograft removed.

(especially lung or liver) or chronic hypercalcemia are unlikely to tolerate or benefit from surgery. Patients with extensive symptomatic skeletal disease are unlikely to benefit, both because their symptoms in other regions will continue to be severe despite symptom control in the pelvis and because generalized skeletal metastases predict a limited longevity. Patients with renal cell carcinoma or thyroid carcinoma frequently present with solitary bony metastases and may have prolonged survival following the appearance of skeletal metastases. Patients with renal cell metastases generally fail to respond to radiotherapy or chemotherapy and, therefore, are good candidates for surgical reconstruction.

In a patient with acetabular metastatic disease being evaluated for surgery, therapeutic angiography with embolization is frequently indicated. Renal cell and thyroid metastases, in particular, are vascular and surgery for these lesions is facilitated and considerably safer following embolization. Embolization of pelvic metastatic tumors requires diligence on the part of the angiographer since multiple vessels frequently feed the lesion (Fig. 7.18).

CT is also performed in our protocol to evaluate the extent of bone lysis and to determine the location of structurally secure bone that will permit fixation of acetabular reconstruction components (Fig. 7.19). The CT scan also assists in determining the optimal surgical approach to the tumor. Lesions that are mainly located in the posterior column with involvement of the acetabular dome are best approached through a posterior or transtrochanteric approach. We tend to use the transgluteal lateral approach for patients with anterior column involvement.

In many patients, periacetabular tumors extend proximally into the ilium toward the sacroiliac joint. These tumors are often complicated by substantial soft tissue extension. Both the safe removal of these lesions and optimal reconstruction is often made easier by utilizing a dual surgical approach. A transacetabular approach is necessary for the distal portion of the reconstruction and placement of the acetabular component. Exposure of the medial or lateral iliac wing and the anterior portion of the sacroiliac joint permits removal of the iliac tumor under direct vision through the acetabulum and through the ilium. The reconstruction implants and fixation screws can be placed under direct vision with increased safety and improved reliability of fixation.

There are three steps to periacetabular tumor reconstruction: tumor removal, filling of the resultant defect, and fixation to the intact bone. Tumor removal should be as complete as possible, curetting the lesion from inside the cavity. Although it is recognized that removal of the lesion is not curative, complete, gross tumor removal both decreases the postoperative tumor-derived pain and improves fixation by removing weak bone that is invaded by cancer cells.

There are three options for filling the defect left by tumor removal: polymethylmethacrylate cement, autogenous femoral head, or allograft acetabulum. No matter which material is used, secure fixation to solid bone must be achieved.

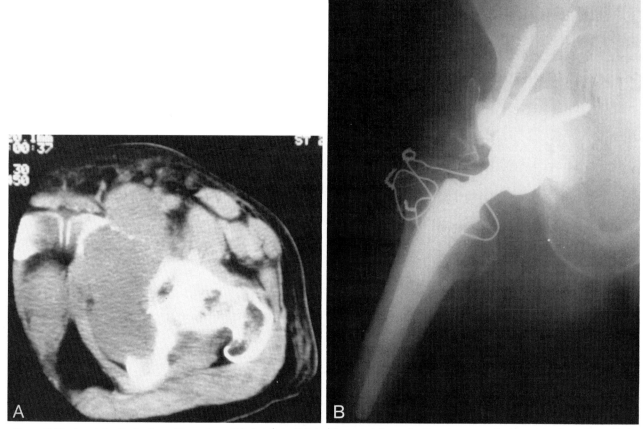

Figure 7.19. A and B. Destruction of the entire acetabulum (type III lesion) by metastatic renal cell carcinoma required reconstruction using a whole acetabular allograft. Excellent fixation is afforded at the iliac osteotomy and intrafragmentary 6.5 screws placed through an acetabular reconstruction ring.

We divide periacetabular metastases into three groups based on evaluation of both the plain x-rays, Judet views, and CT scans. Type I lesions have substantial areas of bone lysis but residual stable bone remains around the periphery of the lytic defect (Fig. 7.20). Type II lesions have lytic lesions that are not contained by residual bone medially and superiorly but do have residual bone in the anterior and posterior columns (Fig. 7.21). Finally, type III defects have unconstrained lytic lesions in the dome as well as destruction of the acetabular columns (Figs. 7.19 and 7.22).

We believe that type I lesions with surrounding intact bone that permits cement to be pressurized should be treated with methacrylate since this methodology provides a rapid, simple type of fixation. Screws should be placed into secure bone prior to cement insertion to provide reinforcement of the cement bone interface. Our preference is to reconstruct the acetabular defect following metastatic curettage in three stages. First, screws are placed proximally into the residual pelvic bone under direction vision. We prefer to use fully threaded 6.5-mm cancellous screws fixed into the proximal ilium or sacrum. Cement is then pressurized into the defect around

the screws and allowed to polymerize. An acetabular roof ring is then attached to the bone, using screws into both the surrounding bone and also into the polymerized cement. Excellent fixation of the roof ring is usually easy to achieve. The acetabular component is then cemented into the roof ring (Fig. 7.20).

If the acetabular defect is unconstrained medially but the acetabular columns remain (type II defect), our preference is to expose the pelvis from above and below and to use the autogenous femoral head (or allograft femoral head if the autogenous bone is weakened by disuse or disease) to fill the defect. The femoral head is fixed to the remaining ilium after first shaping the head to fit the pelvic lesion. Reaming of the femoral head using acetabular reamers should be performed prior to fixation and a roof ring should be utilized in reconstruction (Fig. 7.22).

If the entire acetabulum, including the anterior and posterior columns, has been totally destroyed by tumor (type III), reconstruction may require a total acetabular allograft (Fig. 7.19). If allograft is needed, we prefer to use a donor acetabulum (as opposed to other bones), since we generally restrict allograft bone to lesions that

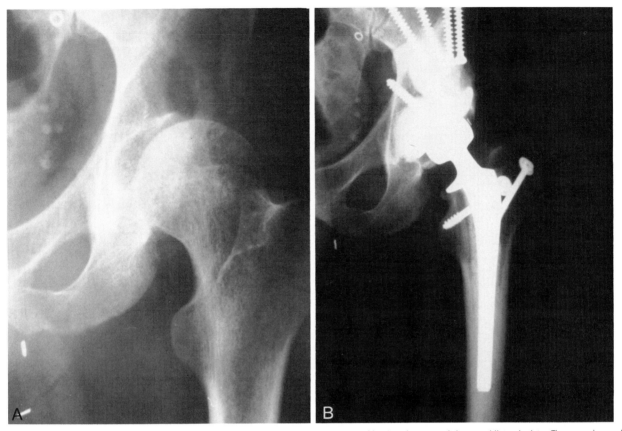

Figure 7.20. A and B. Type I metastatic acetabular destruction with maintenance of both columns and the quadrilateral plate. The superior and lateral defect was reconstructed using cement and screws.

have totally destroyed the socket. The acetabulum is fixed in similar fashion to the reconstruction of the primary tumor. Screws are placed through a roof ring and through the dome of the acetabular allograft to provide rigid fixation. Cemented acetabular components are used in both femoral head autografts and allografts.

RESULTS OF ACETABULAR RECONSTRUCTION FOR METASTATIC TUMORS

In reviewing 27 patients treated for advanced acetabular metastatic disease, we found that 11 were repaired using reinforced cement, five required a femoral head autograft, and 10 received allograft. Patients undergoing allograft reconstruction had larger and more complex regions of bone loss than did patients with less significant reconstruction.

With respect to functional outcome and adequacy of palliation, there was no significant difference between patients reconstructed using allograft and other modalities. There was overall marked improvement in the ability to ambulate and in pain perception in all three groups of patients. There have been no revisions of any allograft reconstructions to date.

The major concern regarding these 27 patients relates to their survival following surgery. Ten of 27 patients are alive at a mean follow-up of 13 months. However, 17 of 27 patients died within 6 months of surgery and it is certainly questionable whether this short-term survival warranted the rehabilitation effort that the patients expended. Better methods are needed to predict longevity in patients with advanced metastatic disease of the acetabulum and prospective analysis of a substantial cohort of patients is being reviewed to permit a better understanding of this problem.

However, if acetabular reconstruction is deemed appropriate, good mechanical restoration of the acetabulum can generally be achieved. We have found that about 30% of patients have defects that have destroyed the medial wall, dome, and the acetabular columns. In these patients, allograft reconstruction offers the best opportunity for restoration of function and relief of pain.

CONCLUSION

Allograft reconstruction for pelvic tumor defects must be considered as a clinical experiment with only short-term follow-up available for analysis. Our data suggest that

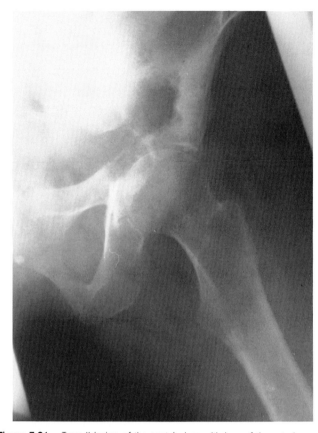

early results are generally acceptable if the complications of tumor recurrence and infection are avoided. However, it should be recognized that many patients with pelvic malignancies have low-grade sacromas that are cured by adequate local surgery. The long-term outcome of pelvic allografts in these patients is currently uncertain and remains a topic of careful clinical and radiographic analysis in our unit.

REFERENCES

1. Ariel IM, Shah JP. The conservative hemipelvectomy. Surg Gynecol Obstet 1977; 144:407–413.
2. Campanacci M, Capanna R. Closing remarks. In: Enneking WF (ed). Limb Salvage In Musculoskeletal Oncology. Churchill Livingstone, New York, 1987; pp. 187–191.
3. Campanacci M, Capanna R. Pelvic malignancies—resections of the pelvic bones. In: Uhthoff H (ed). Current Concepts of Diagnosis and Treatment of Bone and Soft Tissue Tumors. Springer-Verlag, Berlin, Heidelberg, 1984; pp. 359–365.
4. Campanacci M. Opening remarks. In: Enneking WF (ed). Limb Salvage In Musculoskeletal Oncology. Churchill Livingstone, New York, 1987; pp. 103–104.

Figure 7.21. Type II lesion of the acetabulum with loss of the anterior column and the acetabular dome.

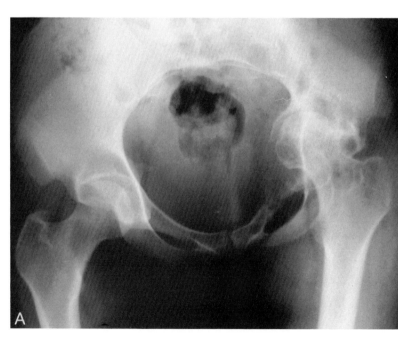

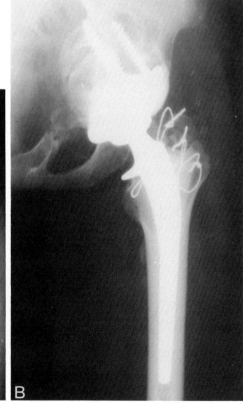

Figure 7.22. A and B. Type III defect with loss of the dome, quadrilateral plate, and both columns. The femoral head was free of tumor and was fixed to the ilium using intrafragmentary screws passed through a protrusio ring. At 51 months, the patient is pain free and disease free (intraosseous round cell tumor treated with chemotherapy and irradiation).

5. Capanna R, Guernelli N, Ruggieri P, Biagini R, Toni A, Picci P, Campanacci M. Periacetabular pelvic resections. In: Enneking WF (ed). Limb Salvage In Musculoskeletal Oncology. Churchill Livingstone, New York, 1987; pp. 141–146.

6. Eilber FR, Grant TT, Sakai D, Morton DL. Internal hemipelvectomy—excision of the hemipelvis with limb preservation: an alternative to hemipelvectomy. Cancer 1979; 43:806–809.

7. Enneking WF, Dunham WK. Resection and reconstruction for primary neoplasms involving the innominate bone. J Bone Joint Surg 1978; 60A:731–746.

8. Enneking WF. Local resection of malignant lesions of the hip and pelvis. J Bone Joint Surg 1966; 48A:991–1007.

9. Enneking WF. Summary. In: Enneking WF (ed). Limb Salvage In Musculoskeletal Oncology. Churchill Livingstone, New York, 1987; pp. 624–626.

10. Erikson W, Hjelmstedt A. Limb-saving radical resection of chondrosarcoma of the pelvis. J Bone Joint Surg 1976; 58A:568–570.

11. Higinbotham NL, Marcove RC, Casson P. Hemipelvectomy: a clinical study of 100 cases with five year follow-up on 60 patients. Surgery 1966; 59:706–708.

12. Johnson JTH. Reconstruction of the pelvic ring following tumor resection. J Bone Joint Surg 1978; 60A:747–751.

13. Karakousis CP. Internal hemipelvectomy. Surg Gynecol Obstet 1984; 158:279–282.

14. O'Connor MI, Sim FH. Salvage of the limb in the treatment of malignant pelvic tumors. J Bone Joint Surg 1989; 71A:481–494.

15. Radley TJ, Liebig CA, Brown JR. Resection of the body of the pubic bone, the superior and inferior pubic rami, the inferior ischial ramus, and the ischial tuberosity: a surgical approach. J Bone Joint Surg 1954; 36A:855–858.

16. Salzer M, Knahr K, Sekera J, Braun O. Resection treatment of malignant pelvic bone tumors. In: Enneking WF (ed). Limb Salvage In Musculoskeletal Oncology. Churchill Livingstone, New York, 1987; pp. 104–111.

17. Shives TC, Sim FH, Pritchard DJ, Bowman WE. Limb salvage for tumors about the pelvic girdle. In: Enneking WF (ed). Limb Salvage In Musculoskepetal Oncology. Churchill Livingstone, New York, 1987; pp. 112–117.

18. Sim FH, Bowman WE Jr. Limb salvage in pelvic tumors. In: Uhthoff H (ed). Current Concepts of Diagnosis and Treatment of Bone and Soft Tissue Tumors. Springer-Verlag, Berlin, Heidelberg, 1984; pp. 367–372.

19. Steel HH. Partial or complete resection of the hemipelvis—an alternative to hindquarter amputation for periacetabular chondrosarcoma of the pelvis. J Bone Joint Surg 1978; 60A:719–730.

20. Xunyuan D, Minsin J. Limb salvage: radical resection of a pelvic bone tumour: report of two cases. Orthopedics 1987; 10:1349–1352.

21. Zatsepin ST. Conservative operations for pelvic bone tumours. Int Orthop 1981; 4:259–268.

22. Eilber FR, Eckardt JJ, Grant TG. Resection of malignant bone tumors of the pelvis: evaluation of local recurrence, survival, and function. In: Enneking WF (ed). Limb Salvage In Musculoskeletal Oncology. Churchill Livingstone, New York, 1987; pp. 136–141.

23. Sundaram M, McGuire MH, Herbold DR, Wolverson MK, Heiberg E. Magnetic resonance imaging in planning limb-salvage surgery for primary malignant tumors of bone. J Bone Joint Surg 1986; 68A:809–819.

24. Mankin HJ, Lange TA, Spanier SS. The hazards of biopsy in patients with malignant primary bone and soft-tissue tumors. J Bone Joint Surg 1982; 64A:1121–1127.

25. Simon MA. Biopsy of musculoskeletal tumors. J Bone Joint Surg 1982; 64A:1253–1257.

26. Enneking WF, Spanier SS, Goodman MA. A system for the surgical staging of musculoskeletal sarcoma. Clin Orthop 1980; 153:106–120.

27. Enneking WF, Spanier SS, Goodman MA. The surgical staging of musculoskeletal sarcoma. J Bone Joint Surg 1980; 62A:1027–1030.

28. Enneking WF. Staging of musculoskeletal neoplasms. In: Uhthoff H (ed). Current Concepts of Diagnosis and Treatment of Bone and Soft Tissue Tumors. Springer-Verlag, Berlin, Heidelberg, 1984; pp. 1–21.

29. Fornasier VL. Classification of bone tumours. In Uhthoff H (ed). Current Concepts of Diagnosis and Treatment of Bone and Soft Tissue Tumors. Springer-Verlag, Berlin, Heidelberg, 1984; pp. 23–27.

30. Eilber FR, Mirra JJ, Grant TT, Weisenburger T, Morton DL. Is amputation necessary for sarcomas? A seven-year experience with limb salvage. Ann Surg 1980; 192:431–438.

31. Gebhart MJ, Lane JM, McCormack RR Jr., Glasser D. Limb salvage in bone sarcomas—Memorial Hospital experience. Orthopedics 1985; 8:626–635.

32. Watts HG. Introduction to resection of musculoskeletal sarcomas. Clin Orthop 1980; 153:31–38.

33. Enneking WF, Menendez LR. Functional evaluation of various reconstructions after periacetabular resection of iliac lesions. In: Enneking WF (ed). Limb Salvage In Musculoskeletal Oncology. Churchill Livingstone, New York, 1987; pp. 117–135.

34. Dunham WK. Acetabular resections for sarcoma. In: Enneking WF (ed). Limb Salvage In Musculoskeletal Oncology. Churchill Livingstone, New York, 1987; pp. 170–184.

35. Harrington KD, Johnson JO, Kaufer HN, Luck JV Jr., Moore TM. Limb salvage and prosthetic joint reconstruction for low-grade and selected high-grade sarcomas of bone after wide resection and replacement by authoclaved (sic) autogenic grafts. Clin Orthop 1986; 211:180–214.

36. Johnson JO. Local resection in primary malignant bone tumours. Clin Orthop 1980; 153:73–80.

37. Lane JM, Duane K, Glasser DB, Kroll M, Otis JC. Periacetabular resections for malignant sarcomas. In: Enneking WF (ed). Limb Salvage In Musculoskeletal Oncology. Churchill Livingstone, New York, 1987; pp. 166–169.

38. Langlais F, Vielpeau C. Allografts of the hemipelvis after tumour resection: technical aspects of four cases. J Bone Joint Surg 1989; 71B:58–62.

39. Enneking WF (ed). Functional results of reconstruction for periacetabular pelvic resections requiring sacrifice of the hip joint

In: Limb Salvage In Musculoskeletal Oncology. Churchill Livingstone, New York, 1987; pp. 103–191.

40. Tomeno B, Languepin A, Gerber C. Local resection with limb salvage for the treatment of periacetabular bone tumors: functional results in nine cases. In: Enneking WF (ed). Limb Salvage In Musculoskeletal Oncology. Churchill Livingstone, New York, 1987; pp. 147–156.

41. Trancik TM, Stulberg BN, Wilde AH, Feiglin DH. Allograft reconstruction of the acetabulum during revision total hip arthroplasty: clinical, radiographic, and scintigraphic assessment of the results. J Bone Joint Surg 1986; 68A:527–533.

42. Mutschler W, Burri C, Kiefer H. Functional results after pelvic resection with endoprosthetic replacement. In: Enneking WF (ed). Limb Salvage In Musculoskeletal Oncology. Churchill Livingstone, New York, 1987; pp. 156–166.

43. Borja FJ, Mnaymneh W. Bone allografts in salvage of difficult hip arthroplasties. Clin Orthop 1985; 197:123–130.

44. Harris WH. Allografting in total hip arthoplasty: in adults with severe acetabular deficiency including a surgical technique for bolting the graft to the ilium. Clin Orthop 1982; 162:150–164.

45. Oakeshott RD, Morgan DAF, Zukor DJ, Rudan JF, Brooks PJ, Gross AE. Revision total hip arthroplasty with osseous reconstruction: a clinical and roentgenographic analysis. Clin Orthop 1987; 225:37–61.

46. Rosenberg AG, Mankin, HJ. Complications of allograft surgery. In: Epps CH Jr. (ed). Complications in Orthopedic Surgery, 2nd Ed. Vol. 2. JB Lippincott, Philadelphia, 1986; pp. 1385–1417.

47. Czitrom AA, Langer F, McKee N, Gross AE. Bone and cartilage allotransplantation: a review of 14 years of research and clinical studies. Clin Orthop 1986; 208:141–145.

48. Mankin H. Allograft implantation. In: Coombs R, Friedlander G (eds). Bone Tumour Management. Butterworths, London, 1987; pp. 227–236.

49. Mankin HJ, Doppelt S, Tomford W. Clinical experience with allograft implantation: the first ten years. Clin Orthop 1983; 174:69–86.

50. Mankin HJ, Fogelson FS, Thrasher AZ, Jaffer F. Massive resection and allograft transplantation in the treatment of malignant bone tumors. N Engl J Med 1976; 294:1247–1255.

51. Miller BJ, Bakirtzian B, Hadjipavlou A, Lander P. Allografts in orthopedic surgery: a case report and literature review. Can J Surg 1987; 30:35–39.

52. Enneking WF. A system for the functional evaluation of the surgical management of musculoskeletal tumors. In: Enneking WF (ed). Limb Salvage In Musculoskeletal Oncology. Churchill Livingstone, New York, 1987; pp. 5–16.

53. Enneking WF. Modification of the system for functional evaluation of surgical management of musculoskeletal tumors. In: Enneking WF (ed). Limb Salvage In Musculoskeletal Oncology. Churchill Livingstone, New York, 1987; pp. 626–639.

54. Miller GJ. The evaluation systems. In: Enneking WF (ed). Limb Salvage In Musculoskeletal Oncology. Churchill Livingstone, New York, 1987; pp. 1–5.

8

REVISION ARTHROPLASTY OF THE HIP USING ALLOGRAFT BONE

Allan E. Gross

The long-term results for the cemented total joint arthroplasty (hip and knee) have had a dramatic impact on the quality of life for patients. The results are extremely impressive for as long as 20 years (1–8) with careful patient selection. The results for the younger, higher demand patient are not as good (5, 9–13) and this had led to the development of uncemented designs, the long-term results of which are still unknown. Ten-year studies for the uncemented hip (14) and 5-year studies for the uncemented knee have been encouraging (15).

There has been controversy about the future role of cemented implants but, at the present time, there is no question that there are still established indications for their use. If anything, their use may have been increasing recently because of improved results with contemporary cementing techniques (16, 17).

Revision surgery for loose hip and knee implants is now a major part of any orthopaedic surgical program and its volume is going to increase. Loose cemented hip and knee prostheses, particularly in the multiply revised implant, are associated with loss of bone stock due to wear particles and the loose cement acting as an abrasive (18–26). Also, each time a revision is carried out, the surgery itself leads to some loss of bone stock. The symptomatic loose knee or hip prosthesis with associated loss of bone stock is going to continue to be a standard orthopaedic problem occupying a significant portion of the surgical resources of any orthopaedic division that performs implant surgery. The problem, therefore, must be dealt with if orthopaedic surgeons are going to continue replacing arthritic joints.

There are surgical alternatives for this problem. Excision arthroplasty may be acceptable but not when the bone loss is extensive (27, 28). Arthrodesis is difficult to achieve and results in excessive shortening if bone loss is extensive (29). The use of tumor or custom implants where bone is replaced by metal may be acceptable in low-demand patients but there are certain disadvantages. The large tumor implants mostly require the use of cement in the host bone, which can no longer provide the rough lattice necessary for good cement techniques. A stress riser is created at the junction of host bone and implant. The prosthesis does not provide a biological anchorage for host bone and muscle.

Restoration of bone stock in association with a relatively conventional implant offers certain advantages. The allograft offers a more normal gradation of forces from the prosthesis to host bone. The reattachment of bone and muscle is possible. The implant may be of a more conventional design and may be less expensive. Restoration of bone stock also allows the surgeon to use uncemented implants and, most importantly, it may allow further revisions if necessary in the future.

Bone stock may be replenished by the patient's own bone or allograft bone. Using the patient's own bone is only applicable where a minimal amount of bone is required. Allograft bone offers quality and quantity and is applicable in certain situations where major defects exist, i.e., proximal femoral or major pelvic column loss. There are also the obvious advantages to leaving the patient's iliac crest intact.

There are, of course, certain disadvantages to using allograft bone. The problems of disease transmission are discussed elsewhere in this book. Banked bone is not always readily available but is becoming increasingly more so. Allograft bone has certain biological problems. It is not as osteoinductive as autograft bone and nonunions may result (30). This can be alleviated by autografting host-allograft junctions and obtaining rigid fixation. Resorption of allograft bone, particularly solid-fragment grafts, may lead to failure (31, 32). This, of course, may also occur with autograft bone but the process probably is slower. There may be problems like fracture or fragmentation of solid-fragment grafts if the biomechanics of the reconstruction are not correct or if the patient is of too high a demand. This problem applies to both auto- and allografts. Whatever the problems are, however, there is no question that

we are facing a large population of patients who are going to need restoration of bone stock before further revision surgery can be performed.

CLASSIFICATION OF BONE DEFECTS

It is important to have a functional and relatively simple classification of bone deficits associated with loose hip implants. There are more complicated classifications in the literature (33, 34) but we have found that all of our grafts can be fitted into the following classification:

Pelvic Side Deficits

1. *Protrusio*— this is a contained cavitary defect with the acetabular walls and columns intact;
2. *Shelf* (minor column)—loss of part of the rim plus the corresponding acetabular wall but less than 50% of acetabulum;
3. *Acetabular* (major column)—one or both columns with corresponding wall defect involving at least 50% of acetabulum.

Femoral Side Defects

1. *Intraluminal*—the canal is widened but the cortex is still intact and thought to be strong enough to support an implant;
2. *Cortical*
   A. Cortical noncircumferential—these are cortical defects that require only strut grafts;
   B. Circumferential—these are subclassified into:
      i. *Calcar*—less than 3 cm in length;
      ii. *Proximal femur (large fragment)*—greater than 3 cm in length.

These bone defects can be classified, in most cases, by plain x-rays (routine views, Judet views). CAT scans may be helpful, particularly when first starting to do these types of reconstructions, but they are not usually necessary.

Infection is determined by routine blood work, gallium and technetium scans, preoperative hip aspiration, and Gram's stains at the time of surgery.

SURGICAL TECHNIQUES

In our hospital, all revisions requiring the use of allograft bone are done in a laminar flow operating room with body exhaust systems. If there is preoperative evidence of infection or any suggestion at the time of surgery (even with a negative Gram's stain), the surgery is staged for any revision requiring the use of allograft bone.

Any allograft bone is brought into the operating room at the beginning of the case, unwrapped, cultured, and immersed in warm Betadine. The bone is obtained from our own bone bank, where it has been deep frozen at −70°C after being irradiated with 2.5 megarads.

SURGICAL APPROACH

The surgical approach is either transgluteal (35) or transtrochanteric. The transtrochanteric approach is used most commonly because of the need for extensive exposure and also because, in many cases, there is a pre-existing trochanteric nonunion.

The large-fragment proximal femoral grafts should be done via the transtrochanteric approach and the trochanteric fragment should be kept as long as possible so that it will unite and so it will also reinforce the allograft. The proximal femur is exposed by reflecting the vastus lateralis off the septum anteriorly, being careful not to strip any residual bone off of its soft tissue completely.

A Steinmann pin is inserted into the iliac crest as a reference point to adjust leg lengths. The distance from the pin to the rough line (insertion of the vastus lateralis) is recorded prior to dislocation.

Acetabulum

The acetabulum is prepared after the hip has been dislocated. After the acetabular prosthesis and the cement are removed, the membrane is excised carefully because of possible complete bony defects that instruments could penetrate through into the pelvis. The defect is then defined by visualization, palpation, and using a trial cup. At this point, the defect must be defined so the allograft can be prepared. If the defect is a contained cavity (protrusio), then morsellized bone can be used. If the defect is a minor or major column defect, then a bulk allograft is indicated. If a bulk allograft can be avoided by raising the acetabulum 1 or 2 cm to get into better bone stock, then this alternative should be used because better contact with the host bone is obtained (36). Bulk allografts on the pelvic side should be avoided, if possible, and in the majority of cases, the acetabulum can be seated in host bone supplemented by morsellized allograft (protrusio graft). If a major or minor column defect does exist and cannot be compensated for by raising or centralizing the acetabular bed, then a bulk allograft should be used. For bulk allografts, we prefer to fashion true acetabular allografts but male femoral heads or even distal femurs can be used. If morsellized bone is used, then female femoral heads should be used rather than sacrificing strong structural bone. We prefer not to use a bone mill because the bone is made too mushy. The bone can be easily morsellized by hand using currettes and rongeurs and is fine enough to pack into cavities but still has some structural

integrity (Fig. 8.1). Moresellized bone can be packed into cavities using the acetabular reamers in reverse.

Minor and major column grafts can be fixed by cancellous screws or reinforcement rings or reconstruction pelvic plates. It is best not to ream these grafts but, if it is necessary, the cartilage is reamed off leaving the subchondral bone intact. It is done very lightly with the grafts fixed in position. If possible, do not expose cancellous surfaces of the allograft to anything but host bone (Figs. 8.2 and 8.3).

There are several options for the acetabular prosthesis (see Table 8.1). In the protrusio situation, morsellized bone, a reinforcement ring, and a cemented cup is a good reconstruction for the moderate- to low-demand elderly patient (Fig. 8.4). The best reconstruction for a protrusio defect in the higher demand patient is morsellized bone with an uncemented, fixed, large-diameter, metal-backed, porous coated cup with direct contact with at least 50% host bone (Figs. 8.1 and 8.5). Bipolar or biarticulating cups are only used if nothing else is technically or biologically possible, or if, because of the patient's health, a more extensive procedure is not indicated (Figs. 8.6).

A shelf or minor column defect will allow contact with at least 50% host bone and, here, we prefer to use an uncemented, porous coated cup, press-fit or fixed by screws (Fig. 8.7). A major column graft involves more than 50% of the acetabulum, which means that the cup is mainly in contact with dead allograft bone. Under these circumstances, the cup should be cemented (Figs. 8.8 and 8.9).

We attempt to obtain fixation of the porous coated cups by press-fit antirotation lugs, if possible. If not, we use screws to fix the metal backing in place. We have had no experience with screw-in cups. Bipolar cups are only used in the extreme salvage situation where nothing else is possible, for technical reasons, or because the patient's health will not tolerate a more extensive operative procedure (see Table 8.1).

Femur

We use long-stem femoral components and, therefore, we do not hesitate to cut a window for controlled cement removal and reaming. If a proximal femoral allograft is to be performed, then the residual proximal femur is split distally to good bone. As much soft tissue as possible is left attached to the residual bone for later use as a vascularized bone graft. The cement is then removed.

The distal host femur is then reamed gently over a guide-wire to assess canal size for the implant rather than

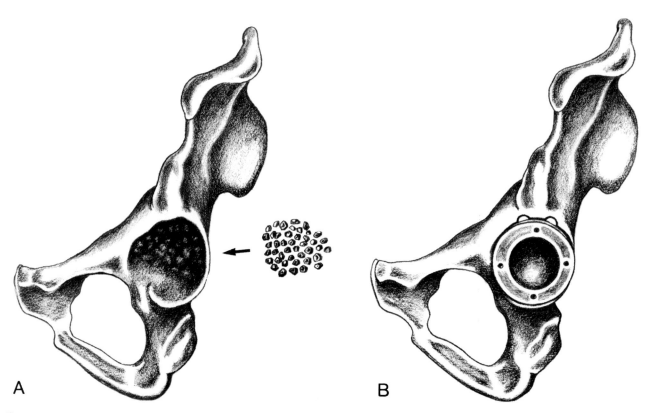

A   **B**

Figure 8.1. Protrusio reconstruction. *A.* Cancellous bone, morsellized by hand instruments rather than a mill, is packed into a contained cavitary (protrusio) defect. *B.* A metal-backed, porous coated uncemented cup is inserted. This may be press-fit or fixed with screws.

to enlarge the canal. When the reamers are at a size that definite reaming is taking place, then the diameter of implant is selected. The allograft, which is either proximal femur or tibia, is then reamed and broached until a good fit for the implant is achieved. The length of the allograft necessary is assessed in vivo by placing the femoral implant into the host bone and reducing it into the trial cup. The selected length depends on stability and leg length discrepancy. A Steinmann pin is inserted into the iliac crest and the distance from it to a fixed point on the femur is measured prior to dislocation of the hip. A step-cut of about 2 cm × 2 cm is carried out in the allograft (positive step) and in the host (negative step) for the grafts longer than 3 cm. This is not usually necessary for the calcar grafts.

When the correct length of allograft is obtained and the stability of the reconstruction is acceptable, the implant is cemented into the allograft after drill holes are made and wires are passed for trochanteric reattachment. It is very important to keep the cement off of the interface that will oppose host bone. The allograft with the long-stem femoral component cemented in place is inserted into the host and cerclage wire is used to stabilize the step-cut. The junction of host and allograft is also auto-

grafted by reamings or other host bone that is available. The residual host proximal femur is wrapped around the allograft and held by cerclage wires. An attempt is made to bring these vascularized pieces distally to wrap around the osteotomy junction to encourage union (Figs. 8.10–8.16). Cortical strut grafts are fixed with wires and autografted at the junction with host bone (Figs. 8.17 and 8.18).

We attempt to obtain a press-fit of the long-stem femoral component but this is not crucial for success because, once union is achieved at the osteotomy and the implant is cemented to the allograft, the femoral reconstruction is stabilized. In order to obtain a press-fit or, at least, a tight fit distally, a range of diameters of long-stem prostheses should be available. It is our opinion that bone ingrowth is impossible to obtain in these multiply revised femoral reconstructions and, therefore, porous coating on the femoral component is not necessary (*see* Table 8.1).

Postoperative Care

Prophylactic intravenous antibiotics are used for 5 days followed by 5 more days of oral antibiotics. We prefer a cephalosporine. If the patient is catheterized intraoperatively, we use gentamycin during the surgery and for the

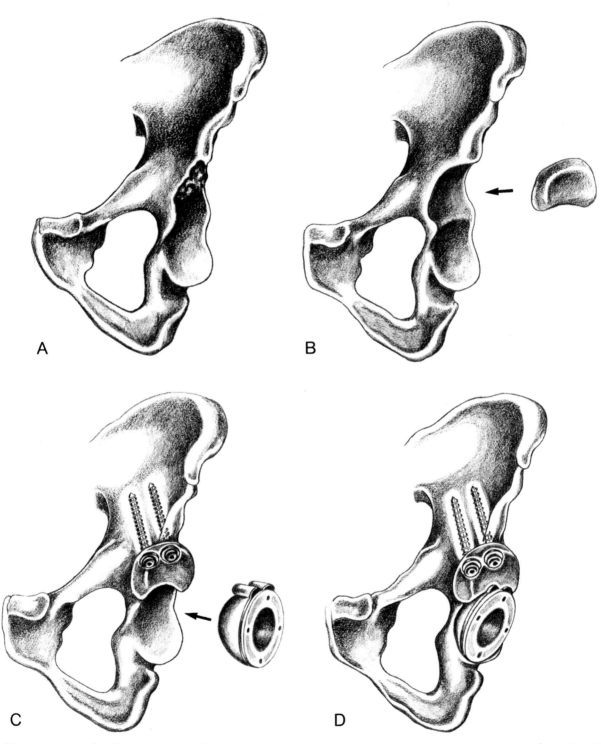

Figure 8.2. Minor column (shelf) reconstruction. *A.* Minor column (shelf) defect. *B.* A minor column allograft (portion of male femoral head allograft or a portion of a true acetabular allograft) is cut to fit the defect. *C.* Allograft is fixed with two screws and washers. Cancellous surfaces are not exposed. *D.* Uncemented press-fit cup in place and in contact with more than 50% of host bone.

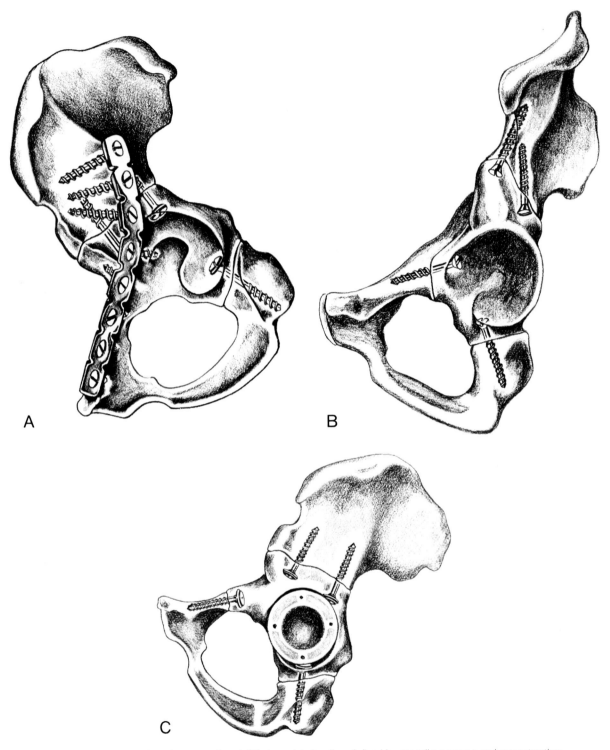

Figure 8.3. Major Column Reconstruction. *A.* Whole acetabular allograft fixed by cancellous screws and reconstruction plate. *B.* Whole acetabular allograft fixed by cancellous screws. *C.* Cemented cup in whole acetabular allograft.

Table 8.1.
Summary of Bone Deficits and Reconstructions

Small Defect
  Autograft
  Modified implant
Large Defect (Allograft)
  Pelvic side
    Contained Cavitary Defect (Protrusio)
      Low-demand patient
        Morsellized bone and protrusio ring and cemented cup
      High-demand patient
        Morsellized bone and large diameter uncemented metal backed cup (porous coated press-fit or held with screws)
    Structural defect (major or minor column defect)
      Solid graft
        Uncemented cup if less than 50% of acetabulum (porous coated press-fit or held with screws)
        Cemented cup if more than 50% of acetabulum
  Femoral side
    Cavitary defect
      Intralumenal graft with long-stem press-fit femoral component
    Structural defect
      Noncylindrical: cortical strut graft
      Cylindrical: proximal femoral allograft with press-fit femoral component; cement may be used in allograft but not in host

first 24 hours but then switch to Septra until the catheter is removed. Because of the extent of the surgery, we usually keep the patients on bed rest and in abduction for 5 days and then they are ambulated in a nonweight-bearing manner. The patients are not allowed any weight bearing until union is obtained between allograft and host, usually at 3–6 months.

PRINCIPLES OF SURGERY

1. Preoperatively, decide on the type of bone, internal fixation, and type of implant on pelvic and femoral sides.
2. If wide exposure is needed, use a transtrochanteric approach and reflect the vastus lateralis off the septum down to the tip of the old prosthesis.
3. Do not hesitate to cut a window at the tip of the old prosthesis since a long-stem prosthesis is going to be used. The window, in addition to allowing safe and rapid cement removal, allows controlled reaming.
4. Do not devascularize residual host femur that can be used later as a wrap-around vascularized bone graft.
5. If possible, do not use cement in the host, but cement can be used in the femoral allograft or in the pelvic allograft if it involves more than 50% of the acetabulum.

6. Rigid fixation of allografts must be achieved.
7. Always autograft host-allograft junctions.

REVIEW OF CLINICAL MATERIAL

Donor selection conformed to the guidelines recommended by the Musculoskeletal Council of the American Association of Tissue Banks. Cadaveric bone was harvested under sterile conditions with appropriate bacteriological examination. Bacteriological and viral sterility is ensured through irradiation with 2.5 megarads. Following the irradiation, the grafts are maintained at $-70°C$ until used.

The patients were followed prospectively with subjective and objective measurement of their hip functions recorded through a modification of the Harris hip scoring system (Table 8.2). Radiographic examination was performed on preoperative and all subsequent postoperative visits (Table 8.3). All surgery was performed by or under the direct supervision of the author (A.E.G.). Failure of the procedure was defined as failure to increase the postoperative hip score by 20 points above the preoperative value or the need for subsequent reoperation as a result of problems with the allograft.

From November 1979 until January 1990, 199 patients have had 212 revision arthroplasties of the hips using allograft bone. There were 325 allografts performed. There have been 111 protrusio grafts with an average follow-up of 5 years; 38 shelf (minor column) grafts with an average follow-up of 5 years; 44 acetabular grafts (major column) with an average follow-up of 4 years; and 132 proximal femoral allografts with an average follow-up of 4 years. The following allograft types had a minimum 2-year follow-up enabling them to be included in this study: 31 calcar grafts, 40 large-fragment proximal femoral allografts, seven femoral cortical strut allografts, 22 minor column acetabular grafts, 28 major column acetabular grafts, and 58 morsellized protrusio allografts. In bilateral cases, both grafts were considered individually as were concomitant femoral and acetabular grafts in the same hip.

RESULTS

Analysis of the results of this type of surgery must include not only clinical parameters but also radiological ones. Many of these patients have had grafts on both the pelvic and femoral sides, which makes the analysis more complex in that some patients are in both series.

The clinical and radiological results will be divided into the following groups: protrusio grafts; minor column

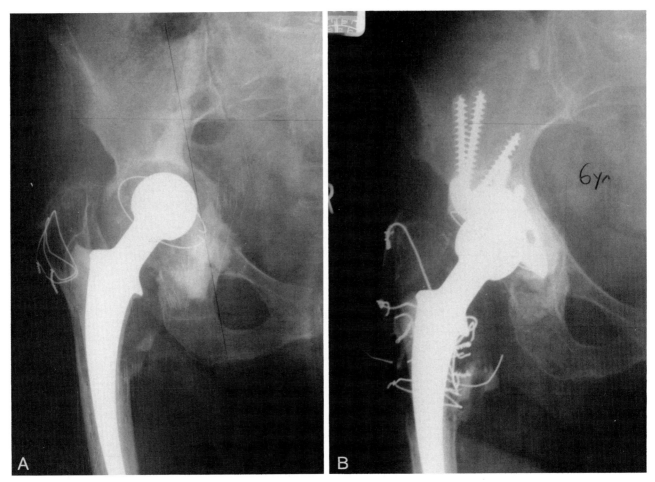

Figure 8.4. Protrusio reconstruction. *A.* Anteroposterior x-ray of the right hip demonstrating severe superomedial protrusio. *B.* Anterioposterior x-ray of the right hip 6 years after revision with morsellized bone, a protrusio ring, and a cemented cup.

or shelf grafts; major column grafts; calcar grafts; proximal femoral grafts; cortical strut grafts.

General Information of Femoral Allografts

This group consisted of 51 females and 18 males. Four patients had bilateral procedures, producing a total of 73 hips. The average age at surgery was 59 years, with a range of 29–83 years. The average time to follow-up was 33.6 months, with a range of 24–65 months. The initial indication for arthroplasty was osteoarthritis in 24 cases; post-traumatic arthrosis in 18 cases; congenital hip dysplasia in nine cases; Legg-Perthes disease in three cases; rheumatoid arthritis in seven cases; avascular necrosis in four cases; achondroplasia in two cases; and one case of each of the following: fibrosarcoma, childhood septic arthritis, proximal femoral cyst, hemophilia, spina bifida, and pigmented villonodular synovitis. As this series was composed of multiply revised patients, the acetabular bone stock was often deficient as well. In this group of patients, 83% underwent concomitant acetabular allografting. Of

these, 41% were for protrusio acetabulae, 21% received minor column allografts for a deficiency of less than 50% of the circumference of the acetabulum, and an additional 20% received a major acetabular allograft for a deficiency of greater than 50% of the circumference of the acetabulum. Previous procedures averaged 2.6, with a range of 1–7. Blood loss was considerable with a mean value of 2249 ml with a range of 900–5600 ml. This necessitated an average blood replacement of 4.6 units with a range of 1–12 units. The actual surgical operating time averaged 4.2 hours, with a range of 3.0–6.5 hours. For proximal femoral allografts as a group, the mean preoperative hip score was 39; the postoperative score was 68.

Specific Results of Femoral Allografts

CALCAR ALLOGRAFTS

There were 31 Calcar allografts, measuring less than or equal to 3 cm in the longest length. The average preoperative hip score was 37, with a range of 7–84. Postoperatively, the scores averaged 77, with a range of 47–

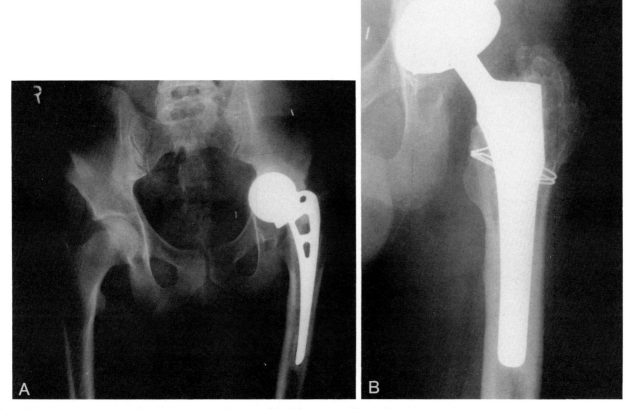

Figure 8.5. Protrusio reconstruction. *A.* Anteroposterior x-ray of the left hip showing a severe superomedial protrusio in a 35-year-old man 9 years after a Moore arthroplasty was performed for osteonecrosis of femoral head. *B.* Anteroposterior x-ray of the left hip 5 years after revision with morsellized allograft bone and an uncemented cup. Note the cup's large diameter and horizontal position. The allograft bone has consolidated and remodeled.

99. The average improvement in the score was 40. The average length of the allograft was 2.4 cm, with a range of 1–3 cm. Nonunion occurred in 17% of calcar allografts; however, only one of these was judged to be an unstable and symptomatic nonunion. Fracture or fragmentation occurred in two cases or 6% of these grafts. Resorption between one-third and one-half occurred in 10% and, in 40% of cases, there was resorption of greater than one-half of the initial allograft. Subsidence was seen in 43% of these calcar allografts with an average subsidence of 1.1 cm, ranging between 0.3 and 3.0 cm. Polymethylmethacrylate in the calcar allograft lessened the risk of significant resorption and fracture. Resorption of greater than one-third of the graft was seen in 79% of allografts without cement compared with only 10% of allografts cemented to the prostheses.

Radiological osseous trochanteric union occurred in 54% (seven of 13 cases) whereas stable fibrous union was seen in 31% (four of 13 cases). Trochanteric escape greater than 1 cm was seen in 15% (two of 13 cases).

Seven cases were classified as failures by our strict definition of failure. Five hips in four patients were classified as failures due to failure of the hip score to improve by 20 points postoperatively. There was one case of deep infection requiring an excisional arthroplasty and one case of a femoral fracture through a screw-hole beneath the prosthesis, which required reoperation. This was treated with open reduction and internal fixation, and, subsequently, resulting in a good outcome. By our strict definition of success, 77.4% of the calcar grafts had a successful outcome. One patient with a high preoperative hip score (69 on the scale) failed to increase by 20 points (a postoperative score of 83) was included as a failure. Most would accept this as a successful clinical outcome, thereby increasing the success rate to 81%.

LARGE-FRAGMENT PROXIMAL FEMORAL ALLOGRAFTS
There were 40 cases of large-fragment proximal femoral allografts. The average preoperative score was 30, with a range of 6–58. Postoperatively, the average score was 66,

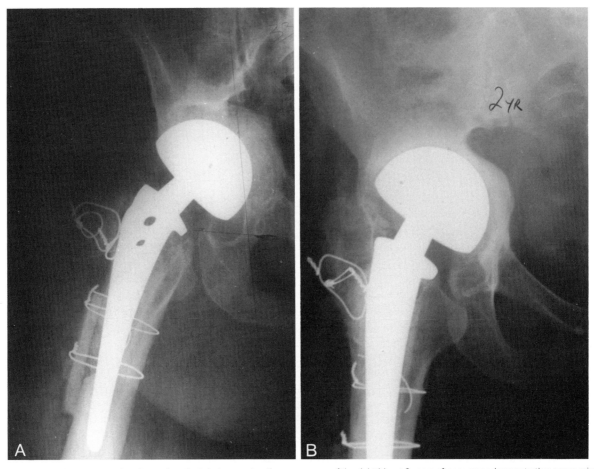

Figure 8.6. Protrusio reconstruction, femoral cortical strut reconstruction. *A.* Anteroposterior x-ray of the right hip, 1 week postoperatively after revision of severe protrusio by inserting morsellized allograft bone and a bipolar cup. Note also the cortical strut femoral graft. *B.* Anteroposterior x-ray of the right hip at 2 years after surgery demonstrating some migration of the cup but excellent remodeling of the morsellized bone and also showing remodelling of the femoral cortical strut.

with a range of 21–100. The average incremental increase in score was 36. The average length of these grafts was 10.4 cm, with a range of 3.5–17.0 cm. Primary radiographic osseous healing between the allograft and host bone was seen in 30 of 40 cases (75%). Bridging union with a persistently identifiable junction was seen in three of 40 cases (7.5%). A stable nonunion was seen in 2.5% (one of 40 cases) and an unstable nonunion was seen in 7.5% (three of 40 cases). One graft (4 cm in length) was seen to fragment. Resorption of the large allografts was not seen. Of 37 cases, four showed subsidence (11%). This ranged from 0.5–1.5 cm, averaging 1 cm. There were no cases of gross mechanical failure of the construct.

Radiographic osseous trochanteric union was seen in nine of 24 cases (38%), with 10 of 24 (42%) obtaining a stable fibrous union. In 21% of cases (five of 24), there was trochanteric escape of greater than 1 cm. There were four failures due to failure to increase the hip score postoperatively by 20 points. This included one patient with

chronic pain and venous insufficiency who subsequently underwent hip disarticulation and one person with a symptomatic nonunion. Three patients underwent resection arthroplasty for deep infection and one further patient underwent resection arthroplasty for recurrent dislocation. This patient had spina bifida and paralytic hip dysplasia. There was one death in this group. This was not related to the proximal femoral allograft but, instead, to acetabular reconstruction with laceration of the external iliac vein at the time of acetabular reconstruction. The overall success rate of proximal femoral allografts by our strict definition was 79%; however, if two patients with high postoperative hip scores who also had high preoperative hip scores were included in the successful group, the success rate is improved to 85%.

CORTICAL STRUT ALLOGRAFTS

There were seven cortical strut allografts performed in this series. The average preoperative hip score was 37,

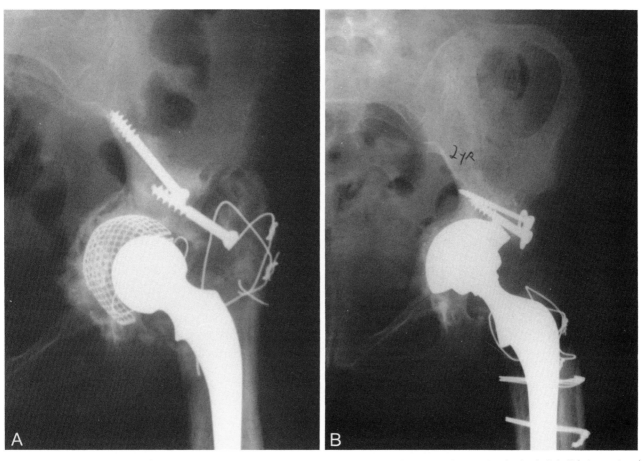

Figure 8.7. Shelf (minor column) reconstruction. *A.* Anteroposterior x-ray of the left hip with combined minor column and protrusio defect.

B. Anteroposterior x-ray at 2 years showing healed shelf (minor column) allograft. The loose washers indicate stress shielding.

with a range of 20–47. The postoperative hip score averaged 79, with a range of 43–78. The average increase of the hip score was 42. The mean length of the cortical strut was 5.8 cm, with a range of 3–8 cm. All cortical struts showed union as well as changing of their external contour, indicating revascularization and remodeling. There was no incidence of subsidence of the prosthesis nor were there any mechanical failures. There were no failures due to reoperation in this group and only one patient failed to increase his or her hip score by 20 points. The overall clinical success rate was, therefore, 86%. Mechanically, all of these grafts were successful.

General Information of Solid-Fragment Acetabular Allografts

The average preoperative hip score for the solid-fragment acetabular group as a whole was 30 (range of 4–60). Five patients were confined preoperatively to a wheelchair. Postoperatively, the hip score averaged 74, with a range of 55–98. Failure occurred in 10 patients (one patient bilaterally). There was one failure by score alone. Seven patients required additional surgery for major column

acetabular allograft complications and three patients needed surgery for minor column (shelf) allograft complications. Of the eight reoperated arthroplasties, six are now considered to have successful clinical scores, despite this setback.

Specific Results of Pelvic Allografts

MINOR COLUMN ACETABULAR ALLOGRAFTS (SHELF GRAFTS)

In the minor column reconstruction group, 19 patients underwent 22 acetabular allograft procedures. All of these patient were female. The mean age was 54.8 years (range, 29–75). The follow-up period ranged from 29–68 months, with a mean of 40.8 months. On each patient, one to five previous procedures had been performed, with an average of 2.5 procedures. The initial indication for arthroplasty was congenital hip dysplasia in 14 cases; osteoarthritis in five cases; and one case each of septic arthritis, pigmented villonodular synovitis, and juvenile rheumatoid arthritis. The mean preoperative hip score was 31 and the mean postoperative score was 72.

The defect was reconstructed using male femoral heads in 21 cases and a male femoral condyle in one case. In

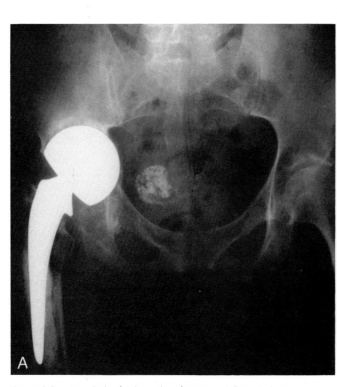

Figure 8.8. Acetabular (major column) reconstruction. A. Anteroposterior x-ray of the right hip with large superomedial defect involving the post column. B. Anteroposterior x-ray of the right hip 4 years following complete acetabular allograft fixed with two cancellous screws and a cemented cup.

one patient with an exceptionally large superior graft, a Mueller protrusio ring (Synthes Canada, Ltd.) was utilized to increase fixation. Polymethylmethacrylate was used as an adjunct to acetabular fixation in nine cases. In 13 cases, cementless prostheses were used. The femoral prosthesis was not changed in four patients; six patients had uncemented femoral prostheses inserted at revision; and seven patients required concomitant femoral allografts. The remainder of the patients had revision of the femoral component utilizing cemented femoral components.

In the 22 cases of minor column allografts, union and incorporation of the allograft was clearly seen in 19 cases. One case demonstrated only partial union and two cases had complete graft resorption by 8 and 12 months. All 19 united cases, along with the partially healed graft, had normal density, with only four of the 20 grafts demonstrating small areas of sclerotic radiodensity. There were two cases showing graft fracture or fragmentation. One of these was an undisplaced fracture seen on the shoot-through lateral, still an excellent clinical result. The other led to acetabular component dislocation necessitating revision of the acetabulum. Two grafts completely resorbed

and eight others showed a stress-shielding type of remodeling process in which the unloaded portion of the graft underwent lysis without affecting that portion of the graft involved in acetabular component support. This lateral lysis usually involved 3–7 mm of resorption of the lateral most edge of the acetabular component. This is a well-recognized phenomenon.

Acetabular implant migration was involved in three of the 22 cases. Two cases of migration involved bipolar prostheses. The third case of migration was associated with sudden dislocation of the acetabular component after 50% graft resorption.

In summary, of the 22 minor column acetabular reconstructions performed, three were failures: two from deep sepsis requiring excision and one from a dislocated acetabular component. The overall success rate was 86%.

MAJOR COLUMN ACETABULAR ALLOGRAFTS

In the major column acetabular reconstruction group, 26 patients underwent 28 major column or whole acetabular allograft procedures. Seven were male patients and 19 were female patients. The mean age was 74.8 years, with

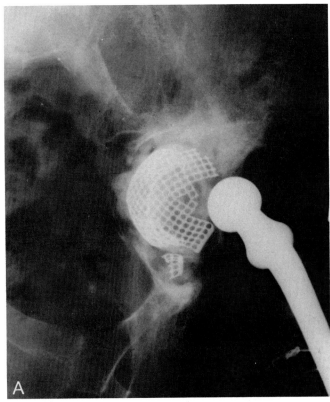

Figure 8.9. Acetabular (major column) reconstruction. A. Judet view of the left hip showing combined anterior and posterior column bone deficit. B. Anteroposterior view of the left hip at 6 years. The whole acetabular allograft was fixed with an acetabular reinforcement ring that went from host bone to host bone.

a range of 27–85 years. Follow-up ranged from 24–71 months, with a mean of 36 months. A range of one to eight previous procedures had been performed, with an average of 2.9 procedures. The initial indication for arthroplasty was rheumatoid arthritis in seven cases; congenital hip dysplasia in five cases; osteoarthritis in five cases; Legg-Perthes disease in four cases; post-traumatic arthritis in three cases; and one case each of chondrosarcoma, fibrosarcoma, fibrous dysplasia, and myelomeningocele. The mean preoperative hip score was 29; the mean postoperative score was 75.

Twelve patients had complete acetabular reconstructions, 11 of them using whole acetabuli from cadaveric hemipelvises, and one using femoral heads. The remaining 16 acetabular deficiencies involved reconstruction of greater than 50% of the acetabular surface area, often whole anterior or posterior column defects. Ten of those were reconstructed using male femoral heads and five used portions of acetabuli from cadaveric hemipelvises. Polymethylmethacrylate was used for 13 of the 28 cases, 12 of which also utilized a reinforcement ring. Fifteen cementless components were used. The femoral prosthesis was not changed in eight pa-

tients; nine patients had uncemented femoral components inserted; and 11 patients had concomitant circumferential proximal femoral allografts inserted for femoral bone stock deficiency.

There was one case of deep sepsis requiring excision in a reconstruction using femoral heads. A patient with flaccid paralysis (myelomenigocele) reconstructed with an acetabular allograft required further surgery for recurrent dislocation.

Six of the remaining 14 true acetabular allografts (i.e., reconstruction with acetabular allograft bone) required further surgery due to fracture or fragmentation of the graft. The subsequent reconstruction was greatly facilitated by the restored bone stock. Five of these six reoperated acetabular allografts have a successful clinical score 2 years after reoperation. The last patient with a bipolar reconstruction remains a failure due to the minimal increase in her clinical score after reoperation.

Six allografts were associated with implant migration and five of these cases involved a bipolar prosthesis that had eroded the allograft in varying amounts of 5–15 mm in a proximal medial direction. Only one of the six bipolar reconstructions was not associated with migration. The

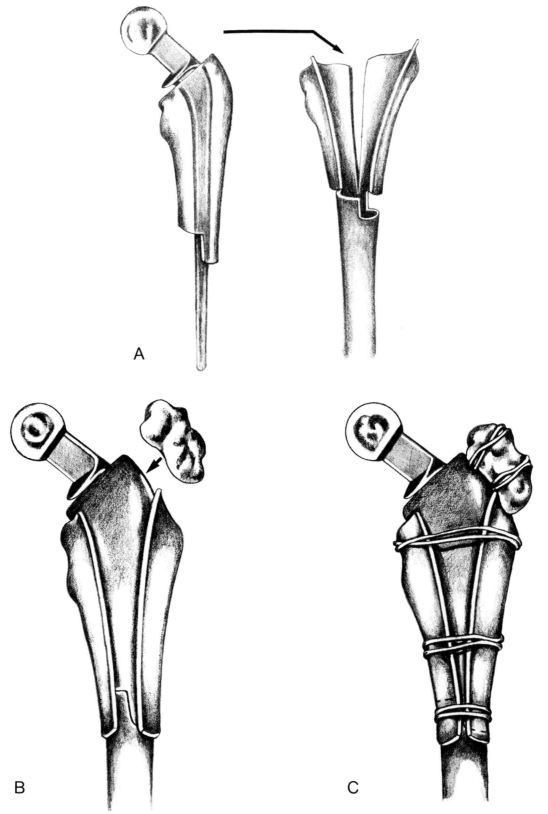

Figure 8.10. Proximal femoral reconstruction. *A.* Proximal femoral allograft, prepared with step-cut, is to be inserted into the host femur with the residual host bone split and retracted to form the host bed. Cement is used between the allograft and implant, but not in the host femur. *B.*

Allograft and implant are in place with residual host bone wrapped around the allograft and pulled down to cover the junction of allograft and host femur as a living bone graft. *C.* Greater trochanter and host bone are wired to the allograft.

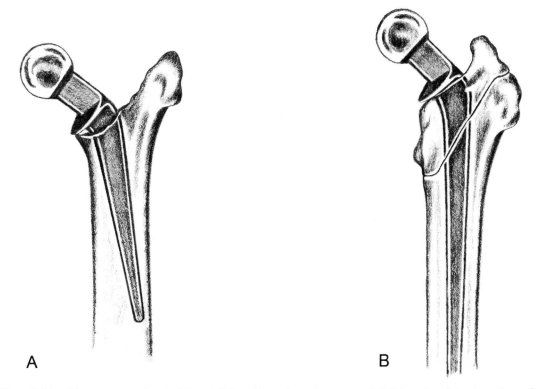

Figure 8.11. Calcar reconstruction. *A.* Calcar deficit and loose femoral component. *B.* Calcar allograft in place. The graft should be cemented to component.

overall success rate for major column allografts was 71% (20 of 28 cases).

MORSELLIZED PROTRUSIO ACETABULAR ALLOGRAFTS

This series consisted of 58 contained cavitary defects. The 19 male and 39 female patients had an average age of 60.9 years (31–87 years). The predominant indication for the initial surgery was osteoarthritis in 27 cases (four of these were bilateral). Other indications include inflammatory arthritis in nine cases; post-traumatic arthritis in 11 cases; congenital hip dysplasia in three cases; post-tumor resection in two cases; and one case each of hemophilia and Legg-Perthes disease. There were an average of 2.4 prior procedures, ranging from one to six. Follow-up averaged 46.4 months (26–87 months). The femoral component was revised in 90% of cases and 57% of the cases underwent revision using proximal femoral allograft.

Morsellized allograft bone was used in all protrusio reconstructions. In 32 hips, an uncemented, porous coated, fixed cup was used; in 15 procedures, a Mueller reinforcement ring and a cemented cup were used; and in 11 hips, a biarticulating device was used. Based on clinical assessment alone, a successful outcome was seen in 100% of reconstructions using a reinforcement ring and a cemented

cup, 93.7% using a noncemented cup, and 63.6% using a bicentric device.

Radiographic review demonstrates probable loosening (circumferential lucent lines of more than 2 mm) in 57% and definite loosening (migration or change of orientation) in 14% of reconstructions using reinforcement rings (average follow-up, 63 months). Possible loosening was seen in 5% of the uncemented cups at an average follow-up of 39 months. Of the bicentric reconstructions, fifty seven percent showed significant migration and less satisfactory pain reduction. Overall, the average medial migration of the bicentric devices was 3.2 mm (range, 0 = 10 mm) and superior migration averaged 17.0 mm (range, 0–60 mm). The superior lateral corner of the obturator foramina served as landmarks utilizing horizontal and vertical lines from the center of the femoral head to determine superior and medial migration (Fig. 8.19). In contrast, cemented implants with reinforcement rings averaged 0.1 mm of medial migration (range −1 to +1 mm) and 1.7 mm of superior migration (range, −6 to +12 mm). The fixed noncemented implants averaged 0.9 mm of medial migration (range, −3 to +4 mm) and 1.1 mm of superior migration (range, −9 to +9 mm).

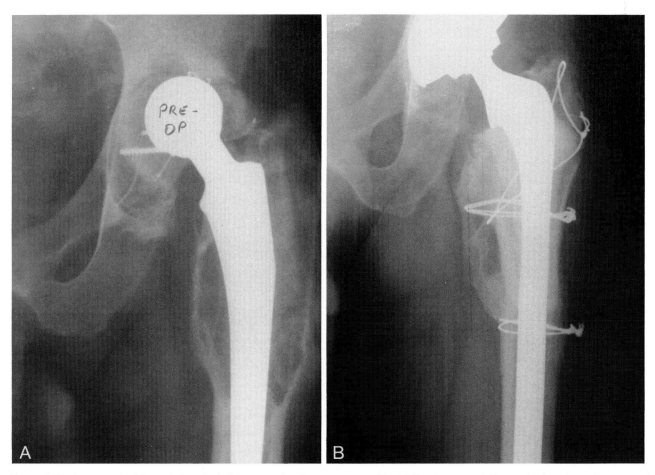

Figure 8.12. Large proximal femoral allograft. *A.* Anteroposterior view of the left hip showing massive osteolysis of proximal femur after total hip replacement. *B.* Anteroposterior view of the left hip 3 years after reconstruction with a proximal femoral allograft. The distal cerclage wire was used to stabilize the step-cut. The proximal cerclage wire was used to wrap the residual host femur around the allograft. Note how the residual host femur reinforces the graft and also helped gain union at the host-allograft junction.

Remodeling and resorption of the morsellized graft were observed. The final width of the bone graft was noted to be diminished compared with the immediate postoperative width. Percentage resorption was 5.7% (range, 0–27%) in the cemented cups, 50.6% (range, 17–100%) in the bicentric devices, and 26.4% (range 0–83%) in the noncemented cups. Table 8.4 includes a summary of the mean preoperative, postoperative, and incremental hip scores for the various allograft groups.

Complications

Complications in this series were significant. There were three dislocations; two of these were managed with closed reduction and one case with spina bifida required excisional arthroplasty for recurrent dislocation.

There were two cases of superficial wound infection that resolved with local wound care and antibiotics. There were five episodes of deep sepsis, four of which required

excisional arthroplasties. One of these has subsequently been reconstructed with a good result. One patient with a late deep infection in a massive allograft is satisfied to continue on long-term antibiotic suppression. The overall deep sepsis rate for the solid-fragment allografts was 6.8%; and for the morsellized allograft group, it was 3.4%.

There were seven episodes of deep venous thrombosis and two cases of pulmonary thromboembolism resolving uneventfully. There was one femoral fracture occurring after plate removal. There were three cases of symptomatic trochanteric nonunion, managed nonoperatively, and one case of trochanteric bursitis, which required operative intervention. There were two cases of peroneal nerve palsy, both resolving spontaneously; one case of postoperative ileus; and one case of depression requiring psychiatric management. Two hips in one patient developed grade IV heterotopic ossification, which adversely affected the end result. There were two cases of *clostridium difficile* enteritis, which were related to

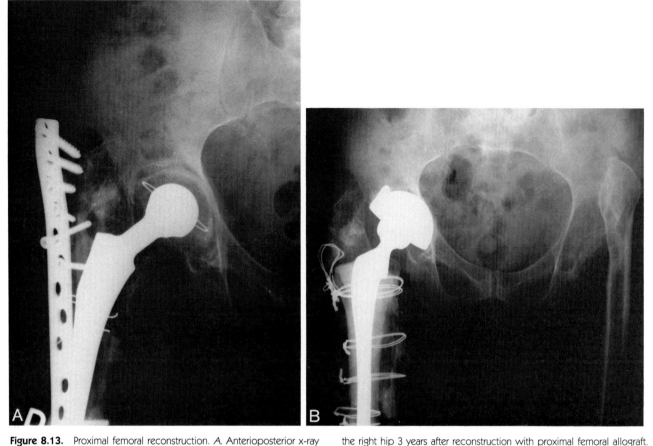

Figure 8.13. Proximal femoral reconstruction. *A.* Anterioposterior x-ray of the right hip of a 55-year-old man with loss of bone stock proximal femur after multiple procedures on right hip. *B.* Anteroposterior x-ray of the right hip 3 years after reconstruction with proximal femoral allograft. Note the stable fibrous union of greater trochanter. The implant is cemented to the allograft but not to the host.

prophylactic antibiotics and subsided uneventfully. There were two cases of symptomatic femoral loosening. Only one of these has required revision surgery.

There were two deaths related directly to surgery. One was a case of postoperative aspiration pneumonia and bowel obstruction. The second case was secondary to laceration of an iliac vein during reconstruction of the acetabulum. There was one further case of vascular injury in a hemophiliac in which an injury of the superior gluteal vessels resulted in a severe intraoperative bleed that was successfully embolized. This patient went on to develop chronic venous insufficiency and pain and, eventually, underwent hip disarticulation elsewhere. There were three unrelated deaths during the course of follow-up. Sufficient data were available prior to death to include these patients in this study.

In the large-fragment proximal femoral allograft group, there were three nonunions at the allograft-host junction requiring bone grafting and internal fixation. All cases united with good clinical results.

Six patients had fracture and/or fragmentation of a portion of the acetabular allograft. These patients were reoperated and five of the six reconstructions are now successful.

Discussion

The results of this study strongly support the use of solid-fragment femoral allografts to reconstruct substantial bony loss. Large allografts undergo slow and incomplete revascularization. Even over a period of years, the large allografts tend to maintain their original structural integrity. Long-term results of allografts used in numerous circumstances are becoming evident in the literature (36–44). The primary benefit is the reconstruction of the osseous architecture to normal or near-normal levels utilizing material that comes as close as possible to mimicking the original tissue. Allografts will heal to the host bone at the areas of contact by a process of creeping substitution (45–47). This gives rise to a "biological weld" at the interface between the host and allograft bone. Union of the allograft to the host bone was not a problem. Primary osseous union occurred in the majority of cases.

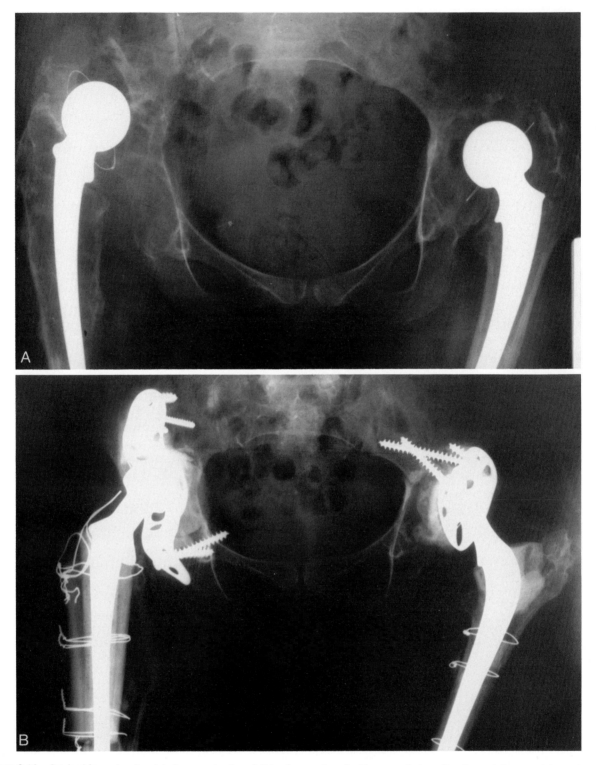

Figure 8.14. Proximal femoral and acetabular reconstructions (bilateral). A. Preoperative x-ray showing bilateral loose implants at 11 years in a 30-year-old juvenile rheumatoid patient. B. Six years after revision arthroplasty with restoration of bone stock. On the right side, there is a major column allograft with a cemented cup fixed by a reinforcement ring and a proximal femoral allograft. On the left side, there is a major column allograft fixed by a reinforcement ring with a cemented cup and cemented calcar graft.

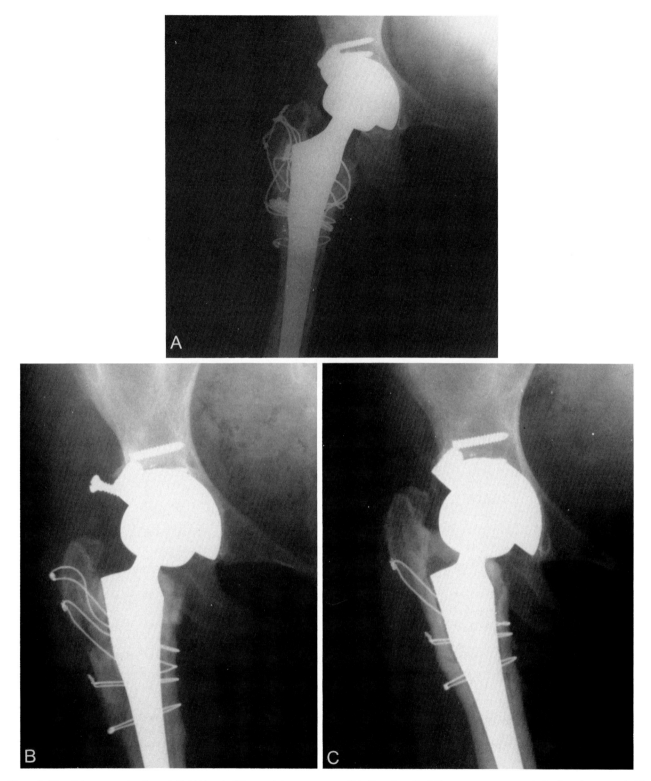

Figure 8.15. Calcar reconstruction. *A.* Right hip of a 30-year-old woman 3 months following a revision arthroplasty with an uncemented calcar allograft. *B.* One year postoperatively, there is subsidence of the implant within the allograft. *C.* Three years postoperatively, there is more subsidence with resulting loss of function necessitating further revision.

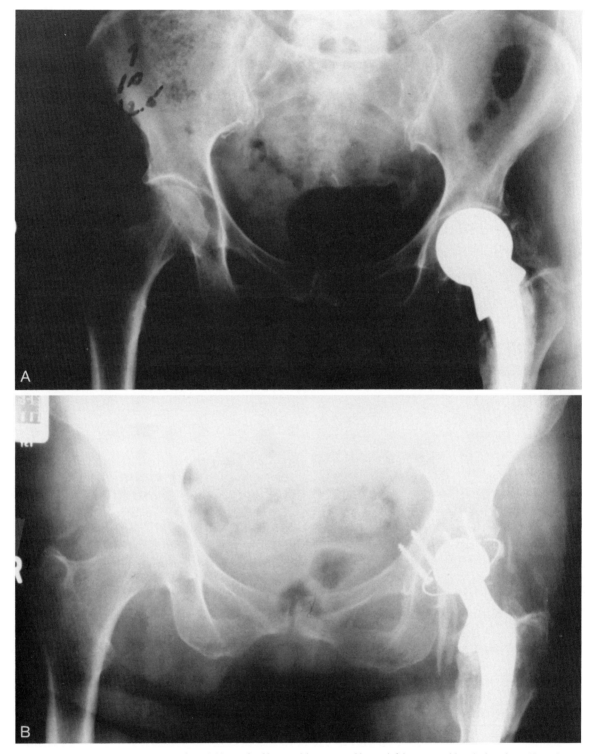

Figure 8.16.   Calcar reconstruction. *A.* X-ray of a 60-year-old woman with a painful cemented hemiarthroplasty. Note the loss of calcar due to stress shielding. *B.* Five years after revision arthroplasty, with a cemented calcar allograft.

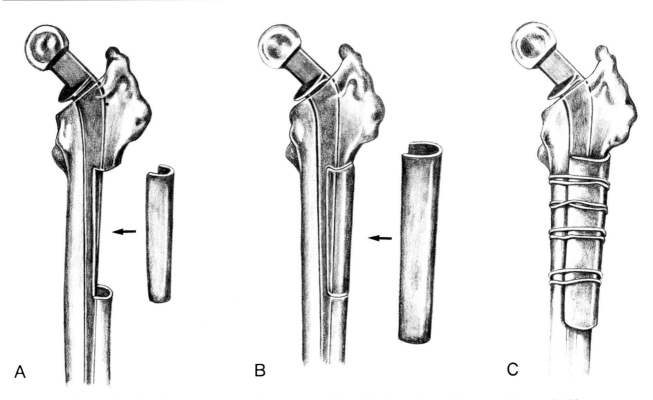

Figure 8.17. Cortical strut graft. *A.* Noncylindrical cortical defect. *B.* Cortical strut allograft is inserted. The strut should overlap the defect. *C.* Cortical strut allograft wired in place.

On occasion, nonunion occurs and, should an unstable situation develop, union is readily achieved through open reduction internal fixation and autogeneous bone grafting.

Soft tissue attachment to the allograft also occurs. This may decrease the stresses on the implants leading to a stable, more durable reconstruction. The structural integrity of an allograft is greater than that of available autogenic grafts and the process of revascularization is significantly retarded and random. Potentially, the failure of an allograft as a mechanical construct occurs when the process of revascularization results in increased porosity of the graft. This may lead to gradual fragmentation or sudden failure through a stress-riser phenomenon. In future long-term follow-up, if the revascularization and remodeling process leads to late construct failure, perhaps further revision surgery can begin on a bed of greater bone stock.

As outlined by others, reconstruction using cemented components in the face of massive osteolysis is only a short-term solution leading to more rapid bone loss and destruction (18–21, 23–26, 48–50).

Performance of allograft surgery of the hip requires certain prerequisites to be met. Not only must the availability of massive allograft bone be ensured, but the assistance of a second surgeon is required. The deep infection rate of 6.8% must also be borne in mind. Undoubtedly, the number of previous revisions and the long operating time with the implantation of a large foreign body contributes to the high infection rate. Every effort must be made to maintain the optimum operating environment. The use of laminar flow and total body exhaust is recommended, as is the use of prophylactic antibiotics and local wound irrigation with topical antibiotic. The incidence of thromboembolic disease may be minimized through the use of prophylactic low-dose warfarin.

CALCAR ALLOGRAFTS

This study cast some doubt on the use of calcar allografts. Calcar allografts measuring less than 3 cm contribute little to the overall stability of implants and their indication for use must be questioned. Alternatives, such as leaving the component proud or utilizing a long prosthetic neck length, may obviate the need for small calcar grafts. The incidence of resorption and fracture of these small grafts is dramatically lessened when the allograft is secured to the prosthesis with polymethylmethacrylate. Not only does the cement enhance the overall strength of the allograft but it is theorized that it may decrease the surface area available for revascularization and, thus, retard this process.

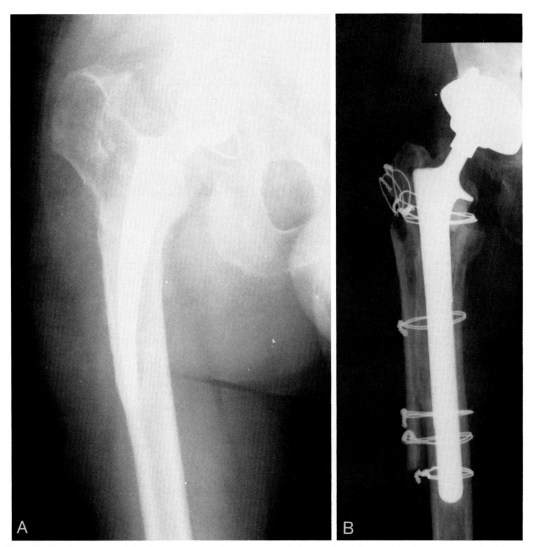

Figure 8.18.   Cortical strut graft. *A,* X-ray of a 40-year-old man with a loose femoral component causing erosion of lateral femoral cortex. *B.* One year following cortical strut allograft.

CORTICAL STRUT ALLOGRAFTS

It would appear that cortical strut grafts unite to host bone and eventually revascularize by virtue of the apparent remodeling of the allograft. The continuity of the femoral cortex is restored. The use of these allografts is, in effect, prophylactic to prevent a stress riser effect and subsequent fracture through a cortical defect. Some surgeons have utilized cortical strut allografts as an alternative to long-stem prostheses or as a means of internal fixation of periprosthetic femoral fractures. Cortical struts are also used, on occasion, to bridge the allograft host junction in some cases of large-fragment allografts.

LARGE FRAGMENT FEMORAL ALLOGRAFTS

These allografts uniformly maintained their overall structural integrity. We believe that it is important to cement these allografts proximally to the implant because it is impossible to shape the allograft perfectly to conform to the geometry of the prosthesis. The cement fills the voids, enhancing the strength of the construct, and may retard revascularization by diminishing the surface area of exposed bone. Cement is always excluded from the allograft-host junction and only rarely is used in the host bone.

Union to the host bone distally has not proven to be a significant problem. Trochanteric nonunion, although common, rarely is symptomatic because significant migration rarely occurs. Union could possibly be enhanced by utilizing a long oblique osteotomy to increase the surface area available for union. The use of an implant of sufficient diameter to permit a press-fit into the host bone gives the most reliable stability to bending forces.

Table 8.2.
Hip Rating

Pain	Deformity
44 = None	Fixed Adduction
40 = Slight	1 = < 10
30 = Moderate, occa-	0 = > 10
sional	Fixed Internal Rotation
20 = Moderate	1 = < 10
10 = Marked	0 = > 10
0 = Disabled	Flexion Contracture
Function	1 = < 15
Limp	0 = > 15
11 = None	Leg Length Discrepancy
8 = Slight	1 = < 3 cm
5 = Moderate	0 = > 3 cm
0 = Severe	Range of Motion
Support	Flexion
11 = None	1 = > 90
7 = Cane, long walks	0 = < 90
3 = 1 Crutch	Abduction
2 = 2 Canes	1 = > 15
0 = 2 Crutches	0 = < 15
Distance walked	Adduction
11 = Unlimited	1 = > 15
8 = 6 Blocks	0 = < 15
5 = 3 Blocks	External Rotation
2 = Indoors	1 = > 30
0 = Bed and chair	0 = < 30
Activities	Internal Rotation
Stairs	1 = > 15
4 = Normally	0 = < 15
2 = Without railing	Trendelenburg
1 = Any manner	1 = Negative
0 = Unable	0 = Positive
Shoes and socks	
4 = With ease	
2 = With difficulty	
0 = Unable	
Sitting	
4 = Any chair, 1 hour	
2 = High chair	
0 = Unable to sit com-	
fortably	
Public transportation	
1 = Able to use	
0 = Unable to use	

The use of a step-cut and cerclage wiring gives rotational stability to the construct. The interface should be generously bone grafted with autogeneous cancellous bone. In several cases, cortical strut allografts have also been utilized to increase the stability. Every effort should be made to wrap remaining host bone circumferentially about the allograft to enhance its stability. Host bone with soft

Table 8.3.
Radiological Parameters

Host/Donor Union

Radiodensity
  Sclerotic
  Normal
  Lytic
Resorption
Fracture/fragmentation
Migration/collapse of allograft alone
Migration/collapse of allograft/implant
Trochanteric union/migration

tissue attachment can also be drawn distally to bridge the site of junction. Although there were no cases of fracture or significant resorption of large-fragment allografts, one case was seen to have some cortical scalloping at 4-year follow-up. This raises concern about the potential for long-term failure of this construct should this process continue.

MINOR COLUMN ACETABULAR ALLOGRAFTS

This form of allograft procedure is known to be successful (31, 37, 51–53). The resorption of the unstressed lateral portion of the graft is expected (52, 53). Technically, fixation can be adequately achieved using interfragmentary compression screws (31, 37). The allograft shelf often must be made slightly larger than needed to prevent fragmentation when it is rigidly secured to the pelvis in compression. Ideally, the graft should be fixed to the pelvis with as large a contact area as possible. This will minimize shear and speed union. Excluding bipolar components, there was no appreciable difference between the clinical and roentgenographic assessments of the cementless versus the cemented prostheses. We feel confident that a well-fixed uncemented component will provide a dependable construct if it is seated on at least 50% live bleeding bone. Male femoral heads should be used and, if possible, cancellous surfaces should not be exposed to host soft tissue.

MAJOR COLUMN ACETABULAR ALLOGRAFTS

The union rate of large and total acetabular allografts is equivalent to that displayed by femoral head allografts (31). The total acetabular construct must be solidly fixed to the recipient's pelvis to achieve union. Often, this must be done with large pelvic protrusio rings or reconstruction plates in common with interfragmentary screws. Fracture or resorption of portions of the acetabular al-

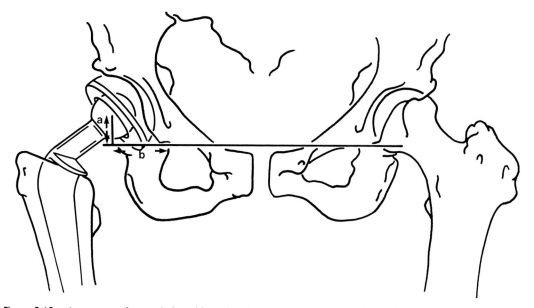

Figure 8.19. Assessment of protrusio in revision arthroplasty of the hip. Reference line is drawn through the superolateral corners of both abturator foramina. *a* = superior migration. *b* = medial migration.

Table 8.4.
Hip Scores for Allograft Reconstruction

Allograft Designation	Mean Preoperative Score	Mean Postoperative Score	Mean Increment Score
Calcar	37	77	40
Proximal femur	30	66	36
Cortical femoral strut	37	79	42
Minor column	31	72	41
Major column	29	75	46
Protrusio cemented	32	74	42
Protrusio noncemented	42	80	38
Protrusio bicentric	33	59	26

lograft may occur and can often be salvaged with repeat allografting.

The type of fixed acetabular component does not seem to matter. The predictability of a cemented cup in a whole acetabular allograft would seem attractive. There was a definite and progressive bone loss in a proximal and medial direction with the use of the mobile bipolar cups. Technically, the surgery related to the true acetabular allografts is simpler than that of a multiple segment femoral head reconstruction. It allows for easier component location in the allograft with the advantage of

bicortical structural integrity with a union rate similar to femoral head grafts (31).

It is clearly evident that the construct of whole or nearly whole acetabular allografts is far from a proven technique. As seen in this small review, it is associated with a relatively high level of complications due specifically to the acetabular allograft. With the elimination of the complications of deep sepsis, femoral component loosening, and improper patient selection, there were six acetabular allografts in the series that required revision surgery. Of these six failures, five have been salvaged to become clinical successes, with all of them having 2 or more years of follow-up. This must be discussed in light of the fact that all of these patients had been referred by other orthopaedic surgeons and many had been told they were no longer candidates for further reconstructive hip surgery. The severity of their conditions is represented by their preoperative scores and modes of ambulation. Many were transported by stretcher, by wheelchair, or were functioning with two crutches or two canes as household ambulators. Therefore, the high revision rate of these acetabular allografts must be assessed, keeping all of these factors in mind. We believe, based on our results to date, that there are certain indications for this type of complex reconstruction.

It is our feeling that if a bulk allograft can be avoided on the pelvic side by moving the cup superiorly or superomedially to gain contact with host bone, then this is the procedure of choice. There are, however, difficult multiply revised hips where contact with host bone is impossible and a bulk acetabular graft is needed. We believe that our present success rate justifies an ongoing study of this type of complex reconstruction.

MORSELLIZED PROTRUSIO ACETABULAR ALLOGRAFTS

Morsellized allograft appears to undergo rapid revascularization as demonstrated by radiographic appearance of incorporation, consolidation, and remodeling. Despite the good clinical results of cemented implants with reinforcement rings, we are concerned with the high incidence of radiolucent lines. These suggest impending implant loosening and, therefore, we prefer to utilize this form of reconstruction only in elderly, low-demand patients. Noncemented cups gave consistently good clinical and radiographic results and are the preferred method of reconstruction. Bicentric devices generally should not be used due to problems with significant migration and less satisfactory pain relief.

CONCLUSIONS
Cortical Strut Grafts

1. Mechanically successful in all cases;
2. Cortical strut grafting is an alternative method of bridging and reconstituting isolated cortical defects of the femur;
3. These small grafts appear to undergo revascularization and subsequent remodeling and virtual 100% union to host bone.

Calcar Allografts

1. Clinically successful in 77% but greater than 50% show significant resorption;
2. The use of calcar allografts of less than 2–3 cm should be abandoned; if necessary to utilize small proximal allografts one should ensure that these grafts are circumferential and be of strong cortical bone; they should definitely be cemented to the prosthesis to enhance its strength and to minimize the chance of resorption.

Large-Fragment Allografts

1. Successful in 85%;
2. Large-fragment allografts must be cemented proximally to the prosthesis with the prosthesis press-fit distally into the host bone;
2. A step-cut should be employed to ensure rotational stability and to increase the surface area of bony contact;
3. Host-allograft junctions should have the cement excluded from the interface and should be generously grafted with autogenic bone;
4. Every attempt should be made to avoid breaking the cortical

integrity of the allograft with drill holes, especially at its distal load-bearing area; small diameter drill holes can be used proximally for trochanter reattachment;
5. By 4 months, the majority of the allografts have undergone bony healing; nonunions managed with open reduction and internal fixation with bone grafting have good results.

Minor Column Acetabular Allografts

1. Successful in 86%;
2. Resorption of the unstressed lateral portion of the graft is common;
3. Fixed, uncemented acetabular components gave a dependable construct if seated on at least 50% host bone.

Major Column Acetabular Allografts

1. Successful in 71%;
2. Of 16 whole acetabular allografts, six were associated with fractures or resorption within 2 years;
3. Of six failed allografts, five were salvaged with repeat auto- and allografting;
4. Of 10 multiple femoral head acetabular allografts, two had radiographic evidence for resorption and nonunion but were still clinically successful;
5. Of six bipolar cups, five were associated with significant migration and should not be used;
6. Major complex deficiencies of the acetabulum are technically easier to reconstruct with total acetabular allografts than with femoral head segments.

Morsellized Protrusio Acetabular Allografts

1. Morsellized allograft incorporates and remodels well;
2. Fixed cemented and noncemented cups function well clinically; however, radiographically, the cemented cups demonstrate 57% possible loosening and 14% definite loosening compared to 5% possible loosening in the noncemented group;
3. Noncemented cups are the preferred method of protrusio reconstruction (94% successful), reserving reinforcement rings and cemented implants for elderly, low-demand patients (100% clinically successful);
4. Bicentric devices are associated with significant implant migration and less satisfactory pain reduction and probably should only be used when fixed devices cannot be used for technical reasons; the overall success rate was only 64%.

REFERENCES

1. Beckenbaugh RD, Illstrup DM. Total hip arthroplasty. A review of three hundred and thirty three cases with long term follow-up. J Bone Joint Surg 1978; 60A:306.
2. Stauffer RN. Ten year follow-up study of total hip replacement with particular reference to roentgenographic loosening of the components. J Bone Joint Surg 1982; 64A:983.

3. Harris WH, McCarthy JC. Jr, O'Neill DA. Femoral component loosening using contemporary techniques of femoral cement fixation. J Bone Joint Surg 1982; 64A:1063.

4. Wroblewski BM. Fifteen to twenty one year results of the Charnley low friction arthroplasty. Clin Orthop 1986; 211:30.

5. Halley DK, Wroblewski BM. Long term results of low friction arthroplasty in patients thirty years or younger. Clin Orthop 1986; 211:43.

6. Eftekhar NS. Long term results of cemented total hip arthroplasty. Clin Orthop 1987; 225:207.

7. Charnley J. Long term results of low friction arthroplasty: the hip. Proceedings of the 10th Open Scientific Meeting of the Hip Society 1982, C.V. Mosby, St. Louis, 1982; p. 42.

8. Hamilton HW, Joyce M. Long term results of low fraction arthroplasty performed in a community hospital including a radiologic review. Clin Orthop 1986; 211:55.

9. Chandler HP, Reinech FT, Wixson RL, McCarthy JC. Total hip replacement in patients younger than thirty years old. A five year follow-up study. J Bone Joint Surg 1991; 63A:1426.

10. Ranawat CS, Atkinson RE, Salvati EA, Wilson PD Jr. Conventional total hip arthroplasty for degenerative joint disease in patients between the ages of 40 and 60 years. J Bone Joint Surg 1984; 66A:745.

11. Gustilo RB, Burnham WH, Long term results of total hip arthroplasty in young patients. The hip. Proceeding of the 10th Open Scientific Meeting of the Hip Society. C.V. Mosby Co., St. Louis, 1982; p. 34.

12. Collis DK. Cemented total hip replacement in patients who are less than 50 years old. J Bone Joint Surg 1984; 66A:353.

13. Ranawat CS, Atkinson RE, Savati EA, Wilson PD, Jr. Conventional total hip arthroplasty for degenerative joint disease in patients between the ages of 40 and 60 years. J Bone Joint Surg 1984; 66A:745.

14. Engh CA, Bobyn JD, Glassman AH. Porous coated hip replacement. J Bone Joint Surg 1987; 69B:45.

15. Hungerford DS, Krackow KW. Total joint arthroplasty of the knee. Clin Orthop 1985; 192:23.

16. Harris WH, McCann WA. Loosening of the femoral component after use of a medullary plug cementing technique. Follow up note with a minimum 5 year follow up. J Bone Joint Surg 1986; 68A:1064.

17. Russotti GM, Coventry MB, Stauffer RN. Cemented total hip arthroplasty with contemporary techniques. A five year minimum followup study. Clin Orthop Relat Res 1988; 235:141–147.

18. Freeman MAR, Bradley GW, Revell PA. Observations upon the interface between bone and polymethylmethacrylate cement. J Bone Joint Surg 1982; 64B:489.

19. Goldring SR, Schiller AL, Roelke MS, Rourke CM, Bringhurst FR, Harris WH. Formation of a synovial-like membrane at the bone cement interface. Arthritis Rheum 1986; 29:836.

20. Goldring SR, Schiller AL, Roelke M, Rourke CM, O'Neill DA, Harris WH. The synovial-like membrane at the bone cement interface in loose total hip replacements and its proposed role in bone lysis. J Bone Joint Surg 1983; 65A:575.

21. Goodman SB, Schatzker J, Sumner-Smith G, Fornasier VL, Geften N, Hunt C. The effect of polymethylmethacrylate on bone: an experimental study. Arch Orthop Trauma Surg 1985; 104:150.

22. Howie D, Oakeshott R, Manthy B, Vernon-Roberts B. Bone Resorption in the presence of polyethylene wear particles. J Bone Joint Surg 1987; 69B:165.

23. Jasty MJ, Floyd WE, Schiller AL, Goldring SR, Harris WH. Localized osteolysis in stable, non-septic total hip replacement. J Bone Joint Surg 1986; 68A:912.

24. Linder L, Lindberg L, Carlsson A. Aseptic loosening of hip prostheses. Clin Orthop 1983; 175:93.

25. Pazzaglia UE, Ceciliani L, Wilkinson MJ, Dell'Orbo C. Involvement of metal particles in loosening of metal-plastic total hip prostheses. Arch Orthop Trauma Surg 1985; 104:164.

26. Revell PA, Weightman B, Freeman MAR, Vernon-Roberts B. The production and biology of polyethylene wear debris. Arch Orthop Trauma Surg 1978; 91:167.

27. Harris WH, White RE Jr. Resection arthroplasty for non-septic failure of total hip arthroplasty. Clin Orthop 1982; 171:62.

28. Grauer JD, Amstutz HC, O'Carroll F, Dorey FJ. Resection arthroplasty of the hip. J Bone Joint Surg 1989; 71A:669–678.

29. Kostuik J, Alexander D. Arthrodesis for failed arthroplasty of the hip. 1984; 188:173.

30. Czitrom A, Gross A, Langer F, Sim F. Bone banks and allografts in community practice. Instructional Course Lectures American Academy of Orthopaedic Surgeon. 1988; 37:24–31.

31. Oakeshott RD, Morgan DAF, Zukor DJ, Rudan JF, Brooks PJ, Gross AE. Revision total hip arthroplasty with osseous allograft reconstruction. Clin Orthop 1987; 225:37–61.

32. Oakeshott RD, McAuley JP, Gross AE, Morgan DAF, Zukor DJ, Rudan JF, Brooks PJ. Allograft reconstruction in revision total hip surgery. In: Aebi N, Regazzoni P (eds). Bone Transplantation. Springer-Verlag, Berlin, Heidelberg, 1989; pp. 265–273.

33. Gustilo RD, Pasternak HS. Revision total hip arthroplasty with a titanium ingrowth prosthesis and bone grafting for failed cemented femoral component loosening. Clin Orthop 1988, 235:111–119.

34. D'Antonio JA, Capello WN, Borden LS, Bargar WL, Bierbaum BF, Boettcher WG, Steinberg ME, Stulberg D, Wedge JH. Classification and management of acetabular abnormalities in total hip arthroplasty. Clin Orthop 1989; 243:126–137.

35. Hardinge K. The direct lateral approach to the hip. J Bone Joint Surg 1982; 64B:17.

36. Harris WH, Krushell RJ, Galante JO. Results of cementless revisions of total hip arthroplasties using the Harris-Galante prosthesis. Clin Orthop 1988; 235:120–126.

37. Gross AE, Lavoie MV, McDermott AGP, Marks P. The use of allograft bone in revision of total hip arthroplasty. Clin Orthop 1985; 197:115.

38. Borja FJ, Mnaymneh W. Bone allografts in salvage of difficult hip arthroplasties. Clin Orthop 1985; 197:123.

39. Gross AE, McKee N, Farine I, Czitrom A, Langer F. Reconstruction of skeletal defects following en-bloc excision of bone tumours. In: Current Concepts of Diagnosis and Treatment of

Bone and Soft Tissue Tumours. Springer-Verlag, Berlin, 1984; p. 163.

40. Mankin HJ, Doppelt SH, Sullivan TR, Tomford WW. Osteoarticular and intercalary allograft transplantation in the management of malignant tumours of bone. Cancer 1982; 50:613.

41. Parrish FF. Allograft replacement of all or part of the end of a long bone following excision of a tumor. J Bone Joint Surg 1973; 55A:1.

42. Scott RD. Use of a bipolar prosthesis with bone grafting in acetabular reconstruction. Contemp Orthop 1984; 9:35.

43. Trancik TM, Stulberg BN, Wilde AH, Feiglin DH. Allograft reconstruction of the acetabulum during revision total hip arthroplasty. J Bone Joint Surg 1986; 68A:527.

44. Volkov M. Allotransplantation of joints. J Bone Joint Surg 1970; 52B:49.

45. Burchart H. The biology of bone graft repair. Clin Orthop 1983; 174:28.

46. Friedlaander GE, Mankin HJ, Sell KW (eds). Osteochondral Allografts. Biology, Banking and Clinical Applications. Little Brown, Boston, 1983; p. 223.

47. McDermott AGP, Langer F, Pritzker KPH, Gross AE. Fresh small-fragment osteochondral allografts. Clin Orthop 1985; 197:96.

48. Dohmae Y, Bechtold JE. Reduction in cement-bone interface shear strength between primary and revision arthroplasty. Clin Orthop 1988; 236:214.

49. Hungerford DS, Robertson DD. The rationale of cementless revision of cemented arthroplasty failures. Clin Orthop 1988; 235:12.

50. Ling RSM. Observations on the fixation of implants to the bony skeleton. Clin Orthop 1986; 210:80.

51. Gordon SL, Binkert BL, Rashkoff ES, Britt AR, Esser PD, Stinchfield FE. Assessment of bone grafts used for acetabular augmentation in total hip arthroplasty. Clin Orthop 1985; 201:18.

52. Harris WH, Crothers O, Oh I. Total hip replacement and femoral head bone grafting for severe acetabular deficiency in adults. J Bone Joint Surg 1977; 59A:752.

53. Ritter MA, Traucik RM. Lateral acetabular bone graft in total hip arthroplasty. Clin Orthop 1985; 193:156.

9

ALLOGRAFT RECONSTRUCTION IN TOTAL KNEE ARTHROPLASTY

Ian Stockley and Allan E. Gross

Deficient bone stock is often the major determining factor in deciding what treatment options are available in salvaging a failed knee arthroplasty. This is particularly so with constrained implants with long intramedullary stems where, after initial resection of the articular surfaces, the loss of bone stock often makes exchange arthroplasty impossible or makes arthrodesis difficult to achieve.

The ultimate success of total knee arthroplasty depends upon preservation of the subchondral plate of the tibial plateau (1). In patients with severe valgus or varus deformities, the proximal tibia should not be cut to the level of the bone defect because the bone at this level is much weaker (2). In addition to preserving the stronger subchrondral plate, it is important to maintain the location of the joint line at the correct level (3). The amount of bone cut should approximately equal the thickness of the proposed tibial insert.

Although the use of allograft bone for the reconstruction of osseous defects following failed hip surgery is well documented (4–6), there is a relative paucity of reports in the literature concerning the use of allograft bone in revision knee surgery. Samuelson (7) reported his experience with allograft bone in revision knee surgery, but gave little detail regarding the type and distribution of allograft used. More recently, Wilde et al. (8) presented their results on the incorporation of allografts in the proximal tibia; none being used in the distal femur. Indeed, the majority of papers to date appear to relate only to proximal tibial reconstruction (8–10). This is probably related to the fact that tibial bone is more at risk than femoral bone because femoral bone is twice as strong as tibial bone (11).

We have addressed the need for distal femoral reconstruction along with that of the proximal tibia using frozen irradiated allograft bone and we wish to present our experience with these techniques.

CLASSIFICATION OF BONE DEFECTS

Defects in the distal femur or proximal tibia were simply classified into contained or uncontained defects. Contained

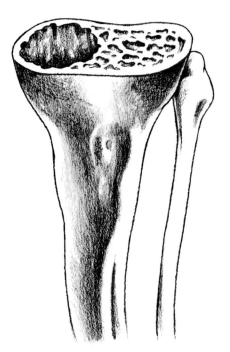

Figure 9.1. Small contained tibial defect.

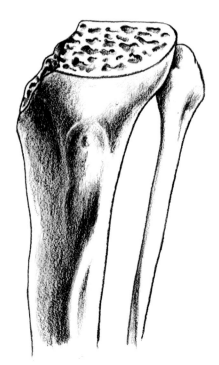

Figure 9.3. Uncontained defect of the medial tibial plateau.

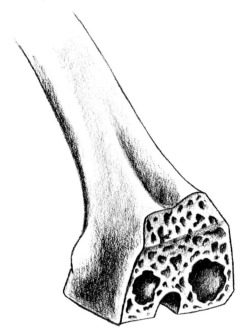

Figure 9.2. Small contained femoral defect.

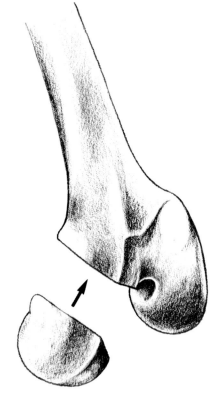

Figure 9.4. Uncontained defect of the lateral femoral condyle.

defects (Figs. 9.1 and 9.2) are surrounded by an intact rim of cortical bone whereas those that are uncontained (Figs. 9.3 and 9.4) extend to the periphery of the bone.

ALLOGRAFT RECONSTRUCTION

Cadaveric allograft bone was harvested under sterile conditions from donors who conformed to the guidelines recommended by the Musculoskeletal Council of the American Association of Tissue Banks (12). The bone was then irradiated with 2.5 megarads from a cobalt 60 source and deep frozen at −70°C until required.

The type of allograft used for reconstruction can be divided into three subtypes: large-fragment or bulk grafts, cortical strut grafts, and morsellized grafts. Large-fragment grafts consisted of distal femora including condyles, diaphyseal segments, or metadiaphyseal segments. Cortical strut grafts are longitudinal grafts used to bridge cortical

Table 9.1.
Methods of Reconstruction Using Allograft Bone

Deficit	Allograft	Fixation to Host
Contained		
Small	Morsellized	
Large	Metadiaphyseal	Either by stem of prosthesis with or without cement or by screws
Uncontained		
Femur	Distal femur including condyles	Screws
Tibia	Proximal tibia including plateau	Screws

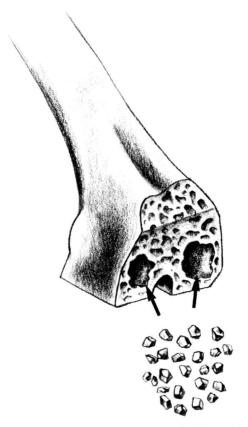

Figure 9.5. Morsellized bone for a small contained femoral defect.

defects in the host bone; these grafts are not circumferential. Morsellized bone consists of corticocancellous chips. Having classified the deficits into contained and uncontained, they were reconstructed using allograft bone according to the formula outlined in Table 9.1.

When cement was used with an allograft, the allograft was cemented to the stem of the prosthesis, thereby making an allograft-prosthesis construct. Care was taken to avoid cement interposing at the host-allograft junction.

Optimal results require good preparation of the recipient bed, press-fitting of the graft with sound fixation, where indicated, and coverage of the graft by the implant. Preparation of the bone defect is done with curettes, gouges, or high speed burrs to remove fibrous membrane and all cement. Dense sclerotic bone must be breached to expose viable bleeding bone. However, host bone must be preserved at all costs, particularly at the periphery, because it will act as support for the graft and or component. It is mandatory that the rim be completely exposed. All allograft-host junctions must be supplemented with autogenous bone and any voids between allograft and host must be packed with morsellized graft.

DISTAL FEMUR RECONSTRUCTION

Small Contained Defects

These defects (Fig. 9.2) are simply treated by impacting morsellized corticocancellous bone into the holes (Fig. 9.5). If autogenous bone is readily available, e.g., as in a primary arthroplasty or if further bone cuts have been made at revision, this can be used by itself or in combination with

allograft bone. If possible, it is better to try and add autograft to the allograft because allograft by itself has little osteoinductive potential. A standard total condylar prosthesis can then be inserted with or without cement, depending upon the individual surgeon's preference.

Large Contained Defects

These defects obviously present a greater challenge to the surgeon. When there is major loss of cancellous bone from the metaphysis leaving a funnel-shaped cortical tube, a distal femoral allograft is trimmed accordingly and invaginated into the residual cortical shell (Figs. 9.6 and 9.7). Residual voids between allograft and host are packed with a mixture of morsellized allo- and autograft. Appropriate bone cuts are then made and the prosthesis is inserted (Fig. 9.8). We recommend a stemmed implant because this will decrease the load on the cancellous bone and transmit the load more directly to the host cortical bone (13, 14). Depending upon graft stability, the allograft can be cemented to the stem of the prosthesis or, if the host bone is strong, then the graft can be fixed to the cortex with cancellous screws.

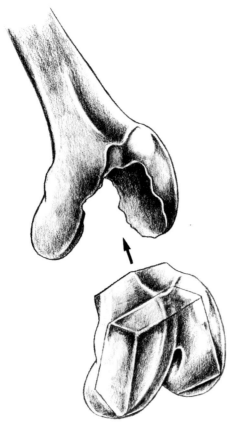

Figure 9.6. Reconstruction of a large contained femoral defect with a distal femur allograft.

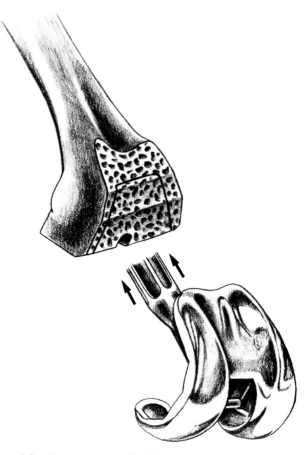

Figure 9.8. The reconstructed distal femur is recut using the appropriate jigs and a stemmed component is inserted.

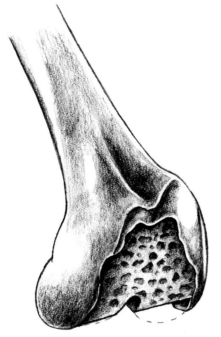

Figure 9.7. Allograft inside shell of distal femur.

Figure 9.9 shows aseptic loosening of a Guepar femoral component and a large contained defect in a 79-year-old female patient. Reconstruction was performed with a distal femoral allograft and a semiconstrained prosthesis. Three years later, the knee is functioning well and the radiograph (Fig. 9.10) shows a well-preserved allograft and a stable implant.

Uncontained Defects

Uncontained defects of the distal femur involve loss of one or both femoral condyles (Figs. 9.4 and 9.11) with or without a segment of diaphysis. Reconstruction of the anatomy is achieved by screwing allograft condyles to the host remnant (Figs. 9.12 and 9.13). Having reconstructed

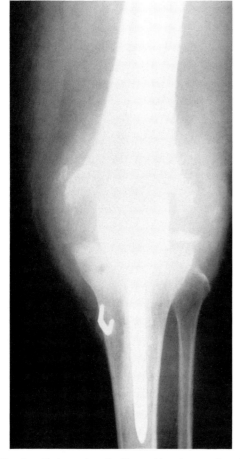

Figure 9.9. Aseptic loosening of a Guepar hinge has produced a large contained defect in the distal femur.

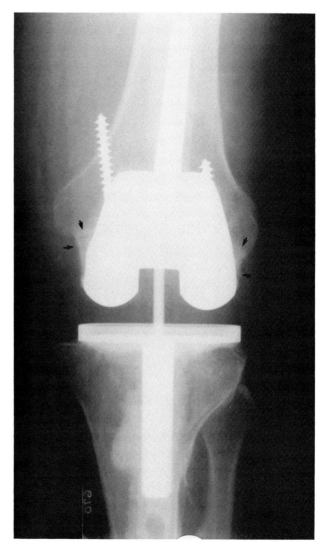

Figure 9.10. Radiograph taken 3 years after reconstruction with a distal femoral allograft (*arrows*) and semiconstrained implant.

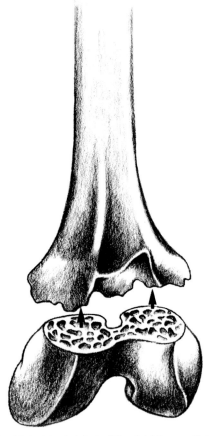

Figure 9.11. Uncontained defect of the distal femur with loss of both condyles.

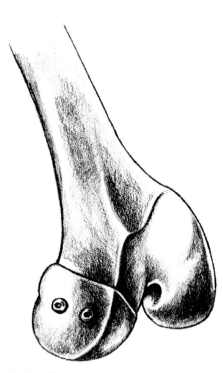

Figure 9.12. Allograft condyle screwed on to host femur.

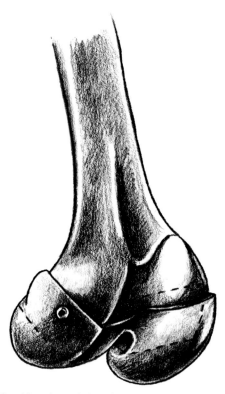

Figure 9.13. Allograft consisting of two condyles screwed to the host femur.

the distal femur, bone cuts are made and the chosen prosthesis is inserted (Fig. 9.14).

Two previous arthroplasties and a loose-linked prosthesis have led to loss of bone stock in the distal femur of a 37-year-old male patient (Fig. 9.15). Restoration of the anatomy with an allograft consisting of both femoral condyles was achieved and, 3 years later, the patient has a good clinical score with radiographs showing a well-aligned prosthesis and union of the allograft to host (Figs. 9.16 and 9.17).

The patient with a supracondylar fracture and poor quality bone presents a difficult bone loss problem (Fig. 9.18). In these instances, bone stock in the metaphysis is often insufficient for internal fixation devices and we have used distal femoral allografts complete with a segment of diaphysis for reconstruction. Step-cuts are made in the diaphyses of allograft and host to achieve rotational stability, with the junction reinforced with cerclage wire and autogenous bone graft (Fig. 9.19). When using complete distal femora, prostheses with intramedullary stems must be used, extending into the host bone to provide further stability at the host-allograft junction.

Often, the soft tissue attachments of the ligaments are still present on a thin shell of distal femur and, then, they can be attached to the allograft.

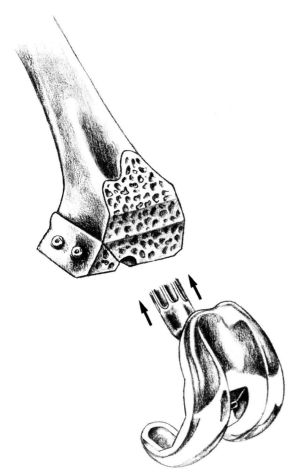

Figure 9.14. The femoral condyle allograft is fixed to the host with screws. Bone cuts are then made and the prosthesis is inserted.

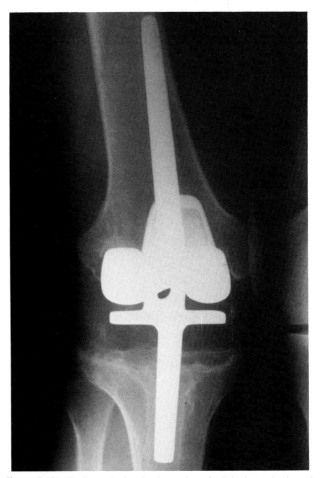

Figure 9.15. Radiograph showing loosening of a linked prosthesis and loss of femoral and tibial bone stock.

PROXIMAL TIBIA RECONSTRUCTION

Small Contained Defects

As with the femur, small contained defects in the tibia can be treated with morsellized allograft, autograft, or a mixture of the two and a regular tibial component (Figs. 9.20 and 9.21). Coverage of the tibia should be as complete as possible because optimum loading across the implant occurs only in the presence of tibial component-cortical rim contact (15).

Large Contained Defects

In the case of massive central bone deficiency (Fig. 9.22), implant fixation can be severely compromised. Having identified the margins of the defect, a metadiaphyseal segment of allograft proximal tibia is prepared (Fig. 9.23). A long-stemmed implant to achieve fixation in intact host diaphyseal bone is indicated in these cases because this will partially unload the proximal bone due to load transfer between the stem and the cortical shell. Depending upon the fit of the graft within the host and the quality of the remaining host bone, the graft can be press-fitted into the defect (Fig. 9.24), fixed with screws (Fig. 9.25), or cemented to the stem of the prosthesis (Fig. 9.26).

Figure 9.27 shows a loose Attenborough prosthesis with large contained defects in the tibia and femur. Reconstruction with bulk allografts and cementless components was performed and, 6 years later (Figs. 9.28 and 9.29), the allograft has maintained its structural integrity with union to host bone.

Uncontained Defects

The principles of reconstruction for small and large uncontained defects are similar. The most common deformity to be corrected in osteoarthritic patients is that of varus. In these instances, the defect is peripheral and posteromedial with the area and depth of defect related to the duration of arthritis, instability of the knee, and strength of bone. In revision situations, defects are often secondary to fracture of the plateau or subsidence of the component without fracture.

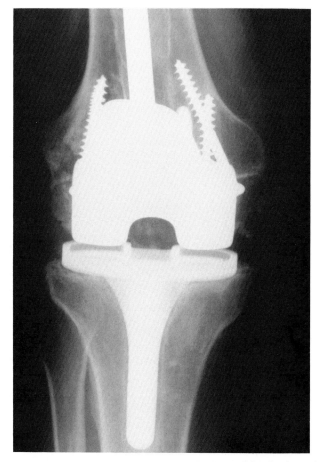

Figure 9.16. Anteroposterior radiograph taken 3 years following femoral reconstruction with a distal femoral allograft. Note union to host bone.

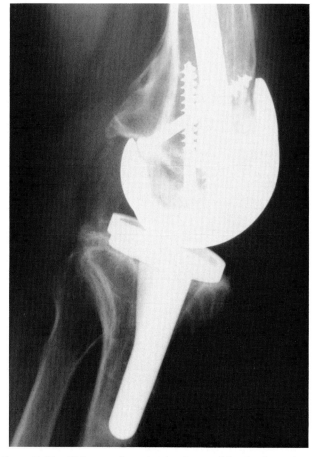

Figure 9.17. Oblique radiograph taken 3 years following femoral reconstruction with a distal femoral allograft.

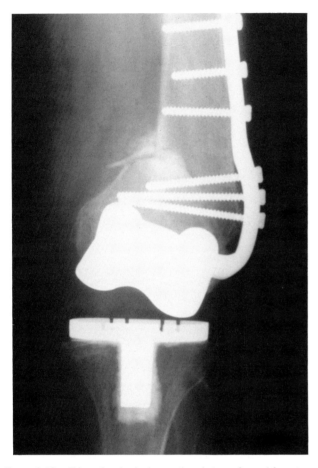

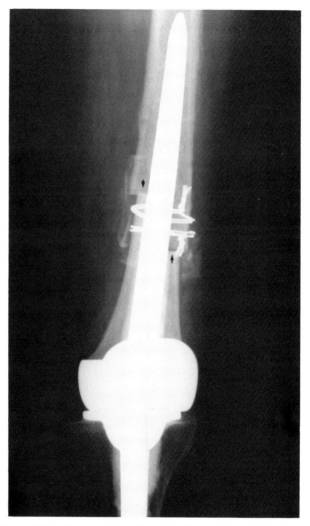

Figure 9.18. This patient had a knee arthroplasty performed for osteo-necrosis. One week following surgery, a supracondylar fracture occurred, which was treated with a condylar blade plate. Unfortunately, the fracture did not unite.

Figure 9.19. Reconstruction with a distal femoral allograft. A step-cut osteotomy (*arrows*) has been performed in the diaphyses of host and allograft for rotational stability.

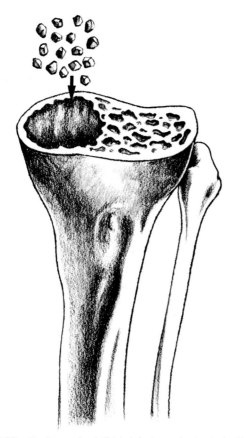

Figure 9.20. Small contained tibial defects can be treated with morsellized bone.

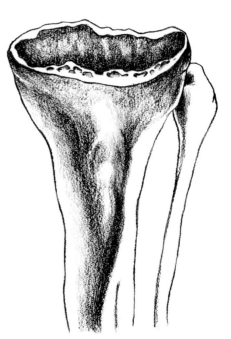

Figure 9.22. Large contained tibial defect.

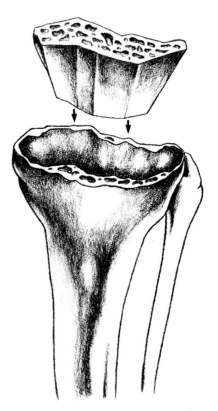

Figure 9.23. Metadiaphyseal allograft cut for contained tibial defect.

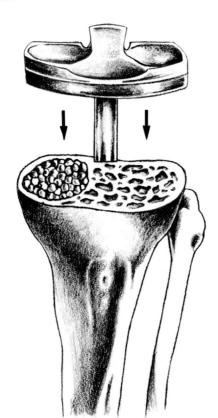

Figure 9.21. The defect has been filled with graft and a regular tibial component inserted.

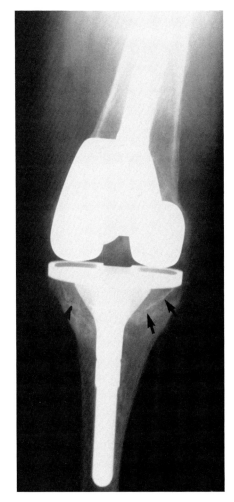

Figure 9.24. Allograft (*arrows*) press-fitted into large contained tibial defect.

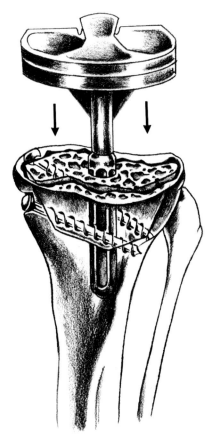

Figure 9.25. Allograft fixed with screws and an uncemented stemmed component.

For primary knees with bone loss restricted to one plateau, local bone from the femoral condyle is often adequate. If not, allograft proximal tibia may be used, with the graft cut to accommodate the defect. Reconstruction of a medial plateau defect is shown diagrammatically in Figures 9.30 and 9.31 and with radiographs in Figures 9.32 and 9.33. The defect is removed by obliquely sawing the bone; this provides a flat surface against which the

graft is easily fitted and rigidly fixed with two cancellous screws perpendicular to the bony surface.

For larger defects, as seen with revision knees (Fig. 9.34), reconstruction is similar. The host bone is cut to provide a bed for the allograft (Fig. 9.35), the allograft is secured to the tibia with screws, appropriate bone cuts are made, and the prosthesis is inserted (Figs. 9.36 and

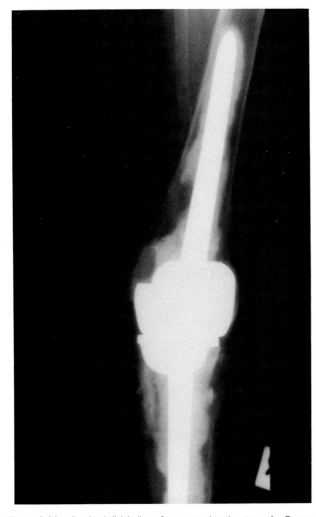

Figure 9.26. Proximal tibial allograft cemented to the stem of a Guepar prosthesis.

9.37). A long-stemmed component is indicated to achieve distal fixation and it is our present practice to use cementless components. However, the prosthesis can be cemented into the allograft.

POSTOPERATIVE CARE

Protection of the bone graft from full weight bearing is necessary. Small grafts of morsellized bone require only 6–8 weeks, whereas large-fragment grafts often need 3–4 months. The type of revision procedure, area of graft, quality and quantity of remaining bone stock, and rigidity of fixation are all factors to be taken into account when considering the time period for limited weight bearing. To try and maximize range of motion, continuous passive motion (CPM) machines are frequently used in the early postoperative period.

Over the last 8 years, we have used the above principles for reconstruction of the distal femur and proximal

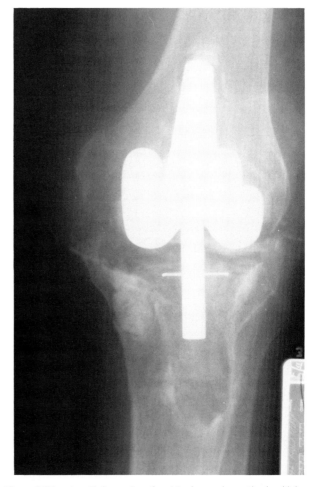

Figure 9.27. Aseptic loosening of an Attenborough prosthesis with large contained defects in the femur and tibia.

tibia in 22 patients, during primary and revision knee arthroplasty. Eighteen of these patients have a minimum 2-years of follow-up and will be discussed further.

MATERIAL AND METHODS

There were 11 female patients and seven male patients, with an average age of 69.4 years (range, 37.9–83.3 years). The primary indication for surgery was osteoarthritis in

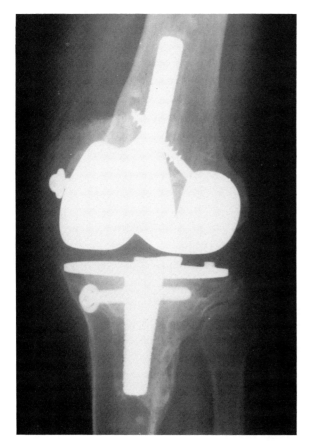

Figure 9.28. Six years following reconstruction with bulk allografts and cementless implants.

13 patients, rheumatoid arthritis in three patients, osteonecrosis in one patient, and psoriatic arthropathy in one patient. Two patients required bilateral knee arthroplasty surgery with allograft reconstruction; the other 16 needed unilateral reconstruction only. Two knees necessitated allograft reconstruction during a primary arthroplasty

whereas the other 18 knees underwent allograft reconstruction as part of a revision procedure. The average time to follow-up was 4.2 years with a range of 2.0–7.2 years.

Patient assessment was both clinical and radiographic according to protocols determined by the University of Toronto Bone Transplant Unit. A modified Hospital for Special Surgery knee evaluation sheet was used for clinical assessment preoperatively and at review. This evaluation produces a clinical score based on subjective and objective criteria (Table 9.2).

Failure of the procedure was defined as (*a*) failure to increase the preoperative score by a minimum of 20 points or (*b*) the need for subsequent reoperation related to the allograft.

The radiographic assessment includes sequential anteroposterior, lateral, oblique, and 3-ft standing anteroposterior views. In particular, the allografts were evaluated for union to host bone, as evidenced by trabecular bridging of the host-donor interface, and structural integrity. In addition, periprosthetic lucencies were evaluated as were prosthetic migration and alignment.

Distal Femur Reconstruction

Twelve of the 16 allografts were bulk allografts, three were morsellized bone, and one was a cortical strut graft (Fig. 9.38). In seven knees where a large-fragment graft was necessary, allograft distal femora were used. These grafts were either screwed to the host bone or secured with a step-cut osteotomy and cerclage wire.

The other five bulk grafts were fashioned from metadiaphyseal bone. Three of these were initially cemented to the stem of a Guepar prosthesis to form an allograft-prosthesis construct and, then, the remaining stem was

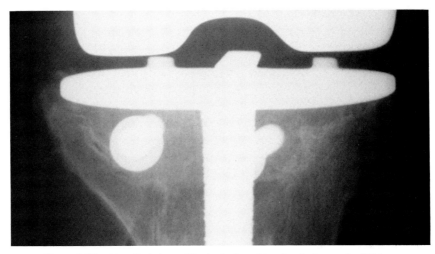

Figure 9.29. Magnified view of the host-allograft junction in the proximal tibia.

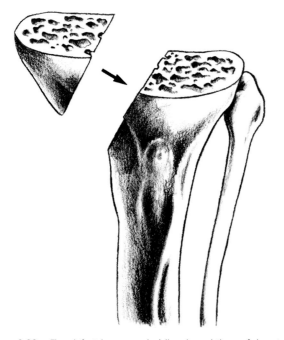

Figure 9.30. The defect is removed obliquely and the graft is cut to size.

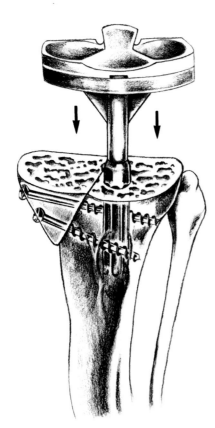

Figure 9.31. The graft is fixed with two cancellous screws perpendicular to the bone.

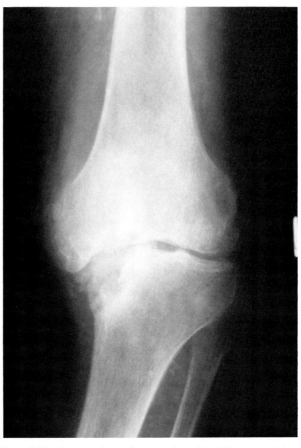

Figure 9.32. Preoperative radiograph of medial tibial plateau defect.

cemented to the host. One of the remaining two grafts was treated in a similar fashion, but without cement fixation. The final case was one in which the allograft was screwed to the host.

The cortical strut allograft was used to fill a large femoral cortical defect produced by the stem of a Guepar prosthesis (Fig. 9.39).

Proximal Tibial Reconstruction

Nine of the eleven bulk (large-fragment) allografts were fashioned from proximal tibiae (Fig. 9.40). Seven of these nine allografts were screwed on to the host directly; the other two were cemented to the stems of the prosthesis. The remaining two large-fragment grafts were metadiaphyseal segments. One graft was press-fitted into the proximal tibia; the other was cemented to the stem of the prosthesis.

Four of the remaining five allografts used in the tibia were morsellized bone for small contained defects and the last case was a cortical strut graft. The strut graft was used where a fracture had occurred at the level of the

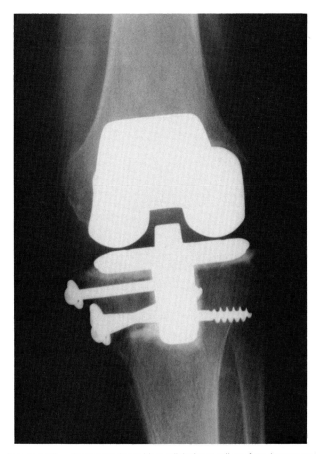

Figure 9.33. Reconstruction with medial plateau allograft and cemented tibial component.

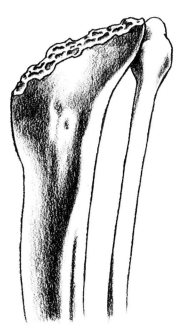

Figure 9.34. Large uncontained defect involving the majority of the tibial plateau.

peg of the tibial component. The stem of the revision prosthesis extended beyond the fracture and the graft was used to reinforce the junction.

Several types of prostheses were used in the study (Table 9.3). The Guepar hinge prosthesis was used at the beginning of the series because this was the only type of implant available for revision reconstruction at that time. Our preference now is to use modular, long-stemmed, semiconstrained implants and aim for a cementless press-fit with a fluted rod in both the tibia and femur diaphyses. This will decrease the load on the cancellous bone and transmit the load more directly to the host cortical bone.

Eleven knees were inserted with antibiotic-impregnated polymethylmethacrylate cement and nine knees were operated without the use of cement. To each 40-g bag of Simplex bone cement, 500 mg of cefamandole was added.

All surgery was performed in an operating room equipped with laminar flow utilizing body exhaust suits for the operating team. Administration of prophylactic antibiotics commenced preoperatively and continued for 5 days

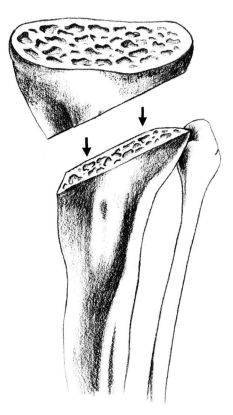

Figure 9.35. Host bone is cut to provide a bed for the allograft.

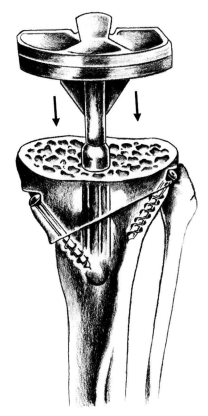

Figure 9.36. The graft is fixed with cancellous screws.

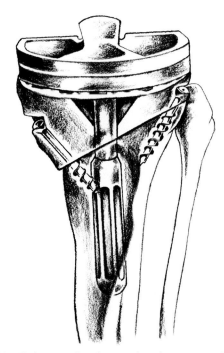

Figure 9.37. The bone cuts have been made and an uncemented stemmed component is inserted.

Table 9.2.
Mount Sinai Hospital Knee Evaluation Sheet

Pain Intensity	
None	35
Mild	25
Moderate (occasional analgesics)	15
Severe (regular analgesics)	5
At rest	0
Feeling of Instability	
None	10
Occasional	7
Moderate with decreased activity	4
Severe, uses braces	0
Walking Distance	
1 mile or more	10
1–5 blocks	6
1 block	3
House confinement	1
Bed confinement	0
Walking Aids	
None	5
Cane	3
Crutches (2 canes)	1
Walker	0
Flexion Deformity	
10°	10
<5°	7
5–10°	4
10–20°	2
>20°	0
Active Flexion	
>120°	20
90–120°	15
45–90°	8
<45°	0
Effusion	
None	10
Moderate	5
Severe	0
Maximum	100

intravenously, followed by 5 additional days of oral therapy. In addition, patients were routinely anticoagulated with warfarin, unless there were any contraindications.

RESULTS

In 20 knees, 32 allografts were used for reconstituting bone stock at the time of total knee arthroplasty; 16 for femoral reconstruction and 16 for the proximal tibia. In 12 knees, allografts were required for both the femur and tibia.

DISTAL FEMUR RECONSTRUCTION

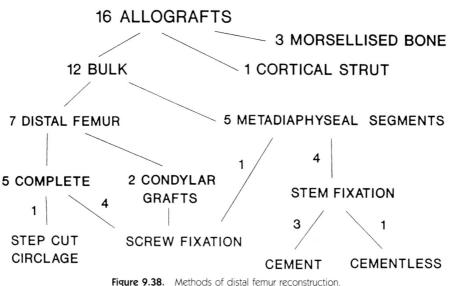

Figure 9.38. Methods of distal femur reconstruction.

Clinical Assessment

The average preoperative knee score was 35, with a range of 18–49. Three knees have required further surgery following allograft reconstruction and will be discussed in detail later. The remaining 17 knees (85%) have all increased their scores by a minimum of 22 to a mean of 74, range of 63–93, and are, therefore, regarded as successful in terms of our assessment criteria.

Clinical Failures

Three knees, all revision arthroplasties, have failed secondary to sepsis. The first was a 70-year-old male diabetic patient who presented with a painful knee pseudoarthrosis having had a loose, infected constrained prosthesis removed 1 year previously. Allograft reconstruction of the distal femur and proximal tibia was performed for extensive bone loss, with bulk allografts being used to make allograft-prosthesis constructs with a Guepar prosthesis. Unfortunately, soon after surgery, an infection recurred and, despite antibiotic therapy and surgical drainage, the infection did not resolve. The patient had an above-knee amputation 3 years after the allograft.

The second patient was a 64-year-old rheumatoid male patient who, 4 years before his revision, had had a total condylar arthroplasty performed for osteonecrosis of the medial tibial plateau. Reconstruction with autogenous bone and cement failed to correct the deformity and the prosthesis loosened. A large medial plateau allograft was screwed to the proximal tibia and an Insall Burstein total condylar prosthesis cemented in. Two years later, he again presented with progressive deformity and pain. Radiographs of the knee showed loosening of the tibial component with dissolution of the allograft. *Streptococcus viridans* was cultured from the knee and, 1 year after a two-stage exchange procedure with a hinge prosthesis, he has a good range of pain-free motion with no evidence of recurrent infection.

The final patient, a 73-year-old man had reconstruction of a large uncontained medial plateau defect with a bulk allograft and cemented Porous Coated Anatomic (PCA) revision prosthesis for aseptic loosening of a total condylar prosthesis. Two years later, a further revision was necessary for tibial loosening and dislocation of the patellar button. At operation, the allograft had incorporated with no evidence of collapse. The PCA components were replaced with a cemented Press Fit Condylar (PFC) knee arthroplasty. Eighteen months on, the patient was admitted in a toxic state with a painful, swollen knee. Debridement of the joint was performed with *Staphylococcus aureus* being grown from the knee. At the present time, the patient is left with a pseudarthrosis.

Radiographic Assessment

CORTICAL STRUT GRAFTS

The two cortical strut grafts have united. In addition, their external contour has changed indicating revascularization and remodeling (Figs. 9.39 and 9.41).

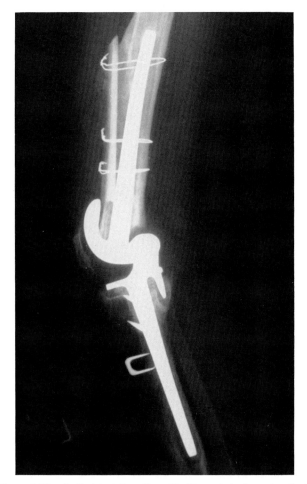

Figure 9.39. Cortical strut allograft used to fill an anterior femoral cortical defect produced by the stem of a loose Guepar prosthesis.

MORSELLIZED BONE

Collapse of allograft occurred in one patient who had revision of a failed cemented Guepar prosthesis for aseptic loosening. Morsellized bone was packed into a large contained tibial defect into which an uncemented component was inserted (Fig. 9.42). Six months after surgery, radiographs showed subsidence of the graft with the prosthesis now in contact with host bone. Radiographs show no progression of tibial subsidence 5½ years later, but, on the femoral side, there is lucency around the stem (Fig. 9.43). However, the patient is asymptomatic with a good clinical result.

BULK ALLOGRAFTS

Two bulk allografts have fractured. A metadiaphyseal allograft was used to reconstruct a large, contained defect in the proximal tibia. The graft was put on to the stem of a Guepar prosthesis and inserted into the proximal

tibia without cement. As a result of inadequate support for the graft, it soon fractured and the prosthesis subsided into the bone. Despite radiographic failure, the patient has a good clinical score. With exception of the previously reported case, all the other allografts have united to the host bone.

The second fracture was in a 13-cm long distal femoral allograft that had been used to restore bone stock in a patient who had sustained a supracondylar fracture immediately proximal to the femoral component of a total condylar prosthesis. The primary arthroplasty was performed for osteonecrosis of the distal femur. The fracture occurred 6 months after surgery and subsequently healed without operative intervention. The patient has an excellent clinical result 3½ years after surgery.

PERIPROSTHETIC LUCENCIES

Eleven knees were reconstructed with cemented components. Six have nonprogressive, incomplete, narrow (less than 2 mm) radiolucencies at the bone-cement interface. In four of these knees, lines are around only one component whereas, in the other two, both the tibial and femoral components are involved.

DISCUSSION

The results of this study support the use of allograft bone for restoring osseous defects following failed knee arthroplasty. Whereas other workers (7, 8) have advocated allograft bone use for tibial reconstruction, we have shown its usefulness in restoring the distal femur also.

The goals of revision arthroplasty surgery include the relief of pain, restoration of stability, and a functional range of motion. All of these can only be achieved by arthroplasty surgery and the available bone stock is often the determining factor as to whether such surgery can be performed.

Bone loss can be dealt with by four mechanisms:

1. Cement with or without reinforcement;
2. Bone grafting;
3. Augmented prostheses;
4. Shift of the implant away from the bone defect.

Cement is a poor substitute because it does not give secure support (13). In addition, cement reconstruction is regarded only as a short-term solution because it can lead to more rapid bone loss and destruction (16–18). Metal wedges, although biomechanically superior to cement (11) do not always fit as well as initially planned; it is difficult to size-match accurately from the preoper-

PROXIMAL TIBIA RECONSTRUCTION

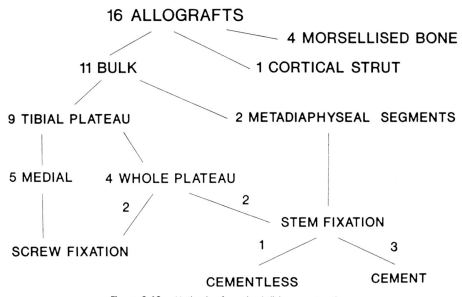

Figure 9.40. Methods of proximal tibia reconstruction.

Table 9.3.
Prostheses Used in the Study

Total Condylar III	5
Revision PCA (porous coated anatomic)	5
Guepar	7
Insall Burstein	2
PFC modular (press-fit condylar)	1

ative radiographs. In addition, wedges are only good for small bone defects. Similar problems can arise with custom implants, which may take a long time to manufacture and can be expensive. The use of modular components will alleviate the need for customized implants.

Bone grafting allows for a more physiological load transfer to the underlying tibia than metal customized components or high cement columns (19).

Shifting of the implant away from the side of a tibial defect with or without cement filling of the defect that is less than 50% of the tibial surface has been reported to provide satisfactory results (20). In revision knees, bony defects are often much greater and, thus, there is a need for large-fragment reconstruction.

The long-term survival of massive grafts has been confirmed in this study. Their use in revision hip surgery and after resection of tumor is well supported (4, 6, 21, 22).

Large grafts maintain their structural integrity be-

cause they only undergo a slow and incomplete revascularization. We do not support the fixation techniques of Mnaymneh et al. (23) utilizing plates and screws to fix the allograft to the host. Multiple drill holes can only lead to the development of vascular channels within the allograft and, subsequently, faster revascularization. This may then lead to collapse of the graft. Union to host bone is achieved by creeping substitution at areas of contact (24, 25).

Alternatives to revision arthroplasty for salvaging a failed knee arthroplasty include arthrodesis, excision arthroplasty, and even amputation. Arthrodesis can be difficult to achieve after failed knee replacement of any kind due to lack of bone stock (26–28). In addition, there are disadvantages in having an arthrodesed knee in elderly patients who spend a lot of time sitting (29). Excision arthroplasty has been proposed as a method of salvaging an infected arthroplasty and both Falahee et al. (30) and Lettin et al. (31) advocate this technique in preference to arthrodesis or to amputation for the management of chronic infection.

Infection was the major complication in our series. Obviously, the number of previous operations and the long operating time contribute to the high infection rate, but every effort should be made to rule out sepsis prior to allograft reconstruction. Allografts, being nonvascularized organic tissue, present little resistance to, and provide an excellent nidus for, the growth of organisms.

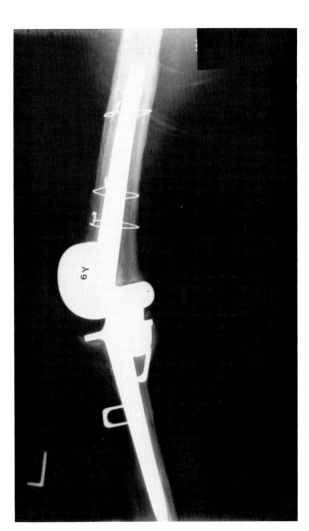

Figure 9.41. Six years later, the graft has remodeled.

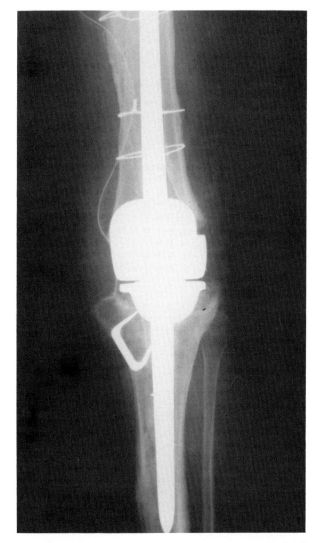

Figure 9.42. Morsellized bone was used to fill a large contained defect in the proximal tibia.

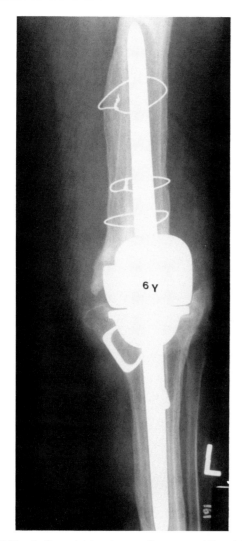

Figure 9.43. Radiograph taken 6 years after surgery. Although the graft subsided 6 months after surgery, there has been no further subsidence.

Despite the three clinical failures, the 17 remaining knees continue with good clinical scores reflecting the durability of allograft bone for the reconstruction of distal femora and proximal tibiae following failed knee arthroplasty.

ACKNOWLEDGMENT

As a clinical fellow at Mount Sinai Hospital, I. Stockley was funded by the John Charnley Trust.

REFERENCES

1. Sneppen O, Christensen P, Larsen H, Vary PS. Mechanical testing of trabecular bone in knee replacement. Int Orthop 1981; 5:251.
2. Hvid I, Hansen SC. Cancellous bone strength patterns at the proximal tibia epiphysis. Orthop Trans 1985; 9:262.
3. Figgie HE III, Goldberg VM, Heiple KG, Moller HS III, Gordon NH. The influence of tibial patellofemoral location on function of the knee in patients with posterior stabilized condylar knee prostheses. J Bone Joint Surg 1986; 68A:1035.
4. Borja FJ, Mnaymneh W. Bone allografts in salvage of difficult hip arthroplasties. Clin Orthop 1985; 197:123.
5. Oakeshott RD, Morgan DAF, Zukor DJ, Rudan JF, Brooks PJ, Gross AE. Revision total hip arthroplasty with osseous allograft reconstruction. A clinical and roentgenographic analysis. Clin Orthop 1987; 225:37.
6. Allan DG, Lavoie GJ, McDonald S, Gross AE. The use of proximal femoral allografts in revision total hip arthroplasty. J Bone Joint Surg (Br) 1991; 73B:235.
7. Samuelson KM. Bone grafting and noncemented revision arthroplasty of the knee. Clin Orthop 1988; 226:93.
8. Wilde AH, Schickendantz MS, Stulberg BN, Go RT. The incorporation of tibial allografts in total knee arthroplasty. J Bone Joint Surg 1990; 72A:815.
9. Dorr LD, Ranawat CS, Sculco TA, McKaskill B, Orisek BS. Bone graft for tibial defects in total knee arthroplasty. Clin Orthop 1986; 205:153.
10. Windsor RE, Insall JN, Sculco TP. Bone grafting of tibial defects in primary and revision total knee arthroplasty. Clin Orthop 1986; 205:132.
11. Brooks PJ, Walker PS, Scott RD. Tibial component fixation in deficient tibial bone stock. Clin Orthop 1984; 184:302.
12. Tomford WW, Mankin HJ. Cadaver bone procurement. In: Fawcett KJ, Barr AR (eds). Tissue Banking. American Association of Blood Banks, Arlington, 1987, pp. 97–107.
13. Bartel DI, Burstein AH, Santaville EA, Insall JN. Performance of the tibial component in total knee replacement. Conventional and revision designs. J Bone Joint Surg 1982; 64A:1026.
14. Murase K, Crowninshield RD, Pedersen DR, Chang TS. An analysis of tibial component design in total knee arthroplasty. J Biomech 1983; 16:13.
15. Bourne RB, Finlay JB. The influence of tibial component intramedullary stems and implant-cortex contact on the strain distribution of the proximal tibia following total knee arthroplasty. An in vitro study. Clin Orthop 1986; 208:95.
16. Freeman MAR, Bradley GW, Revell PA. Observations upon the interface between bone and polymethylmethacrylate cement. J Bone Joint Surg 1982; 64B:488.
17. Goodman SB, Schatzker J, Sumner-Smith G, Fornasier VL, Geften N, Hunt C. The effect of polymethylmethacrylate on bone: an experimental study. Arch Orthop Trauma Surg 1985; 104:150.
18. Hungerford DS, Robertson DD. The rationale of cementless revision of cemented arthroplasty failures. Clin Orthop 1988; 235:12.
19. Shrivastava SC, Ahmed AM, Shiraze-Adl A, Burke DL. Effect of cement-bone composite layer and prosthesis geometry on stresses in a prosthetically resurfaced tibia. J Biomed Mater Res 1982; 16:929.
20. Lotke PA, Wong R, Ecker M. The management of large tibial defects in primary total knee replacement. Orthop Trans 1983; 9:425.
21. Mankin HJ, Doppelt SH, Sullivan TR, Tomford WW. Osteoartic-

ular and intercalary allograft transplantation in the management of malignant tumours of bone. Cancer 1982; 50:613.

22. Gross AE, McKee N, Farine I, Czitrom AA, Langer F. Reconstruction of skeletal defects following en-bloc excision of bone tumours. In: Current concepts of diagnosis and treatment of bone and soft tissue tumours. Springer-Verlag, Berlin, 1984; pp. 163–173.

23. Mnaymneh W, Emerson RH, Borja J, Head WC, Malinin TI. Massive allografts in salvage revisions of failed total knee arthroplasties. Clin Orthop 1990; 260:144.

24. Burchart H. The biology of bone graft repair. Clin Orthop 1983; 174:28.

25. Friedlaender GE, Mankin HJ, Sell KW (eds). Osteochondral Allografts. Biology, Banking and Clinical Applications. Little Brown, Boston, 1983.

26. Deburge A. Guepar hinge prosthesis: complications and results with two years' follow-up. Clin Orthop 1976; 120:47.

27. Hagemann WF, Woods GW, Tullos HS. Arthrodesis in failed total knee replacement. J Bone Joint Surg 1978; 60A:790.

28. Shea JG, Wynn Jones CH, Arden GP. A study of the results of removal of total knee prostheses. J Bone Joint Surg 1981; 63B:287.

29. Waugh W. The knee. In: Harris NH (ed). Postgraduate Textbook of Clinical Orthopaedics. Wright PSG, Bristol, 1983; pp. 586–594.

30. Falahee WF, Mathews LS, Kaufer H. Resection arthroplasty as a salvage procedure for a knee with infection after a total arthroplasty. J Bone Joint Surg 1987; 69A:1013.

31. Lettin AWF, Neil MJ, Citron ND, August A. Excision arthroplasty for infected constrained total knee replacements. J Bone Joint Surg 1990; 72B:220.

10

SOFT TISSUE ALLOGRAFT RECONSTRUCTION: THE KNEE

Douglas W. Jackson, Mark Rosen, and Timothy M. Simon

Allografts have been used in knee surgery to replace a single structure, as composite transplants replacing por-tions of the knee, and for total replacement of the knee. The initial experience with allografts in knee surgery was primarily for cases involving defects created by the sur-gical excision of tumors and by damage secondary to severe trauma. During the past decade, the use of allo-grafts for ligament replacement in the physically active population has gained more widespread use. The most frequently performed reconstruction using an allograft in knee surgery presently is for replacement of the an-terior cruciate ligament. Meniscal and osteochondral al-lografts are being utilized on a more limited basis. This chapter will be limited to discussion of the use of tendon, ligament, and meniscal allografts in knee surgery. Be-cause the transplantation of these allografts often includes their bony attachments, its fate will also be discussed.

Allografts as an alternative to autografts offer the po-tential to reduce donor site morbidity and, at the same time, preserve the patient's own tissues. In addition, there are times when no biological alternative exists because the pa-tient's own tissues are not available or cannot be compro-mised further. Another potential benefit from the use of an allograft is a reduction in surgical time and improved cos-mesis by eliminating the step of harvesting an autograft.

Allografts have some limitations in that an acceptable one may not be available. Potential disadvantages include disease transmission and immunogenicity. These two im-portant areas are factors to be considered in choosing an allograft.

STERILIZATION (POTENTIAL FOR DISEASE TRANSMISSION)

Discussions with a potential recipient of an allograft for a knee reconstruction should include the possible transmission of infectious diseases and requires that special consideration be given to the sterility of the allograft. For example, the anterior cruciate ligament (ACL) graft recipients are young and healthy and are seeking an elective procedure to improve the quality of life. They are usually able to be employed without surgery and have a normal life expectancy. The women often are going to enter or are in their child-bearing years. These patients must consider the risks of disease transmission differently than a patient with less potential for a normal life expectancy and no other real alternative to an allograft in their knee surgery.

The ideal allografts for cruciate ligament reconstructions are obtained from younger donors, 15–30 years of age. Donors in this age group are usually victims of motor vehicle or penetrating trauma and are predominantly young men. The incidence of homosexuality and drug abuse in this population increases the risk of the potential transmission of disease. While both bacterial and viral infections can be transmitted by an allograft, certainly the most dreaded disease at the present time is the human immunodeficiency virus (HIV). The prevalence of acquired immunodeficiency syndrome (AIDS) varies depending on the authority. C. Everett Koop (1) estimates that, by the year 2000, 100,000,000 people worldwide will be infected with HIV. Presently, sterility is perhaps the most important concern when using an allograft in reconstructive knee surgery.

The relative risk of transmission of AIDS is important not only to the recipient but also of concern to those who procure and process the allograft, the operating room personnel, and the surgeon. Attempts to estimate the risk of transmission of HIV through allografts is hampered by what is not known about the disease. The figures and information on the incidence and methods of sterilization for many viruses is changing. To date, there has been one documented case of transmission of the HIV in an orthopaedic procedure in which infected bone was used for a scoliosis fusion in 1984 (2). In retrospect, the donor had not been adequately screened. The recipient converted in 1988. This case may have been prevented with current safeguards. Although the HIV has not yet been transmitted through tendon, ligament, or meniscal transplantation, one must assume that the possibility exists.

Many factors in donor selection and screening reduce the risk of HIV transmission. There is, however, a window of failed detection between the time that an individual is HIV infected and when that person develops antibodies that are detectable on the enzyme-linked immunosorbent assay (ELISA) or Western blot studies for HIV antibodies. While most people develop detectable antibodies within 6 weeks, longer latency periods have been reported. The risks for disease transmission are effectively reduced when potential donors are carefully screened and have undergone a post mortem autopsy, a lymph node evaluation, and serological screening. Hepatitis or other viruses should be carefully screened for as well and will eliminate some potential donors.

HIV antigen is a relatively new test and has the possibility of detecting individuals during the window period that the infected person tests negative with the ELISA. P-24 antigen, which is the core protein of HIV, is an immunologically distinct antigen. Initially, after the exposure, it can be detected and then drops off as the antibody is produced and complexes with it. It is detected again in the late stages of the disease when the patient starts to decompensate and the antibody production drops off. It is anticipated that the Food and Drug Administration (FDA) will approve one or more antigen detection tests when their usefulness have been established. This should further help minimize the risk of transmission. In addition to the thorough screening, bone and tendon grafts can be held for a relatively long period of time to study the recipients of other organs from the same donor.

Several attempts have been made to estimate the risk of an infected donor going unrecognized (3–5). Factors such as disease prevalence, the doubling time of the disease, time from infection until detectable antibody develops, age of the donor, medical history, and serological screening procedures all enter into a calculation of risk. Buck et al. (4, 6) calculated the risk of transmission to be as high as 1/161 and as low as 1/1,667,600 if all of the presently available safeguards were employed. They have also demonstrated that freezing or freeze-drying may reduce the risk of transmission. Data are still absent on the presence of the virus in tendon, ligament, articular cartilage, and menisci of a clinically undetected but infected donor. These screening factors, which contribute to acquiring a low-risk graft, are made on the assumption that there is no human error in the handling and labeling, no clerical errors in acquiring the laboratory results, nor any misinterpretation of screening tests.

SECONDARY STERILIZATION OF SOFT TISSUE ALLOGRAFTS

Many of the early workers using nonviable allografts, such as tendon and ligaments, in knee surgery decided to use secondary sterilization as a back up. Less was known about the risks of viral transmission and it also reduced the chance of bacterial contamination during graft procurement and storage. In an effort to minimize any bacteria or viral transmission, some tissue banks started to sterilize the grafts secondarily in addition to aseptic procurement. Two of the more popular methods of secondary sterilization included the use of ethylene oxide (ETO) and γ-irradiation. ETO had been used to sterilize bone without apparent problems in the recipient and was one of the first choices for secondary sterilization of soft tissues. As the number of recipients of ETO-processed tendon allografts increased, complications began to be encountered. Paulos and associates (7, 8) and Curtis et al. (9) reported a delayed response in a high incidence of ETO-sterilized allografts at 6–24 months. They described its appearance as an applesauce reaction. Their initial interpretation was that it was a toxic giant cell response, typical of foreign bodies, and not a lymphocytic immunological response. Jackson et al. (10) reported a similar reaction in 6.4% of the 107 patients who had chronic ACL reconstructions. Synovial biopsies in these patients showed hyperplasia, fibrosis, and a mild to severe chronic inflammatory process. There were infiltrates of lymphocytes (and plasma cells in two of seven patients) in the removed grafts. Some infiltrates consisted of giant cells, histiocytes, lymphocytes, and polymorphonuclear leukocytes. There was extensive bone resorption around the femoral tunnel in one patient.

The intra-articular environment of the knee appears to participate in reactions to tendon allografts secondarily sterilized with ETO with little measurable systemic effect. The exact role of ETO in this intra-articular reaction to the graft needs further clarification. There are indications that it is, in part, a nonspecific reaction; however, an immunological basis may exist in some recipients. Among the unanswered questions regarding the nature of the response to the graft is whether this is a foreign body reaction to the residual products of ETO. Among the many possible byproducts, ethylene chlorohydrin and ethylene glycol have been measured.

An alternative explanation could be that the ETO alters the antigenic properties of the graft. Pinkowski et al. (11) showed an allograft failure that elicited a lymphocytic reaction, which presumably was immunogenic. It could be that immunogenic rejection occurs in some individuals while, in others, a nonspecific reaction is responsible for the failure. Until these reactions are explained, the use of ETO-sterilized grafts for intra-articular knee surgery has been stopped by most tissue banks.

Low-dose γ-radiation from cobalt 60 has been reported to give good penetration of soft tissue and is used as a means of secondary sterilization. Questions remain as to the dose of radiation for complete and reliable viral sterility and tissue degradation secondary to the radiation. Data suggest the HIV can be killed with 2.5 megarads but its reliability is not proven in soft tissue and bone allografts. Conway and associates (12) estimated that it would take 3.6 megarads to inactivate the free HIV-1 virus by γ-irradiation and an even higher dose would be required to obtain an acceptable safety margin with cell-associated virus. Withrow et al. (13) studied the feline leukemia virus (FeLV) as a model of HIV. They looked at seven methods of preservation; fresh, frozen 14 days, dimethylsulfoxide (DMSO) and freezing, lyophilization, irradiation with 2.9 megarads, demineralization with 0.6 M HCl, and ETO. They found that these standard methods do not consistently kill the FeLV retrovirus. Additional work must be done to ascertain if there is a dose that is high enough to sterilize a bone tendon bone graft reliably yet not so high as to alter the desired mechanical properties of the graft. Mechanical properties of tendon and ligament have been reported to be altered by 3.0 megarads at an unacceptable level. Whether lower levels give the desired viral kill rate will take further work. Some tissue banks believe that it is useful as a secondary method effective for bacteria and some viral components.

GRAFT PROCUREMENT

In the specialized use of allografts for knee surgery, much of the sizing and shaping can be accomplished at procurement. Therefore, the intraoperative preparation time prior to placing the graft can be shortened. This requires that a knowledgeable person who understands how the allograft will be used be responsible for procurement of the allograft. There have been cases, for example, where the patella tendon insertion into the bone has been damaged at the time of procurement, greatly diminishing the strength to failure of the bone-tendon junction.

We prefer that all tissue be procured and handled aseptically, whether secondary sterilization is used or not. This is an individual bank and surgeon's decision. Ligament and tendon allografts can be stored for up to 6 months when fresh-frozen and for 2 years or longer when freeze-dried. At the present time, the length of time that cryopreservation, as a method, is able to maintain the living fibroblast and chondrocytes is to be demonstrated. In addition, the ability of the cells to duplicate and function following transplantation remains to be delineated. The benefit of living cells in articular cartilage has been shown; however, similar benefits with ligament, tendon, and meniscus have yet to be demonstrated. Potential sources of allografts used for knee ligament reconstructions have included the anterior and posterior cruciate ligament, patellar tendon, quadriceps tendon, fascia lata, Achilles tendon with bone, semitendinosus, gracilis, tibialis anterior, and posterior leg tendons. Shino et al. (14) have stated that one donor can furnish 22 different grafts to be used for anterior cruciate ligament reconstructions.

BIOMECHANICS

The allograft replacement must be incorporated and must remain as a functional replacement. The biomechanical forces seen by the ACL and posterior cruciate ligament (PCL) for various activities are reported in Table 10.1. The strength of the substitute graft at the time of implantation compared to normal ACL is shown in Figure 10.1 and Table 10.2. Once the allograft tissue is implanted within the knee, it appears that its strength decreases over the first month up to one-fourth of the original strength. This fall may be followed by a slow increase in strength to 30–50% of the original strength (9). There is a slower return to strength than would be expected for autogenous tissues but the final mechanical values are roughly equivalent (20). If the inherent strength of the allograft to tensile testing is greater than the ACL, the ultimate strength may approach 80% of its value. However, more data suggest that the strength of most allografts used approaches only about 25–50% of the original ligament. In addition, most animal work suggests that it is difficult to re-establish the normal anteroposterior translation of the joint. In the allograft ligament reconstructions, the knees in animals tested have increased anteroposterior translation in comparison with the contralateral knee. Several studies have

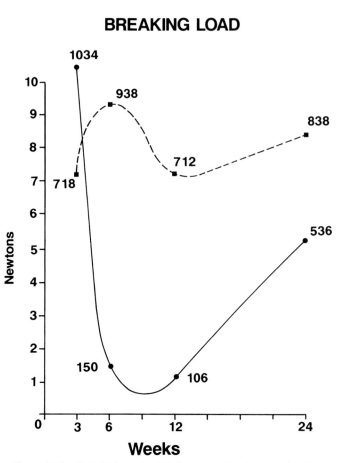

BREAKING LOAD

Figure 10.1. Plot of biomechanical data comparing the mean breaking load for the intra-articular allograft and the contralateral ACL at each time interval. *Closed square* = contralateral; *closed circles* = graft (intra-articular). Reproduced with permission from Curtis RJ, et al. Reconstruction of the anterior cruciate ligament with freeze dried fascia lata allografts in dogs. A preliminary report. Am J Sports Med 1985; 13:408–414.

Table 10.1.
Forces Seen in Newtons Calculated for Daily Activities

Activity	ACL	PCL
Level walking	(169–210)	352
Ascending stairs	67	641
Descending stairs	(113–445)	262
Ascending 9.45° ramp	(27–107)	1215
Descending 9.45° ramp	(93–485)	449
Jogging	630	
Jolting	700	
Sitting and rising	173	
Stress at failure	1700	

[a]Data compiled from references 15–18.

Table 10.2.
Substitute Graft Strength at Time of Implantation

Graft Type	Strength	Maximum Force (Newton)
Bone patellar tendon Bone		
Central ⅓ 13.8 mm	158%	2734
Medial ⅓ 14.9 mm	168%	2900
ACL	100%	1725
Semitendinosus	70%	1216
Gracilis	49%	838
Iliotibial band		
15.6 mm	36%	628
45 mm	44%	1800
Fascia lata	36%	628
Retinaculum	21%	266

[a]Adapted from Noyes (19).

reported that the method of preservation used does not weaken the graft (21–24) but rather the loss of strength is due to the remodeling process. Webster and Werner (23, 24) studied freeze-dried flexor tendons in dogs and found that, although the original strength was equal or greater than the control, there was a significant drop in strength to between one-third and two-thirds of the control at 6–8 months after implantation. Shino et al. (25) studied patellar tendons in dogs and found that, at 30 weeks, the autograft was 29.7% of control while the deep frozen (−20°C) allograft was 27.9% of control. Curtis et al. (9) reconstructed the anterior cruciates of dogs with freeze-dried fascia lata. They reported that, although the freshly reconstructed allograft was 130% of control by 12 weeks, it was only 14% of the control knee. At 24 weeks, it had improved to 67% of control. Jackson et al. (26, 27) studied the Spanish goat and found that ETO-sterilized and freeze-dried ACL allografts had a stiffness of between 35% and 50% of controls and failed at only 25% of control ACL strength at 1 year. The transplanted tissues have the strongest mechanical properties at the time of implantation. Biological alteration by host remodeling of the graft leads to a deterioration of the mechanical properties. Additional studies (28) demonstrated no significant difference between the mechanical properties of ETO freeze-dried, freeze-dried, and control specimens at time zero. Vasseur et al. (29) found the breaking strength of allografts to be 14% and autografts to be 10% of control dogs at 9 months. The one conflicting study was done by Nikolaou et al. (22) who transplanted ACL allografts in mongrel dogs and found that autografts and deep frozen allografts were similar in that both obtained 90% of control strength at 36 weeks. The stiffness of the allograft started at 97% of control, dropped to 89% of control, and returned to 98% of control while the energy to failure was 50% of control at 8 weeks and gradually increased to 90% of control by 36 weeks postoperatively. They compared fresh and cryopreserved bone ACL bone grafts in dogs and found no significant differences on the breaking strength, energy to failure, and ligament stiffness. It is difficult to explain the divergent results in graft strength found in this study when compared with the previous studies; however, some of the discrepancy is probably related to control values and methodology of mechanical testing.

ANTERIOR CRUCIATE LIGAMENT ALLOGRAFTS

At the present time, using ACL (ACL for an ACL) allografts to reconstruct an ACL-deficient knee is of limited use. The sizing problems in substituting an ACL allograft for an injured ACL are considerable. The decrease in strength in the graft make it less desirable than sources of tendon that start inherently stronger. An ACL allograft offers the potential for nonparallel fibers, accommodation for the different lengths of fibers, and the potential to contribute more to controlling rotational stability. At the present time, ACL and PCL ligament allografts are used most often with a composite graft where multiple ligaments and/or capsule, menisci, or articular cartilage are transplanted. This accommodates for some of the sizing problems. Our experience with composite grafts in animals and limited use in humans has been less predictable in attaining the desired stability and knee function. These have represented end stage knees where alternatives have included knee fusion or joint replacement. Fixation of the transplanted composite, sizing, and balancing the ligaments are all factors that affect the success rate.

HISTOLOGY

Both allografts and autografts using tendons for ligament reconstruction in the knee appear to undergo a similar process that is characterized by initial necrosis, which is followed by revascularization, cellular replacement and ingrowth, collagen formation, and collagen fiber realignment. Initially, after harvest and implantation, the graft undergoes avascular necrosis. There is separation of collagen bundles so that they are less tightly packed than the normal ACL and the native fibroblasts die.

At 6 weeks, there is evidence of revascularization (9, 14, 22, 30–35) on the surface of the graft. The central portion of the graft lags behind the periphery and is vascularized at about 16 weeks. This process may continue until an increased vascularity pattern in ACL allografts is seen as compared with the normal ACL (26, 27). The host vascular response subsides and the hypervascularity response has been reported to return to normal between 12 and 18 months (14, 22, 25, 35). The vessels in the fat pad seem to be the main source for the revascularization of the inferior portion of ligament while the superior portion is revascularized from synovial tissues in the intercondylar notch. This revascularization may be accompanied by an increase in graft cross-sectional area. During this time period, it appears that larger diameter collagen fibrils within the graft are replaced by smaller diameter fibrils. The mechanical properties of the graft are weakest between 6 and 12 weeks after implantation and then gradually increase in strength but never regain the original strength.

While the allograft tendon is being incorporated, the bony attachment is also undergoing changes. Bone grafts in rats undergo two stages of osteogenesis (36–40). An early phase of new bone formation lasts 4–8 days and is similar to that seen in autografts but is quantitatively less for allografts. A period of necrosis and resorption ensues and then a slower osteogenesis phase starts at about 28 days. Cellular activity was more pronounced in the autografts than in the allografts (29). The allograft takes longer to incorporate than a corresponding autograft.

Fresh autograft bone represents a different environment than a fresh-frozen bone allograft because the transplanted cells have the potential to remain viable and function. A tendon transplanted into the intra-articular environment brings with it no cells that remain viable, be it an autograft or an allograft. During the necrotic phase, the ACL specific fibroblasts are replaced with cells of synovial and vascular origin. These new fibroblast replacements produce collagen that is longitudinally oriented and resembles normal collagen under the light microscope. However, the regular crimp pattern of collagen fibrils is absent (41). In addition, the replacement fibroblasts may not be able to maintain the larger diameter fibers. When viewed under the electron microscope, at 6 months, the collagen fibers showed an increased number of smaller fibers (500 angstroms), were more numerous than the controls (1000–1500 angstroms), and were less tightly packed (33, 42, 43). Studies of human ACL reconstruction have shown a persistent predominance of small collagen fibers with no demonstrable fiber size increase at 6 years postimplantation (42). The larger fiber size has been correlated with an increase in maximum stress, linear modulus, and energy density to maximum strength. Recently, in situ studies have reported on the biological and mechanical fate of injured ligaments and tendons. Postacchini and Del Martino (44) created partial and complete transections of rabbit Achilles tendon. The partial thickness defect healed in 16 weeks with large-diameter collagen fibers while the complete transection healed with small-diameter fibrils. They believed that the mechanical loading was the stimulus to produce large-diameter fibers. Jackson et al. (33) subjected in situ goat ACLs to five freeze-thaw cycles. The freeze-thaw process devitalized and devascularized the central one-third of the ACL while retaining its collagen fiber orientation, tension, and fixation. After 6 months, the ligaments were tested and compared to control ligaments. No significant differences were found among anteroposterior translation, maximal force (to failure), stiffness, modulus, or strain. There was a 42% increase in cross-sectional area and a separation of the collagen bundles that persisted beyond 6 months. The mean collagen fiber diameter of the control was 841 angstroms while the experimental side was 930 angstroms at 6 weeks and 435 angstroms at 6 months post freeze-thaw. Because this study conflicted with previous allograft studies that had shown a 50–75% reduction in maximum strength, it was concluded that physiological tension and placement of the collagen fiber may alter the effects of the biological response. Others have also documented that early loading influences maturation, remodeling, and leads to larger collagen fiber size (45, 46).

An allograft that attains the same biomechanical parameters as the ACL requires proper orientation and tension. In addition, the fate of the ACL-specific fibroblasts that produce the large-fiber collagen appears to represent a challenge. The change in collagen fiber size may be due to a fibroblast repopulation of the ligament by stem cell fibroblasts that are not capable of maintaining or synthesizing large-diameter fibrils (42, 47). Theoretically, there are two ways to obtain the desirable collagen size. First, one could somehow stimulate the appropriate host fibroblast to repopulate the allograft ligament. This has not been achieved but is an area that is being actively pursued. Second, one could preserve enough of the original cells of the donor ligament so that they could maintain the large-fiber collagen of the graft. Although such capability has yet to be demonstrated with ligaments, O'Brien and associates (48, 49) have suggested this in aortic valve replacement. Viable cells have been shown to be of donor origin by chromosome studies over 9 years after implantation. Histological studies have shown the allograft valve to have the appearance of an essentially normal valve. Whether similar results can be found with ligament and menisci allografts remains to be shown. Another consideration is the role played by the host immune system in the long-term survival of allograft cells. It seems clear, however, that, to obtain optimal results particularly in articular cartilage and meniscal allografts, the appropriate cells must be functioning.

TRANSPLANT IMMUNOLOGY

The histocompatibility is of concern in allograft tissues. While this subject is covered in detail in Chapter 2, a brief summary of aspects especially pertinent to allograft ligaments is presented in this section. The meniscus, ligament, or tendon allograft are often transplanted with bony attachments. The bone carries more antigens than the tendon. While, earlier, our understanding was that deep frozen and freeze-dried tissue did not elicit an immunological or inflammatory response, we now know that the response can be very subtle. Bone tendon bone grafts are not immunologically privileged whether fresh, deep frozen, or freeze-dried.

The immunological response of the host plays a major role in the rate of incorporation and strength of the allograft. Both humoral and cell-mediated immune responses are implicated in allograft rejection (50–53).

Histocompatibility plays a role, especially early, in the incorporation of bone grafts. The ultimate clinical significance is not well delineated and remains controversial. It may vary depending on the animal model. Schachar et al. (53) in cats, Goldberg et al. (54) and Stevenson and Templeton (55) in dogs, and Friedlaender et al. (56) in rabbits showed evidence of an immune response against frozen bone. Bos et al. (57–59) showed that histocompatibility matching improved the incorporation of frozen bone allografts in beagles and mice. A later study (36) of histocompatibility comparing fresh and frozen groups showed early differences in incorporation between closely and disparately matched allografts. After 40 days, however, there were no demonstrable differences between the groups. Halloran et al. (60, 61) using an orthotopic model in mice, and Muscolo et al. (52), using in vitro rat studies, both believed that histocompatibility matching may be desirable. Mankin (34) and Stevenson (62) have suggested that histocompatibility matching may reduce host sensitization and improve graft incorporation. The size of the allograft may also play a role in eliciting an immune reaction. Freezing or freeze-drying prior to use has been shown to decrease or eliminate the antigenicity of the allograft (38–40, 49, 57, 58, 60). Recently, work by Pinkowski and associates (11) has demonstrated lymphocyte reaction in humans to freeze-dried ACL allografts in 50% of the eight patients studied. This contradicts earlier work in the area and is indicative of an increased ability to detect subtle immunological responses. Tendon antigenicity studies show that the collagen carries few antigens (63, 64) whereas the cellular components carry the major antigens (65). The freezing process destroys cellular components and denatures the histocompatibility antigens while leaving the collagen framework intact (66). Adjuvant treatment with radiation, glutaraldehyde, and mitomycin C can fix the cells and preserve the histocompatibility antigens (41, 65–69). While freezing has the advantage of damaging the histocom-

patibility antigens, the process can delay graft incorporation. Bos et al. (36) compared syngeneic fresh and frozen bone grafts in mice and found that freezing reduced the ability of the host to incorporate the graft. A fresh graft elicits an inflammatory rejection response characterized by lymphocytic and plasma cell invasion that can be reduced by processing the graft.

In an effort to decrease the immune reaction by eliminating the bone, Shino and associates (25) studied fresh-frozen tendon without any bony attachments. They could not demonstrate an immune response in their grafts.

The joint, being a separate compartment, can have antibody titers higher than that found in the serum; it can even demonstrate a presence of an antibody when no detectable antibody can be demonstrated in the serum. Local immunity has been shown in dogs (29, 62) and in humans with rheumatoid arthritis (70). Vasseur et al. (29) studied frozen bone ligament bone allografts and detected an antidonor dog leukocyte antibody in the knee that was undetectable in the serum. While freezing may reduce the antigenicity of the graft, the concept of compartmental antibodies challenges the belief that antigenicity is eliminated or reduced to the point of not being important.

A major obstacle exists with the various animal models studied because the results cannot always be extrapolated to humans. Also, the immunological response assay methods vary widely. In some individuals, we may be seeing an allergy to certain types of collagen and not a response to the histocompatibility antigens. Only recently have studies looked at this important area and its significance is not fully understood. In the past, it was believed that immunosuppression had no effect on bone grafting (51). This area needs to be investigated further in light of the new concepts of compartmental immunity and data demonstrating that humans may respond even when the animal model does not. The role of histocompatibility matching for soft tissue allografts is currently under investigation. Immunogenic reactions may account for a small percentage of previously unexplained graft failures.

Two divergent approaches have been tried to solve the conundrum of allograft incorporation. One previously mentioned in the histology section is from O'Brien's work and is centered around trying to maintain the donor cells to maintain the graft collagen. Theoretically, the immunological complications would be higher with this approach. A second approach would be for host cells to invade the graft and to replace it with large-diameter collagen fibers of host origin. This approach would not elicit as much of an immunological response as the first approach. To date, no researcher has demonstrated that host fibroblasts can repopulate the graft and function in the same manner as the original cells.

PRESENT CONSIDERATIONS FOR USING ALLOGRAFTS IN KNEE LIGAMENT RECONSTRUCTION

1. ACL reconstruction where there is no autograft alternative;
2. PCL reconstruction;
3. Patients over age 40 years;
4. Failed autograft reconstruction;
5. Small patella tendon;
6. Pre-existing patella femoral chondrosis or extensor mechanism alignment abnormalities.

We believe that there are indications for use of an allograft in knee reconstructions. These include PCL reconstructions where a large graft is desirable; the knee with multiple injuries that have required multiple grafts; knees that have failed previously attempts at reconstruction, which used potential autograft sources (salvage cases); reconstructions in patients with very elastic tissues; and older patients whose tissues may not have the desired strength. By using a large allograft initially, as the strength drops off, it still has the potential to be adequate.

The results of the use of fresh-frozen allografts in ACL and PCL reconstructions have been encouraging and we continue to use them in selective cases. Several factors have limited our use of them routinely for all ligament reconstruction of ACL and PCL.

1. Inability to meet our patients' needs with reliably procured grafts that meet our specifications;
2. Concern for disease transmission by the patient and the problems of adequate secondary sterilization procedures;
3. Good results with autografts associated with less morbidity to the patient than in the past;
4. Awaiting longer term follow-up on the allografts that are in place.

RESULTS

With over 200 ACL and 50 PCL reconstructions done between 1985 and 1989, results have improved with experience. In this series, there were seven unexpected failures (6.4%) secondary to the use of ETO grafts in 107 consecutive chronic ACL reconstructions. The use of autografts in our clinical practice has constituted the majority of our ACL reconstructions. The autograft and allograft groups are dissimilar by selection factors as listed.

An aseptically procured and carefully screened fresh-frozen allograft is our present preference. We are using patellar tendon-bone for the ACL and Achilles tendon-

bone for the PCL reconstructions. To date, we have not had to remove a fresh-frozen graft because of an intra-articular reaction. We have had failures secondary to trauma in 5% of our PCLs and have significantly improved the posterior instability in 80% of our reconstructions. Over 60% of the PCL reconstructions approach 5-mm side-to-side differences and lose approximately 20° of symmetrical flexion.

The ACL allografts approach 80% with less than 3-mm side-to-side difference if one eliminates the failures we have had related to graft reactions (6.4%) and technical considerations early in our experience.

Our present allograft technique for ACL reconstruction is as follows.

ACL Reconstruction Technique

1. The procedure begins with examination of the injured and contralateral knee under anesthesia. This is followed by an arthroscopic evaluation of the knee and performance of indicated intra-articular procedures.
2. The bone plugs of the adequately thawed allograft are sized to 10 mm in width and 20 mm in length for the proximal end and a 11-mm width and 25-mm length for the distal end (Fig. 10.2). Sizing is confirmed by passing the grafts through an appropriate cylindrical sizer. We prefer three no. 5 sutures through the distal end and one through the proximal end. Once the thawed graft is prepared, it is held under 10-lb tension on a tension board while the bony tunnels are prepared.
3. The superior and lateral side of the notch are debrided (notchplasty).
4. A 2.5-cm incision is made in the skin about 4 cm below the medial joint line. This is just medial to the tibial tubercle. Dissection is carried sharply down to bone. Using a guide, a smooth 3/32-inch Steinmann pin is placed into the joint at the previous tibial insertion of the ACL (Fig. 10.3). A currette placed over the Steinmann pin tip protects as a tibial tunnel is prepared with a 11-mm drill (Fig. 10.3). At least 4 cm of bone is desirable between the joint line and the center of the tibial tunnel.
5. All excess bone is removed from the tunnel and the soft tissue thoroughly debrided where the tunnel enters the joint. A rasp is used to chamfer the entrance tunnel.
6. The anatomic insertion site of the ACL on the femur is located and, with an awl, this spot is marked in the bone.
7. A special canula is passed up through the tibial tunnel and centered in the previously selected site for the center of the femoral tunnel.
8. A Steinmann pin is then drilled into the bone for approximately 20 mm.
9. Protecting the PCL with a retractor, an 11-mm drill is placed by hand over the guide pin. The drill is then advanced for

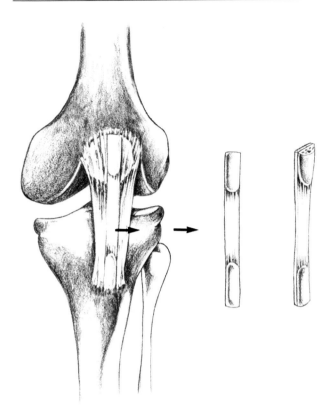

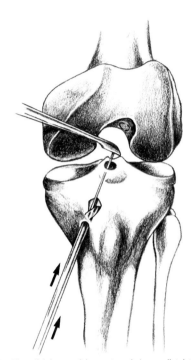

Figure 10.3. The tibial tunnel is centered 4 cm distal to the joint line and medial to the tibial tubercle. The Steinmann pin enters the joint through the residual stump of the ACL. A curette is placed over the tip of the Steinmann pin as it is over drilled with an 11-mm drill.

Figure 10.2. The tissue bank supplying soft tissue allografts may provide a presized patellar tendon allograft or a patella-patellar tendon-tibial bone block that will require further trimming and sizing. Three sutures are placed through the tibial end and one through the femoral end.

25 mm (Fig. 10.4). There should be approximately 1–2 mm of bone comprising the posterior wall of the tunnel (Fig. 10.5).

10. A drill with an eyelet is passed through the tibial and femoral tunnels and out through the quadriceps. Using the tracking eyelet, a suture is then used to pull the graft up into the joint (Fig. 10.6).

11. A small guide pin is placed anteriorly into the femoral tunnel for 1 cm (Fig. 10.7). The graft is pulled into the tunnel with its cortical side posterior. In this position, the tendon portion with the collagen fibers are at the center and posterior portion of the tunnel (Fig. 10.8).

12. The proximal end of the graft is pulled into the femoral tunnel.

13. A cannulated screw and screw driver is placed through a separate portal over the guide pin and a 7.5-mm interference screw is placed while tension is held on the sutures through the proximal bone plug. The screw is placed anterior to the graft. This pushes the graft posteriorly and also the screw will not cut out through the thin posterior cortex (Fig. 10.9).

14. Tension is placed on the femorally fixed graft and, if it withstands 20 lb of load, the knee is taken through a range of motion approximately six times. The bone plug is secured

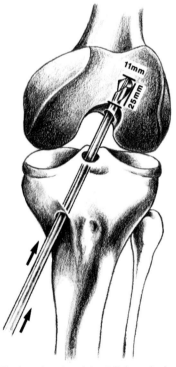

Figure 10.4. The insertion site of the ACL is marked with an awl. Protecting the PCL with a retractor, an 11-mm drill is placed by hand over the guide pin. The drill is then advanced for 25 mm.

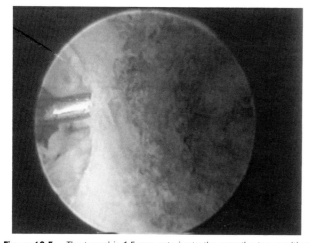

Figure 10.5. The tunnel is 1.5 mm anterior to the over-the-top position marked by the probe.

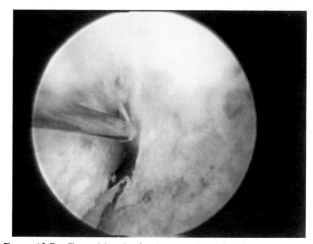

Figure 10.7. The guide wire for the cannulated interference screw is placed into the tunnel as the graft is pulled into the tunnel.

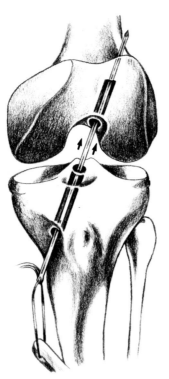

Figure 10.6. Using a tracking eyelet, a suture is used to pull the graft into the tunnel.

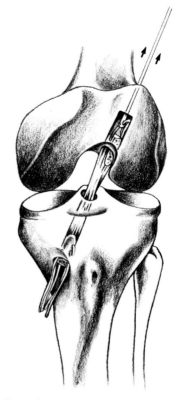

Figure 10.8. The graft is pulled into the tunnel with its cortical side posterior. In this position, the tendon portion with the collagen fibers are at the center and posterior portion of the tunnel.

in the tibia with a 9.0-mm interference screw. The knee is checked for stability. The sutures are removed from the bone plug and the small incisions are closed in the standard fashion (Fig. 10.10).

15. Side-to-side testing following fixation confirms desired stability.

PCL Reconstruction Technique

1. Examination of both knees is performed under anesthesia. Arthroscopic evaluation of the knee and indicated intra-articular procedures are completed.

2. The previous PCL insertion site from the medial side of the notch and the posterior proximal tibia are debrided. Elevating the posterior joint capsular attachments requires good visualization and often requires a posterior medial portal for instrumentation and arthroscopic visualization.

3. An incision in the skin is made approximately 10 cm below the lateral joint line. Dissection is carried sharply down to

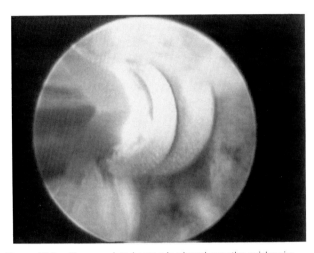

Figure 10.9. The cannulated screw is placed over the guide wire.

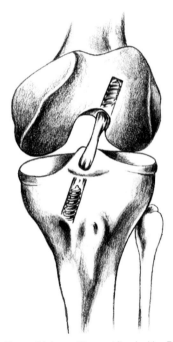

Figure 10.10. The graft is in position and fixed with a 7.5-mm cannulated interference screw proximally and a 9 mm × 25 mm interference screw distally.

bone and the anterior tibial musculature is elevated to obtain adequate exposure for the tibial tunnel (Fig. 10.11).

4. The anatomic insertion site of the PCL on the tibia is located and, with the guide a Steinmann pin is placed from the tibia just below the lateral to the tibia tubercle (about 10 cm distal to the joint line) (Fig. 10.12). We prefer to check the position with image intensification and observe the Steinmann pin and the 10-mm reamer. The position is again checked with the arthroscope and fluoroscopy as the posterior cortex is perforated. The ideal position is just lateral and 10 cm below the joint line.

5. All excess bone is removed and the soft tissue debrided thoroughly from the posterior tibial tunnel.

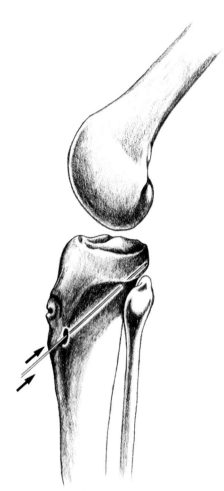

Figure 10.11. An incision in the skin is made approximately 10 cm below the lateral joint line. Dissection is carried sharply down to bone and the anterior tibial musculature is elevated to obtain adequate exposure for the tibial tunnel.

6. The femoral tunnel is prepared by dissecting down to the medial femoral condyle but staying out of the joint capsule. A Steinmann pin is placed entering the joint at the desired femoral insertion for the PCL graft, which is approximately 10 mm proximal to the articular surface and at the superior medial position in the notch (Fig. 10.13).

7. A curette is placed over the Steinmann pin tip in the joint to protect the 11-mm drill as it prepares the tunnel (Fig. 10.14).

8. The Achilles tendon allograft is prepared by sizing the bone plug and tapering it from 12.5 mm to 10.5 mm. An Achilles tendon allograft 10 mm in diameter is preferred. The Achilles tendon has the advantage of being a round tendon and is stronger than the flat patellar tendon. It has bone on one end only and, therefore, lacks the advantage of bony fixation on both sides of the joint (Fig. 10.15). Three Bunnel sutures of nonabsorbable suture are placed through the Achilles tendon (Fig. 10.16). These are then threaded through the fingertrap portion of the Gore smoother (Fig. 10.16).

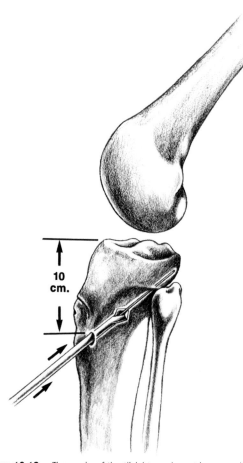

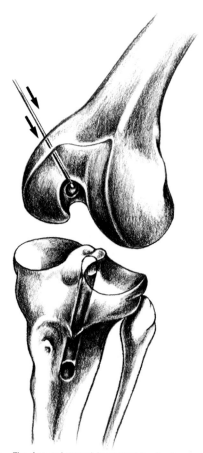

Figure 10.12. The angle of the tibial tunnel must be enough to leave a substantial amount of bone between the tunnel and the joint surface but not so great that too much posterior cortex is removed. The ideal position is just distal and lateral to the tibial tubercle or about 10 cm below the joint line.

Figure 10.13. The femoral tunnel is started by finding a point on the medial wall of the intercondylar notch approximately 9 mm from the articular cartilage and in the one o'clock position for a right knee or an eleven o'clock position for a left knee. A Steinmann pin is placed to enter the joint at the desired femoral insertion for the PCL graft, which is approximately 10 mm proximal to the articular surface and at the superior medial position in the notch.

9. The red rubber catheter is placed through the joint and used to bring a Gore smoother into the joint, which is used to chamfer the tunnel entrances. The graft is then pulled into the joint from the femoral side to the tibia (Fig. 10.17).

10. The tapered bone forms an interference fit within the medial femoral condyle osseous tunnel.

11. The femoral bone plug is impacted into the femoral tunnel.

12. The tibia is held reduced and tension is adjusted. The lateral tibial insertion is fixed under a soft tissue washer (Fig. 10.18). The muscle is used to cover the fixation. If thought to be necessary, the sutures may be tied over a tibial post used to secure fixation further. The incisions are closed in the standard fashion.

Meniscal Transplantation

The meniscus functions both in stress distribution and in stabilizing the knee joint. Degenerative arthritis develops due to altered hoop stresses, cushioning effects, and instability that can occur following complete or even partial meniscectomy (71–77). Meniscal repair, while being a great advancement in the treatment of meniscal tears, is not possible in all patients. Interest in meniscal transplantation centers around ways to avoid the degenerative changes by having an allograft perform the essential meniscal functions. Meniscus is perhaps an ideal tissue for transplantation because it is relatively avascular fibrocartilage that conforms to the articular surfaces of the tibia and femur. The cells in fibrocartilage and articular cartilage grafts have generally been regarded as immunoprivileged partially because of their relative avascular environment. The preservation of graft fibrochondrocytes is thought to be important for the long-term maintenance of the complex extracellular matrix.

Fresh transplants theoretically offer this capability but their use is limited primarily to institutions where there

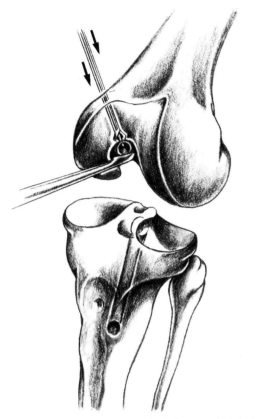

Figure 10.14. A curette is placed over the Steinmann pin tip in the joint to protect the 11-mm drill as it prepares the tunnel.

is an organ transplant service. Availability of fresh transplants remains limited. Sizing consideration of the donor and recipient, and the logistics of matching a surgical team and the recipient on short notice present a problem. An alternative that would allow storage of grafts with living cells is cryopreservation. The studies by Arnoczky et al. (78) in dogs showed that, with a controlled rate for freezing the cell, viability was about 10% over a period of 2 weeks. The cells that survived were hypermetabolic. Our survival rates by dye exclusion and tissue culture viability studies indicate a 30% survival rate for meniscal cells at 1 month. The number of viable cells required in a transplant and the ability of the cells to replicate and maintain long-term extracellular matrix synthesis remains to be established.

Milachowski and associates (79) have transplanted deep frozen and freeze-dried γ-irradiated menisci in sheep and humans. Both tissues healed at their periphery to the host with minimal changes described in the sheep model. The human menisci underwent significant shrinkage and the γ-irradiated menisci underwent a complete remodeling with almost complete resorption. Canham and Stanish (80) performed glutaraldehyde-preserved meniscal

transplants but had difficulties with attachment to the capsule and repeated effusions. We performed meniscal transplants using fresh and cryopreserved allografts in goats. The goats were matched for size and weight. Bone plugs containing the meniscotibial ligament attachments were transplanted to stabilize the menisci. The menisci in this study retained their normal size. At 6 months following transplantation, the water content was elevated in both the fresh and cryopreserved allografts. This was thought to be indicative of early compromise in the fibrillar meshwork of the extracellular matrix. The uronic acid concentration was lower than control in the 6-month allograft groups indicating that the loss of proteoglycan was greater than the rate of synthesis and deposition. Cell viability was tested with Trypan blue exclusion, which demonstrated the fresh and cryopreserved allograft groups to be about 80% of the control at 6 months. The origin of these cells remains to be delineated as well as the fate of the transplanted fibrochondrocytes. Injection studies demonstrated adequate capsular healing and a normal vascular pattern.

The present use of meniscal transplants in humans should be considered investigational until longer term data are available. The indications for meniscal transplants must be clarified because, often, it is thought that the adjacent articular cartilage would also benefit from replacement. It is an unusual clinical setting in which an isolated meniscal transplant would re-establish all of the alterations in the involved compartment of the joint. It appears meniscal transplants will have the greatest benefit as part of a meniscal composite graft. Details of fibrochondrocyte viability, fibrillar meshwork, extracellular matrix, indications, and surgical technique remain to be elucidated before meniscal allografts become part of the armamentarium of the local knee surgeons.

MENISCAL TRANSPLANTATION TECHNIQUE (GOAT MODEL)

Our initial investigation of meniscal transplantation was conducted in the goat model (81). Early attempts at graft fixation consisted of suturing the peripheral rim of the allograft meniscus to the capsule and placing traction sutures through the meniscotibial ligaments. This proved to be an inadequate method of fixation. The menisci using this technique were often forced out peripherally of the joint over time. It became clear that the method of fixation could potentially affect the meniscal function. The cine MRI work of Fu et al. (18) in the human cadaver model demonstrated the magnitude of anterior and posterior excursion that the meniscus undergoes when the knee goes through a full range of

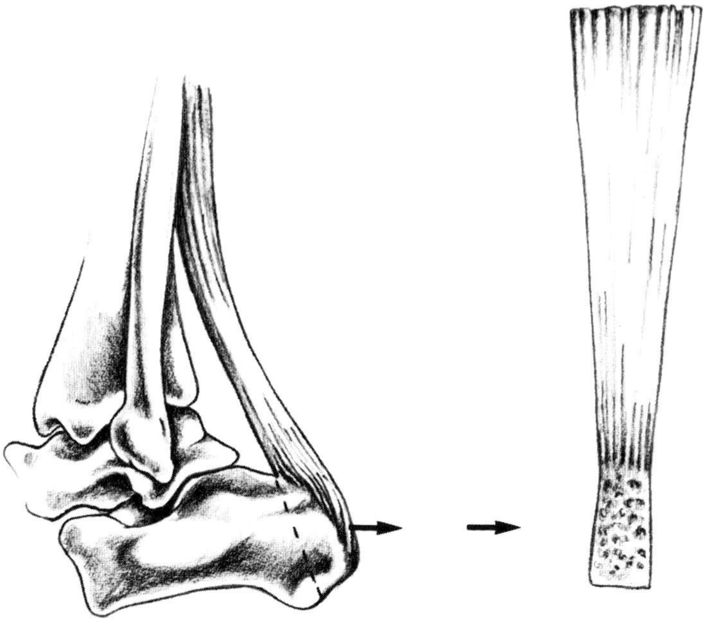

Figure 10.15. Achilles tendon allograft 10 mm in diameter is preferred. The Achilles tendon has the advantage of being a round tendon and is stronger than the flat patellar tendon. It has bone on one end only and, therefore, lacks the advantage of bony fixation on both sides of the joint.

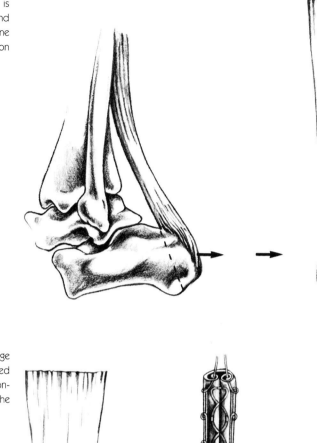

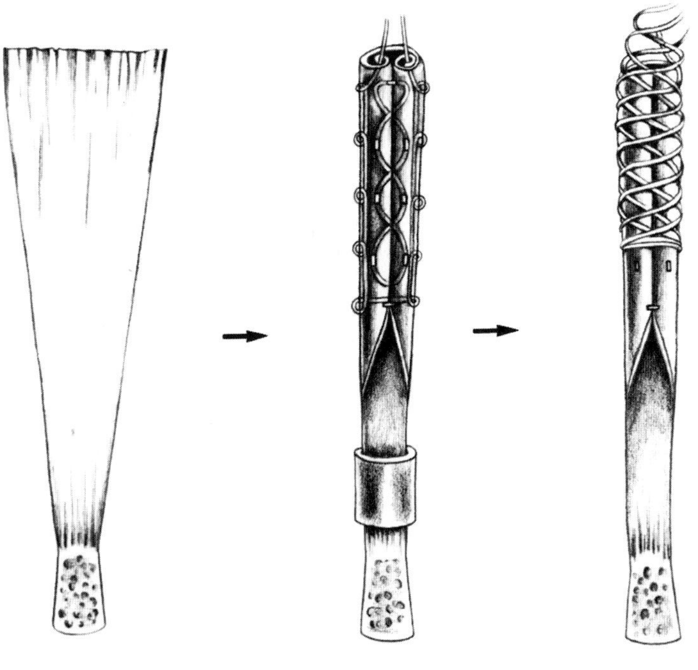

Figure 10.16. The Achilles tendon allograft is shaped into a wedge from 12.5 mm to 10.5 mm and nonabsorbable sutures are placed through the tendon. An appropriate sizer (the graft is slightly conical) is used to check the fit. The tendon is then secured to the Gore smoother in preparation for insertion.

motion. The proper position and motion of the menisci is important to weight-bearing force distribution and joint stability. Impaired motion could potentially alter these functions.

Our approach to establishing better anteroposterior stabilization was to utilize bone plugs attached to the meniscotibial ligaments. This offers the advantages of bone interface for fixation.

POSTOPERATIVE TREATMENT

Postoperatively, the limbs were not immobilized and full weight bearing was allowed as tolerated by each animal.

BIOCHEMICAL INDICATION OF DEGENERATIVE CHANGES IN MENISCAL TRANSPLANTS

The water content of cartilaginous tissue is governed by the capacity of the tensile strength of the collagen meshwork

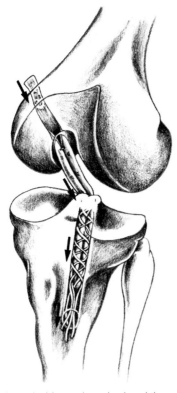

Figure 10.17. The red rubber catheter is placed through the joint and used to bring a Gore smoother into the joint, which is used to chamfer the tunnel entrances. The graft is then pulled into the joint from the femoral side to the tibia.

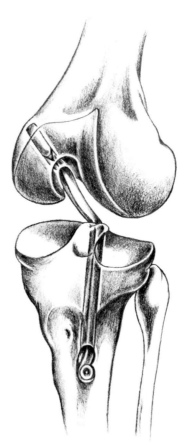

Figure 10.18. Knee with reconstruction PCL in position. There is an interference fit on femur. The tension is adjusted and the distal side is tied over a screw and washer.

to resist the swelling pressure of the underhydrated proteoglycans (82). An increase in water content has been observed previously in osteoarthritic menisci (83). The mechanisms that compromise the integrity of the collagen meshwork leading to an increased water content are unknown. Mechanical rupture of the fibrillar meshwork or proteinase attack, particularly from the enzymes generated from inflammatory cells, could contribute to this effect.

Proteoglycans are usually the first molecules to be degraded in proteinase attack of cartilaginous tissues and their concentrations in the extracellular matrix is an indicator of the balance of synthetic and degradative mechanisms in a tissue. Uronic acid is a constituent sugar of the repeating disaccharide of chondroitin sulfate and hyaluronic acid. Inasmuch as over 90% of the glycosaminoglycan in menisci is chondroitin sulfate (84), uronic acid assays reflect the proteoglycan concentration in the tissue.

REPRODUCIBLE METHODS IN ANIMALS

Meniscal transplantation in the small goat knee is a demanding surgical procedure and requires an extensive exposure. We believe that our attainment of clinically

acceptable transplants in 26 of our 30 animals is encouraging in this small knee model.

Anchoring the bone plugs anteriorly and posteriorly has the potential to re-establish more normal meniscus mobility and to prevent some of the lengthening and extrusion in menisci with only a peripheral attachment.

The transplantation of viable fibrochondrocytes in a fresh or cryopreserved meniscal allograft may protect the joint from some of the degenerative changes seen after total meniscectomy. This assumption requires that the material properties of the transplanted meniscus can be maintained on a long-term basis. Clinically, the menisci in our animal models looked good grossly as did the adjacent articular cartilage; however, the biochemical changes in the extracellular matrix at 6 months raise questions about the long-term function of these transplanted menisci.

While the viability of donor cells and the role of the replacement cells will require genetic probes for further elucidation, the authors believe that the clinical results of these subgroups of meniscal transplants merit serious study as an alternative to total meniscectomy.

HUMAN MENISCAL TRANSPLANT WITH BONE BRIDGE

Garrett has reported his observation of six patients who underwent meniscal transplantation (four medial, two lateral) and were followed from 24–44 months (85). Prior to transplantation, all of the patients had multiple surgeries, including meniscectomy (range, 8 months to 20 years). All of the patients had additional procedures performed; three had ACL reconstruction, two had osteochondral allografts for lateral femoral condyle defects, and one had an ACL reconstruction and bone graft for the lateral femoral condyle.

SURGICAL TECHNIQUE

Eligible donors in their late teens and early 20s were matched within 5% of recipients for skeletal size (anteroposterior roentgenograph of distal femur). Graft procurement was performed under sterile operating room conditions just after kidney removal and life-support termination.

1. Medial menisci transplantation was performed through a medial parapatellar incision.
2. A lateral parapatellar incision and tibial tubercle osteotomy was used for lateral menisci transplantation.
3. The ipsilateral collateral ligament was detached from its femoral origin.
4. Visualization was also improved by forward subluxation of the tibia in the ACL-deficient cases.
5. The meniscal rim was resected to the vascular zone and the allograft trimmed to fit (Fig. 10.19).
6. A modified technique allowed the anterior and posterior horn attachments to be preserved by means of maintaining a 7-mm bony bridge between them.
7. A trough was cut in the host tibia to receive this bone bridge as a press fit (Fig. 10.20).
8. The meniscus was then sutured to the meniscal rim. In four

patients with meniscal/tibial plateau allografts, the entire complex was fixed with 4.0 mm AO cancellous screws (Fig. 10.21).
9. A 6.5-mm AO cancellous screw was used to reattach the collateral ligament.

Tourniquet times averaged 1 hour and 50 minutes. Exercises for range of motion were begun on the first postoperative day with CPM machines. Weight bearing was restricted for 6 weeks.

FOLLOW-UP

Three patients had no complaints of pain. Three claimed occasional minimal pain about the knee and were noted

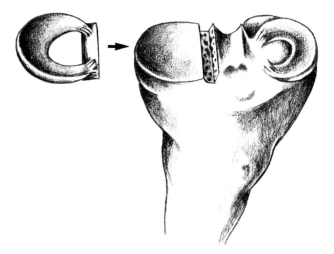

Figure 10.20. A modified technique allowed the anterior and posterior horn attachments to be preserved by means of maintaining a 7-mm bony bridge between them. A trough was cut in the host tibia to receive this bone bridge as a press-fit.

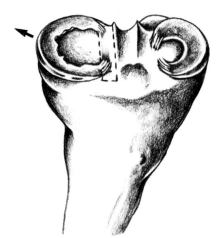

Figure 10.19. The meniscal rim was resected to the vascular zone and the allograft was trimmed to fit.

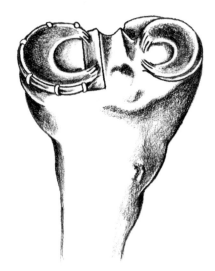

Figure 10.21. The meniscus was then sutured to the meniscal rim. In four patients with meniscal/tibial plateau allografts, the entire complex was fixed with 4.0-mm AO (Society of Internal Fixation) cancellous screws.

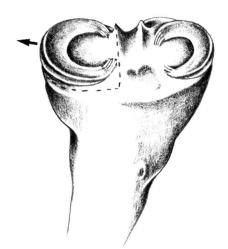

Figure 10.22. Meniscus attachments are resected with a 5-mm thick tibial plateau.

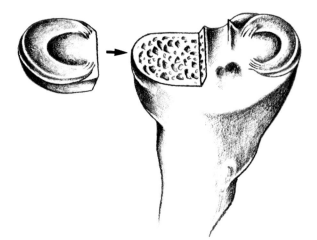

Figure 10.23. A meniscal-tibial plateau allograft, sized to match the recipient, is implanted to the site.

to have occasional clicking sensations but no locking. One patient had intermittent effusion. No "giving out" or "locking" was reported.

Roentgenographs did not show progressive degenerative changes. Five patients had no joint space loss compared with the same compartment of the contralateral knee. The sixth patient had a −4-mm joint space preoperatively, which was reduced to −2 mm after transplantation.

Arthroscopic examination in four cases showed healing to be secure around the meniscal rim at the superior and inferior surface. The anterior and posterior horns appeared to be firmly anchored. The substance of the meniscus was reported to appear normal with no evidence of shrinkage, synovitis, necrosis, or pannus formation.

The results of Dr. Garrett's limited series is encouraging. None of the patients are reported to have undergone further meniscal surgery. The fresh menisci appears to have maintained their shape and size.

In the goat model, we have been able to transplant the meniscus and tibial plateau cartilage as a single complex (Fig. 10.22–10.24). This technique may have future application where the meniscus tibial compartment needs to be replaced.

The role of meniscal transplantation in enhancing joint stability is still undetermined. Only further studies and longer follow-up will ascertain if meniscal allografts will be a durable substitute, prevent degenerative change, and provide joint stability.

MENISCAL TRANSPLANTATION PROBLEMS IN HUMANS

The work, to date, in humans, albeit limited, has been encouraging. The procedure is investigational and tech-

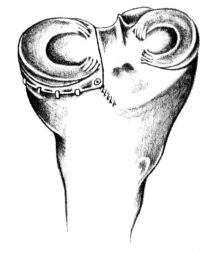

Figure 10.24. The periphery of the meniscus is sutured in place. Additional fixation is accomplished by placing a cancellous bone screw in a nonbearing aspect of the anterior tibial plateau.

nically demanding. The current open technique allows for the greatest visualization to assure proper site preparation, graft placement, and fixation. The open technique carries with it the familiar morbidity, rehabilitation, and cosmesis problems.

The possibility of arthroscopic meniscal transplantation has been demonstrated. Refinement of this technique would be a significant improvement for those rare cases where only a meniscal transplantation is indicated. We believe that the use of bone plugs as we have developed in the goat model as opposed to a trough would be more amenable to arthroscopic techniques.

The availability of suitable donor material is an issue. The demand for these tissues will increase until it exceeds the supply as is the case with most transplantable tissues.

With the potential lack of tissue donors, synthetic composite materials may be developed as meniscal substitutes. Another potential source might involve genetic engineering to generate materials and growth factors that could optimize this technique.

BIOPROSTHESIS

Allograft and Synthetic Material

The ligament augmentation device (LAD, 3M) is a braided polypropylene device intended to augment the strength of a biological graft material. It is not intended to be a permanent prosthetic replacement for the ACL because it will eventually deform. It is intended to augment the weak area of biological grafts used in ligament reconstruction. In this capacity, the LAD provides early joint stability and protects the graft from stress until biological fixation occurs.

From the authors' previous experience with LAD-ACL allografts used for reconstruction of the ACL, it was observed that the LAD enhanced the strength (maximum strength to failure) of the allograft (27). The LAD was placed in the over-the-top position and over the anterior tibia with no direct attachment to the ACL allograft. The LAD was adjacent to the intra-articular portion of the allograft and its bony fixation was released from the tibial fixation site at 3 months. Over the 1-year study interval, the healing of the allograft with the adjacent LAD appeared to form a composite graft.

This work led to the concept of placing the LAD within the substance of the graft. It was hypothesized that the LAD could provide a period of protection while the graft is being incorporated by the recipient. The LAD would protect the repair during the early interval of revascularization and cellular ingrowth. This period of stress protection could prevent the effects of tibial displacement and injury to the collagen fibers being synthesized during the healing phase. The LAD provides joint stability and allows immediate mobility and weight bearing as tolerated. The LAD has been later released from the tibia or allowed to rupture to allow complete stress transfer.

The use of an LAD with an allograft in knee ligament reconstructions is still investigational. Questions to be answered include the ideal load sharing and sparing between the allograft and LAD, timing of load transfer, long-term relationship of a biological and synthetic material, and technical considerations on positioning and tensioning. The concept of a bioprosthesis offers many possible areas for future study.

CONCLUSIONS

In conclusion, the use of allografts in knee surgery is an exciting area with present clinical application. Great strides are being made in the areas of sterility, biomechanics, immunology, and techniques of transplantation. As one looks to the future, allografts will play a substantial role in knee surgery.

REFERENCES

1. Koop CE. Los Angeles Times 1989; November 19.
2. Centers for Disease Control. Transmission of HIV through bone transplantation: case report and public health recommendations. MMWR 1988; 37:597.
3. American Academy of Orthopaedic Surgeons. Recommendations for the prevention of human immunodeficiency virus (HIV) transmission in the practice of orthopaedic surgery. AAOS, Las Vegas, 1989.
4. Buck BE, Malinin TI, Brown MD. Bone transplantation and human immunodeficiency virus. Clin Orthop 1989; 240:129.
5. Goode SM, Hertzmark E, Steinert RF. Adequacy of ELISA test for screening corneal transplant donors. Am J Ophthalmol 1988; 106:436.
6. Buck BE, Resnick L, Shah S, Malinin TI. Human immunodeficiency virus cultured from bone: implications in transmission. Clin Orthop 1990; 251:249.
7. Paulos LE, France EP, Rosenberg TD, et al. Comparative material properties of allograft tissues for ligament replacement, effect of type, age, sterilization, and preservation. Trans Orthop Res Soc 1987; 12:129.
8. Paulos LE, Rosenberg TD, Gurley WD. Prosthetic ligament reconstruction of the knee. In: Anterior Cruciate Ligament Allografts. WB Saunders, Philadelphia, 1988; pp. 25–26.
9. Curtis RJ, DeLee JC, Drez DJ. Reconstruction of the anterior curciate ligament with freeze dried fascia lata allografts in dogs. Am J Sports Med 1985; 13:408.
10. Jackson DW, Windler GE, Simon TM. Intraarticular reaction associated with the use of freeze-dried ethylene oxide-sterilized bone-patella tendon-bone allografts in the reconstruction of the anterior cruciate ligament. Am J Sports Med 1990; 18:1.
11. Pinkowski JL, Reiman PR, Suio-Ling C. Human lymphocyte reaction to freeze-dried allograft and xenograft ligamentous tissue. Am J Sports Med 1989; 17:595.
12. Conway B, Tomford WW, Hirsch MS, Schooley RT, Mankin HJ. Effect of gamma irradiation on HIV-1 in a bone allograft model. Trans Orthop Res Soci 1990; 15:225.
13. Withrow SJ, Oulton SA, Suto TL, et al. Evaluation of the antiretroviral effect or various methods of sterilizing/preserving corticocancellous bone. Trans Orthop Res Soc 1990; 15:226.
14. Shino K, Kimura T, Hirose H, Inoue M, Ono K. Reconstruction of the anterior cruciate ligament by allogenic tendon graft. J Bone Joint Surg 1986; 68B:739.
15. Morrison JB. Bioengineering analysis of force actions transmitted by the knee joint. Bio-Med Eng 1968; 3:164.

16. Morrison JB. The mechanics of the knee joint in relation to normal walking. J Biomech 1970; 3:51.

17. Grood ES, Noyes FR. Cruciate ligament prosthesis: Strength, creep, and fatigue properties. J Bone Joint Surg 1976; 19A:1083.

18. Fu FH, Greenwald AS, Olson EJ, Silvaggro VJ. The science of anterior cruciate ligament implants—1989. AAOS 56th Annual Meeting, Las Vegas, NV, 1989.

19. Noyes FR, Butler DL, Grood ES, Zernicke RF, Hefzy MS. Biomechanical analysis of human ligament grafts used in knee ligament repairs and reconstructions. J Bone Joint Surg 1984; 66A:344.

20. Nasca RJ. The use of freeze-dried allografts in management of global rotator cuff tears. Clin Orthop 1988; 228:218.

21. Barnd S, Cuband HE, Rondrigo JJ. The effect of storage at 80°C as compared to 4°C on the strength of rhesus monkey anterior cruciate ligament. Trans Orthop Res Soc 1982; 7:378.

22. Nikolaou PK, Seaber AV, Glisson RR, Ribbeck BM, Bassett FH. Anterior cruciate ligament allograft transplantation. Am J Sports Med 1986; 14:348.

23. Webster DA, Werner FW. Freeze-dried flexor tendons in anterior cruciate ligament reconstruction. Clin Orthop 1983; 181:238.

24. Webster DA, Werner FW. Mechanical and functional properties of implanted freeze-dried flexor tendons. Clin Orthop 1983; 180:301.

25. Shino K, Kawasaki T, Hitoshi H, Gotoh, I, Inoue M, Ono K. Replacement of the anterior cruciate ligament by an allogeneic tendon graft. J Bone Joint Surg 1984; 66B:672.

26. Jackson DW, Grood ES, Arnoczy SP, Butler DL, Simon TM. Freeze dried anterior cruciate ligament allografts. Am J Sports Med 1987;15:295.

27. Jackson DW, Grood ES, Arnoczky SP, Butler DL, Simon TM. Cruciate reconstruction using freeze dried anterior cruciate ligament allograft and a ligament augmentation device (LAD). Am J Sports Med 1987; 15:528.

28. Jackson DW, Grood ES, Wilcox P, Butler DL, Simon TM, Holden JP. The effects of processing techniques on the mechanical properties of bone-anterior cruciate ligament-bone allografts. Am J Sports Med 1988; 16:101.

29. Vasseur PB, Rodrigo JJ, Stevenson S, Clark G, Sharkey N. Replacement of the anterior cruciate ligament with a bone-ligament-bone anterior cruciate ligament allograft in dogs. Clin Orthop 1987; 219:268.

30. Arnoczky SP, Warren RF, Ashlock MA. Replacement of the anterior cruciate ligament using patellar tendon allograft. J Bone Joint Surg 1986; 68A:376.

31. Cabaud HE, Feagin JAF, Rodkey WG. Acute anterior cruciate ligament injury and augmented repair: experimental studies. Am J Sports Med 1980; 8:395.

32. Clancy WG Jr, Narechania RG, Rosenberg TD, Gmeiner JG, Wisnefske DD, Lang TA. Anterior and posterior cruciate reconstruction in rhesus monkeys: a histological, microangiographic, and biochemical analysis. J Bone Joint Surg 1981; 63A:1270.

33. Jackson DW, Grood ES, Cohn BT, Arnoczky SP, Simon TM, Cummings JF. The effects of in situ freezing on the anterior cruciate ligament. An experimental study in goats. J Bone Joint Surg 1991; 73A:201.

34. Mankin HJ. Allograft transplantation in the management of bone tumors. In: Uhthoff HK (ed). Current Concepts of Diagnosis and Treatment of Bone and Soft Tissue Tumors. Springer-Verlag, Berlin, 1984; pp. 147–162.

35. Shino K, Inoue M, Horibe S, Nakamura H, Uno K. Anterior cruciate ligament reconstruction using allogeneic tendon. A long term follow up. Am J Sports Med 1989; 17:714.

36. Bos GC, Goldberg VM, Gordon NH, Dollinger BM, Zika JM, Powell AE, Heiple KG. The long-term fate of fresh and frozen orthotopic bone allografts in genetically defined rats. Clin Orthop 1985; 197:245.

37. Burwell RG. Studies in the transplantation of bone. V. The capacity of fresh and treated homografts of bone to evoke transplantation immunity. J Bone Joint Surg 1964; 46B:110.

38. Burwell RG, Gowland G, Dexter F. Studies in the transplantation of bone. VI further observations concerning the antigenicity of homologous cortical and cancellous bone. J Bone Joint Surg 1963; 45B:597.

39. Chalmer J. Transplantation immunity in bone homografting. J Bone and Joint Surg 1959; 41B:160.

40. Elves MW. Humoral immune response to allografts of bone. Internat Arch Allergy Appl Immunol 1974; 47:708.

41. Takahashi T, Economou GC, Boone CW. Accelerated regeneration of trypsin treated surface antigens of simian virus 40-transformed BALB/3T3 cells induced by x-irradiation. Cancer Res 1976; 36:1258.

42. Frank C, Woo S, Andriacchi T, et al. Normal ligament: structure, function, and composition. In: Woo S, Buckwalter J (eds). Injury and Repair of the Musculoskeletal Soft Tissues. American Academy of Orthopaedic Surgeons, Park Ridge, IL 1987; pp. 45–101.

43. Oakes B. Personal Communication

44. Postacchini F, De Martino C. Regeneration of rabbit calcaneal tendon maturation of collagen and elastic fibers following partial tenotomy. Connect Tissue Res 1980; 8:41.

45. Date T. The influence of exercise in the healing of the rabbit achilles tendon. Nippon Seikeigeka Gakkai Zasshi 1986; 60:449.

46 Williams IF, Craig AS, Pary DAD, etal. Development of collagen fibril organization and collagen crimp patterns during tendon healing. Int J Biol Macromol 1985;7:275.

47. Scott JE, Hughes EW. Proteoglycan-collagen relationships in developing chick and bovine tendons: Influence of the physiological environment. Connect Tissue Res 1986; 14:267.

48. O'Brien MF, Stafford EG, Gardner MAH, Pohlner PG, McGiffin DC: A comparison of aortic valve replacement with viable cryopreserved and fresh allograft valves, with a note on chromosomal studies. J Thorac Cardiovasc Surg 1987; 94:812.

49. O'Brien MF, Stafford EG, Gardner MAH, et al. The viable cryopreserved allograft aortic valve. J Cariac Surg 1987; 2(Suppl):153.

50. Langer F, Czitrom A, Pritzker KP, Gross AE: The immunogenicity of fresh and frozen allogeneic bone. J Bone Joint Surg 1975; 57A:216.

51. Brown KLB, Cruess RL. Bone and cartilage transplantation in orthopaedic surgery. J Bone Joint Surg 1982; 64A:270.

52. Muscolo DL, Kawai S, Ray RD. Cellular and humoral immune response analysis of bone allografted rats. J Bone Joint Surg 1976; 58A:826.

53. Schachar NS, Fuller TC, Wadsworth PL, Henry WB, Mankin HJ. A feline model for the study of frozen osteoarticular allografts. II Development of lymphocytotoxic antibodies in allograft recipients. Trans Orthop Res Soc 1978; 3:131.

54. Goldberg VM, Bos GD, Heiple KG, Zika JM, Powell AE. Improved acceptance of frozen allografts in genetically mismatched dogs by immunosuppression. J Bone Joint Surg 1984; 66A:937.

55. Stevenson S, Templeton JW. The immune response to fresh and frozen, DLA matched and mismatched osteochondral allografts. Trans Orthop Res Soc 1985; 10:287.

56. Friedlaender GE, Strong DM, Sell KW. Studies of the antigenicity of bone. I Freeze-dried and deep-frozen bone allografts in rabbits. J Bone Joint Surg 1976; 58A:854.

57. Bos GD, Goldberg VM, Powell AE, Heiple KG, and Zika JM. The effect of histocompatibility matching on canine frozen bone allografts. J Bone and Joint Surg 1983; 65A:89.

58. Bos GD, Goldberg VM, Zika JM, Heiple KG, Powell AE. Immune responses to frozen bone allografts. J Bone Joint Surg 1983; 65A:239.

59. Powell AE, Bos GD, Goldberg VM, Zika JM, Heiple K. Immune responses to bone allografts. In: Friedlaender GE, Manin HJ, Sell KW (eds). Osteochondral Allografts, Biology, Banking, and Clinical Applications. Little, Brown, Boston, 1983; p. 259.

60. Halloran PE, Ziv I, Lee EH, Langer F, Pritzker KPH, Gross AE. Orthotopic bone transplantation in mice. Technique and assessment of healing. Transplantation 1979; 27:414.

61. Halloran PE, Lee EH, Ziv I, Langer F, Gross AE. Orthotopic bone transplantation in mice. II. Studies of alloantibody response. Transplantation 1979; 27:420.

62. Stevenson S. The immune response to osteochondral allografts in dogs. J Bone Joint Surg 1987; 69A:573.

63. Steffen C, Timpl R, Wolff I. Immunogenicity and specificity of callagen II. Investigations about specificity of callagen and its derivatives by hemagglutination and hemagglutination-inhibition of anti-callagen and anti-parent gelatine immune sear. J Immunol 1964; 93:656.

64. Steffen C, Timpl R, Wolff I. Immunogenicity and specificity of collagen. Demonstration of three different antigenic determinants on calf collagen. Immunology 1968; 15:135.

65. Minami A, Ishii S, Ogino T, Oikawa T, Kobayashi H. Effect of the immunological antigenicity of the allogeneic tendons of tendon grafting. Hand 1982; 14:111.

66. Graham WC, Smith DA, McGuire MP. The use of frozen stored tendons for grafting: an experimental study. J Bone Joint Surg 1955; 37A:624.

67. Benjamini E, Fong S, Erickson C, Leung CY, Rennick D, Scibienski RJ. Immunity to lymphoid tumors induced in syngeneic

mice by immunization with mitomycin C-treated cells. J Immunol 1977; 118:685.

68. Kataoka T, Oh-hashi F, Tsukagoshi S, Sakurai Y. Induction of resistance to L1210 leukemia in BALB/cxDBA/2CrF1 mice with L210 cells treated with glutaraldehyde and concanavalin A. Cancer Res 1977; 37:964.

69. Oikawa T, Gotohda E, Austin FC, Takeichi N, Boone CW. Temperature-dependent alteration in immunogenicity of tumor-associated transplantation antigen monitored via paraformaldehyde fixation. Cancer Res 1979; 39:3519.

70. Andripoulos NA, Mestecky J, Miller EJ, and Bennett JC. Antibodies to human native and denatured collagens in synovial fluids of patients with rheumatoid arthritis. Clin Immunol Immunopathol 1976; 6:209.

71. Bourne RB, Finlay JB, Papadopoulos P, Andreae P. The effect of medial meniscectomy on strain distribution in the proximal part of the tibia. J Bone Joint Surg 1984; 66A:1431.

72. Fairbank TJ. Knee joint changes after meniscectomy. J Bone Joint Surg 1948; 30B:664.

73. Ferkel RD, Davis JR, Friedman MJ, et al. Arthroscopic partial medial meniscectomy: an analysis of unsatisfactory results. Arthroscopy 1985; 1:44.

74. Krause WR, Pope MH, Johnson RJ, Wilder DG. Mechanical changes in the knee after meniscectomy. J Bone Joint Surg 1976; 58A:599.

75. Lynch MA, Henning CE, Glick KR. Knee joint surface changes: long term follow up meniscus tear treatment in stable anterior cruciate ligament reconstructions. Clin Orthop 1983; 172:148.

76. McGinty JB, Geuss LF, Marvin RA. Partial or total meniscectomy. J Bone Joint Surg 1977; 59A:763.

77. Tapper EM, Hoover NW. Late results after meniscectomy. J Bone Joint Surg 1969; 51A:517.

78. Arnoczky SP, McDevitt CA, Schmidt MB, Mow VC, Warren RF. The effect of cryopreservation in canine menisci: a biomechanical morphologic and biomechanical evaluation. J Orthop Res 1988; 6:1.

79. Milachowski KA, Weismeier K, Erhardt W, Ramberger K. Meniscus transplantation—animal experiment study. Sportverletz Sportschaden 1987; 1:20.

80. Canham W, Stanish W. A study of the biological behavior of the meniscus as a transplant in the medial compartment of a dog's knee. Am J Sports Med 1986; 14:376.

81. Jackson DW, McDevitt CA, Simon TM, Arnoczky AP, Atwell EA, Silvano N. Meniscal transplantation using fresh and cryopreserved allografts. Am J Sports Med 1990; in press.

82. Maroudas A. Swelling pressure versus collagen tension in normal and degenerate articular cartilage. Nature 1976; 260:808.

83. Adams ME, Billingham MEJ, Muir H. The glycosaminoglycans in menisci in experimental and natural osteoarthritis. Arthritis Rheum 1983; 26:69.

84. McDevitt CA, Webber RJ. The ultrastructure and biochemistry of meniscal cartilage. Clin Orthop 1990; 252:8.

85. Garrett JC. Meniscal transplantation in the human knee: a preliminary report. AANA Annual Meeting, Orlando, FL, April 1990.

INDEX

Page numbers followed by "t" denote tables; those in italics denote figures.

217

DATE DUE

DEMCO 38-296